WOMEN'S HEALTH RESEARCH

PROGRESS, PITFALLS, AND PROMISE

Committee on Women's Health Research

Board on Population Health and Public Health Practice

INSTITUTE OF MEDICINE
OF THE NATIONAL ACADEMIES

D0907772

THE NATIONAL ACADEMIES PRESS
Washington, D.C.
www.nap.edu

THE NATIONAL ACADEMIES PRESS   500 Fifth Street NW   Washington, DC 20001

NOTICE: The project that is the subject of this report was approved by the Governing Board of the National Research Council, whose members are drawn from the councils of the National Academy of Sciences, the National Academy of Engineering, and the Institute of Medicine. The members of the committee responsible for the report were chosen for their special competences and with regard for appropriate balance.

This study was supported by Contract HHSP23320042509XI, TO# HHSP2332080003T, between the National Academy of Sciences and the Department of Health and Human Services. Any opinions, findings, conclusions, or recommendations expressed in this publication are those of the authors and do not necessarily reflect the view of the organizations or agencies that provided support for this project.

Library of Congress Cataloging-in-Publication Data

Institute of Medicine (U.S.). Committee on Women's Health Research.
  Women's health research : progress, pitfalls, and promise / Committee on Women's Health Research, Board on Population Health and Public Health Practice.
    p. ; cm.
  Includes bibliographical references.
  ISBN 978-0-309-15389-8 (Book) — ISBN 978-0-309-15390-4 (PDF) 1. Women—Health and hygiene—Research. I. Title.
  [DNLM: 1. Women's Health—United States—Guideline. 2. Clinical Trials as Topic—United States—Guideline. 3. Health Services Research—methods—United States—Guideline. 4. Health Status—United States—Guideline. WA 309 AA1]
  RA564.85.I565 2010
  362.1082—dc22
                                2010040695

Additional copies of this report are available from the National Academies Press, 500 Fifth Street NW, Lockbox 285, Washington, DC 20055; (800) 624-6242 or (202) 334-3313 (in the Washington metropolitan area); Internet, http://www.nap.edu.

For more information about the Institute of Medicine, visit the IOM home page at: **www.iom. edu**.

The serpent has been a symbol of long life, healing, and knowledge among almost all cultures and religions since the beginning of recorded history. The serpent adopted as a logotype by the Institute of Medicine is a relief carving from ancient Greece, now held by the Staatliche Museen in Berlin.

Cover credit: Cover painting is reprinted with permission from the artist, Alberto Schunk.

Suggested citation: IOM (Institute of Medicine). 2010. *Women's Health Research: Progress, Pitfalls, and Promise.* Washington, DC: The National Academies Press.

"Knowing is not enough; we must apply.
Willing is not enough; we must do."

—Goethe

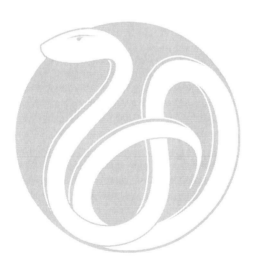

INSTITUTE OF MEDICINE
OF THE NATIONAL ACADEMIES

Advising the Nation. Improving Health.

THE NATIONAL ACADEMIES
Advisers to the Nation on Science, Engineering, and Medicine

The **National Academy of Sciences** is a private, nonprofit, self-perpetuating society of distinguished scholars engaged in scientific and engineering research, dedicated to the furtherance of science and technology and to their use for the general welfare. Upon the authority of the charter granted to it by the Congress in 1863, the Academy has a mandate that requires it to advise the federal government on scientific and technical matters. Dr. Ralph J. Cicerone is president of the National Academy of Sciences.

The **National Academy of Engineering** was established in 1964, under the charter of the National Academy of Sciences, as a parallel organization of outstanding engineers. It is autonomous in its administration and in the selection of its members, sharing with the National Academy of Sciences the responsibility for advising the federal government. The National Academy of Engineering also sponsors engineering programs aimed at meeting national needs, encourages education and research, and recognizes the superior achievements of engineers. Dr. Charles M. Vest is president of the National Academy of Engineering.

The **Institute of Medicine** was established in 1970 by the National Academy of Sciences to secure the services of eminent members of appropriate professions in the examination of policy matters pertaining to the health of the public. The Institute acts under the responsibility given to the National Academy of Sciences by its congressional charter to be an adviser to the federal government and, upon its own initiative, to identify issues of medical care, research, and education. Dr. Harvey V. Fineberg is president of the Institute of Medicine.

The **National Research Council** was organized by the National Academy of Sciences in 1916 to associate the broad community of science and technology with the Academy's purposes of furthering knowledge and advising the federal government. Functioning in accordance with general policies determined by the Academy, the Council has become the principal operating agency of both the National Academy of Sciences and the National Academy of Engineering in providing services to the government, the public, and the scientific and engineering communities. The Council is administered jointly by both Academies and the Institute of Medicine. Dr. Ralph J. Cicerone and Dr. Charles M. Vest are chair and vice chair, respectively, of the National Research Council.

www.national-academies.org

HERBERT PETERSON, M.D., Professor and Chair, Department of Maternal and Child Health, Gillings School of Global Public Health, University of North Carolina, Chapel Hill

ETTA D. PISANO, M.D., Kenan Professor of Radiology and Biomedical Engineering, Director, Biomedical Research Imaging Center, Vice Dean for Academic Affairs, and Director of the North Carolina Translational Research Center, University of North Carolina School of Medicine, Chapel Hill (until June 30, 2010); Vice President for Medical Affairs and Dean, College of Medicine, Medical University of South Carolina, Charleston (after July 1, 2010)

ALINA SALGANICOFF, Ph.D., Vice President and Director, Women's Health Policy and KaiserEDU.org, Kaiser Family Foundation, Menlo Park, CA

LINDA G. SNETSELAAR, R.D., Ph.D., L.D., Endowed Chair, Associate Head for Admissions and Curriculum, and Professor in the Department of Epidemiology, College of Public Health, University of Iowa, Iowa City

Study Staff

MICHELLE C. CATLIN, Ph.D., Study Director
MORGAN A. FORD, Program Officer (until October 2009)
JENNIFER A. COHEN, Program Officer (from June 2010)
ALEJANDRA MARTÍN, Research Assistant (from April 2010)
KATHLEEN McGRAW, Senior Program Assistant
NORMAN GROSSBLATT, Senior Editor
REBEKAH E. GEE, M.D., M.P.H., Norman F. Gant/American Board of Obstetrics and Gynecology IOM Anniversary Fellow (from November 2009)
ROSE MARIE MARTINEZ, Sc.D., Director, Board on Population Health and Public Health Practice

Reviewers

This report has been reviewed in draft form by persons chosen for their diverse perspectives and technical expertise in accordance with procedures approved by the National Research Council's Report Review Committee. The purpose of this independent review is to provide candid and critical comments that will assist the institution in making its published report as sound as possible and to ensure that the report meets institutional standards of objectivity, evidence, and responsiveness to the study charge. The review comments and draft manuscript remain confidential to protect the integrity of the deliberative process. We thank the following for their review of this report:

Chloe E. Bird, Senior Behavioral and Social Scientist, RAND

Johanna T. Dwyer, Professor of Medicine (Nutrition) and Community Health, Tufts University School of Medicine and Friedman School of Nutrition Science and Policy, Director, Frances Stern Nutrition Center, Tufts Medical Center, Senior Scientist, Jean Mayer Human Nutrition, Research Center on Aging at Tufts University

Archondoula (Archelle) Georgiou, Independent Consultant

Daniel F. Hayes, Clinical Director, Breast Oncology Program, Stuart B. Padnos Professor in Breast Cancer Research, University of Michigan Comprehensive Cancer Center

Bernadine P. Healy, Health Editor and Columnist, US News and World Report

Victor W. Henderson, Professor of Health Research and Policy (Epidemiology) and of Neurology and Neurological Sciences, Stanford University

Lewis H. Kuller, Distinguished University Professor of Public Health, Department of Epidemiology, University of Pittsburgh

JoAnn Manson, Chief, Division of Preventive Medicine, Brigham and Women's Hospital, Professor of Medicine and the Elizabeth F. Brigham Professor of Women's Health, Harvard Medical School

Carolyn M. Mazure, Professor of Psychiatry, Associate Dean for Faculty Affairs, Director, Women's Health Research at Yale, Yale School of Medicine

C. Noel Bairey Merz, Chair, Women's Ischemic Syndrome Evaluation Initiative, Director of the Women's Heart Center and the Preventive and Rehabilitative Cardiac Center, Cedars-Sinai Medical Center

David P. Pryor, Medical Director, Aetna

Natalie Rasgon, Professor, Psychiatry and Behavioral Science and Obstetrics and Gynecology, Stanford School of Medicine

Nancy E. Reame, Mary Dickey Lindsay Professor of Nursing, Columbia University

Rita Redberg, Director, Women's Cardiovascular Services, University of California San Francisco Medical Center

Elizabeth L. Travis, Associate Vice President of Women Faculty Programs, Mattie Allen Fair Professor in Cancer Research, and Professor of Experimental Radiation Oncology, The University of Texas M. D. Anderson Cancer Center

Nancy Fugate Woods, Professor, Biobehavioral Nursing and Health Systems, University of Washington

Although the reviewers listed above have provided many constructive comments and suggestions, they were not asked to endorse the conclusions or recommendations, nor did they see the final draft of the report before its release. The review of the report was overseen by **Ellen Wright Clayton**, Vanderbilt University, and **Georges C. Benjamin**, American Public Health Association. Appointed by the National Research Council and Institute of Medicine, they were responsible for making certain that an independent examination of the report was carried out in accordance with institutional procedures and that all review comments were carefully considered. Responsibility for the final content of the report rests entirely with the authoring committee and the institution.

Preface

My colleagues on the committee reviewing progress in women's health research and I each work in our own area of this vast domain and appreciated the opportunity to look at the range of research that has been done and whether it has made a difference in health care delivery, in public health approaches, and in women's health. While frustrated by the impossibility of doing justice to the work, we were privileged to have the opportunity to review much of it and to get the overall outlines of the field. The subtitle of our report on *Women's Health Research: Progress, Pitfalls, and Promise* captures the conflicting evaluations and feelings we all experienced in reviewing the status of research on women's health over the past two decades.

It is not by accident that we listed *progress* first. It was encouraging and gratifying to see how much has been learned. Not only do we know a great deal more about the etiology and course of specific diseases that affect women's health, but our understanding of women's health itself has become more multifaceted and nuanced. The concept of women's health has expanded beyond a narrow focus on disorders associated with the female reproductive system to encompass other diseases that create a significant burden in women's lives. These diseases are more common or more serious in women than in men, have distinct causes or manifestations in women than in men, have different outcomes or treatments in women than in men, or cause high morbidity or mortality in women.

This broader approach to women's health and related research moves toward a woman-centered view rather than a disease-centered view. It highlights the importance of considering quality of life rather than simply survival or mortality in evaluating the success of treatments and interventions. It has also revealed the inequities in the extent of disease among women from different sociodemographic groups, and of the uneven distribution of benefit from research advances and new treatments. Research has also broadened to include studies that take into account not only biological sex as a determinant of disease, but also gender; this expanded view encompasses and highlights the importance of social, psychological and behavioral influences.

The substantial progress in our understanding of the range of determinants of women's health has, in many cases, been translated into better treatments and decreases in incidence and prevalence of some conditions; these are reviewed in this report. In a few instances, there were breakthroughs that the committee considered to be "game-changers," but in most cases there were smaller advances that followed from an accumulation of knowledge from a range of different types of studies.

While impressed by the progress that has occurred, the committee was also distressed by the number of *pitfalls*, particularly in the translation of findings into practice and policy, and in the health disparities among women. Some of these pitfalls derive from problems in the current organization of research (for example, institutes within the National Institutes of Health [NIH] that are primarily focused on specific diseases) and of health care (for example, fragmentation of care, misalignment of financial incentives). Others reside in the many problems of the health delivery system; it is yet too soon to know how well the just-passed reform bill will address these in general or in relation to women's health.

Other challenges arise in the clear communication of complex research findings in a media context that thrives on sound bites and controversy. Because these problems have been the focus of many Institute of Medicine (IOM) reports and are not specific to women's health, we only acknowledge them briefly in the report.

The committee ended its work feeling hopeful about the *promise* of future improvements in the health of women. Some of the changes at NIH (for example, the focus on translational research and cross-institute initiatives) should be particularly helpful for women's health. There is accumulating knowledge of the broad set of determinants of women's health, including data on their risk factors, epidemiology and pathophysiology of diseases, functioning, and well-being. The recommendations made in this report, if implemented, would accelerate those advances.

The committee faced a number of challenges. Given the broad charge to the committee and the large amount of relevant research, we could not conduct a comprehensive review of the literature on all potential health conditions and determinants, or even for any single health condition or determinant. This report, therefore, should not be considered as a comprehensive review of any specific topic, but as a highlight of some of the relevant research which the committee used to draw general conclusions and make recommendations. The absence of a discussion of any condition is not meant to diminish its potential importance for women's health or for the women who are affected by those conditions. Every day new research findings are published, so this report reflects the state of the science when we wrote our report. We realize and, in fact, hope that new results will emerge that we could not capture in this report.

I am extremely appreciative to the members of this committee for their hard work: Eli Adashi, Sergio Aguilar-Gaxiola, Hortensia Amaro, Marietta Anthony, Diane Brown, Nananda Col, Susan Cu-Uvin, Denise Faustman, John Finnegan, William Hazzard, Jaye Hefner, Jeanne Miranda, Lori Mosca, Herbert Peterson, Etta Pisano, Alina Salganicoff, and Linda Snetselaar. This committee faced a challenging task of coming to consensus despite a broad variety of backgrounds and expertise, and it worked diligently to ensure the numerous facets of women's health research were properly covered and addressed. I would also like to thank the IOM staff, especially study director Michelle Catlin and her team, Morgan Ford, Katie McGraw, Alejandra Martín, and Norman F. Gant/American Board of Obstetrics and Gynecology/IOM Anniversary Fellow Rebekah Gee. Without their dedicated work this report would not have been possible. I am grateful as well to those who reviewed the report and provided thoughtful comments that improved the final report.

In addition, I want to thank the individuals who presented to the committee at open sessions: Wanda Jones, US Department of Health and Human Services; Vivian Pinn, National Institutes of Health; Kathleen Uhl, Food and Drug Administration; Shakeh Kaftarian, Agency for Healthcare Research and Quality; Phyllis Greenberger, Society for Women's Health Research; Diana Zuckerman, National Research Center for Women and Families; Cindy Pearson, National Women's Health Network; Mona Shah, Professional Staff Member, United States Senate Committee on Health, Education, Labor, and Pensions; Kerri D. Schuiling, American College of Nurse-Midwives; Linda Lipson, Department of Veterans Affairs; Elizabeth Yano, Department of Veteran Affairs Greater Los Angeles; Jacquelyn C. Campbell, The Johns Hopkins University School of Nursing; Madelyn Fernstrom, University of Pittsburgh Medical Center; Beverly Rockhill Levine, University of North Carolina, Greensboro; and Dennis G. Fryback, University of Wisconsin, Madison. Those individuals provided the committee with background information and expertise that enriched our understanding of the issues.

The committee hopes that this report will foster future research and efforts to continue the excellent work that has already been done, and also to fill present gaps in knowledge. Women's health is fundamental to the overall health of the entire population. Given the multiple roles women play in society, to invest in the health of women is to invest in the well-being and progress of society.

Nancy E. Adler, *Chair*
Committee on Women's Health Research

Contents

APPENDIXES

---

*The contents of Appendix C are provided on the CD in the back of the book and are available online at http://www.nap.edu/catalog.php?record_id=12908.

Summary

BACKGROUND

Women make up just over half the US population and should not be considered a special, minority population, but rather an equal gender whose health needs require equal research efforts as those for men. Historically, however, the health needs of women, apart from reproductive concerns, have lagged in medical research. In 1985, the Public Health Service Task Force on Women's Health Issues concluded that "the historical lack of research focus on women's health concerns has compromised the quality of health information available to women as well as the health care they receive." Since the publication of that report, there has been a transformation in women's health research—including changes in government support of research, in policies, in regulations, and in organization—that has resulted in the generation of new scientific knowledge about women's health. Offices on women's health have been established in a number of government agencies.[1] Government reports and reports from other organizations, including the Institute of Medicine (IOM), have highlighted the need for, and tracked the progress of, the inclusion of women in health research. A number of nongovern-

---

[1]During the preparation of this report the Patient Protection and Affordable Care Act of 2010 (Public Law 111-148) was passed, which formally codifies the Offices of Women's Health within the Department of Health and Human Services (HHS). The act also formally establishes an Office of Women's Health in the directors' office of the Agency for Healthcare Research and Quality, the Centers for Disease Control and Prevention, the Food and Drug Administration, the Health Resources and Services Administration, the Substance Abuse and Mental Health Services Administration; an HHS Coordinating Committee on Women's Health; and the National Women's Health Information Center.

1

ment organizations have also provided leadership in research in women's health. And women as advocates, research subjects, researchers, clinicians, administrators, and US representatives and senators have played a major role in building a women's health movement.

CHARGE TO THE COMMITTEE

Given the research activities occurring in women's health over the last 2 decades, in the Consolidated Appropriations Act of 2008 (Public Law 110-161) Congress provided the Department of Health and Human Services Office on Women's Health (OWH) with funds for the IOM "to conduct a comprehensive review of the status of women's health research, summarize what has been learned about how diseases specifically affect women, and report to the Congress on suggestions for the direction of future research." In response, the OWH requested that the IOM conduct a study of women's health research; the charge to the committee for the project is presented in Box S-1.

In response to that request, the IOM convened a committee of 18 members who had a wide variety of expertise, including expertise in biomedical research, research translation, research communication, disabilities, epidemiology, healthcare services, behavioral and social determinants of health, health disparities, nutrition, public health, women's health, clinical decision making, and such other medical specialties as cardiovascular disease (CVD), mental health, endocrinology, geriatrics, and immunology.

THE COMMITTEE'S APPROACH TO ITS CHARGE

The committee met six times, including two open information-gathering sessions at which the members heard from stakeholders and researchers, and conducted extensive literature searches of publications from the last 15–20 years. The committee approached women's health as a concept that has expanded beyond a narrow focus on the female reproductive system to encompass other conditions

---

BOX S-1
Charge to the Committee

An Institute of Medicine committee will examine what the research on women's health has revealed; how that research has been communicated to providers, women, the public and others; and identify gaps in those areas. The committee will identify examples of successful dissemination of findings paying particular attention to how the communication has influenced women's use of care and preventive services. The committee will make recommendations where appropriate.

that create a significant burden in women's lives. The committee focused on health conditions that are specific to women, are more common or more serious in women, have distinct causes or manifestations in women, have different outcomes or treatments in women, or have high morbidity or mortality in women. Numerous conditions could be included in such a list. The committee could not review all such conditions and, therefore, highlights a number of such conditions as examples that are specific to women; that have differences in prevalence, severity, preferred treatment, or understanding for women; or that the condition is prominent in women or there is a research need regarding women, whether or not there are sex-differences. Searches included research on factors that are determinants of health (biologic, psychologic, environmental, and sociocultural factors), especially factors that might affect women disproportionately or uniquely, and on the translation of research findings into practice and the communication of research findings to the public.

When considering health end points, the committee did not present a comprehensive review of findings of all research on all diseases, disorders, and conditions that are women's health issues. The committee identified a number of conditions that have a large impact on women, reviewed the literature related to them, and categorized them as conditions in relation to which there has been major, some, or little improvement in women's health.

The committee developed a series of questions to focus deliberations and ensure appropriate response to the charge. Those questions and the committee's responses to them are presented below.

IS WOMEN'S HEALTH RESEARCH STUDYING THE MOST APPROPRIATE AND RELEVANT DETERMINANTS OF HEALTH?

Determinants can range from a woman's genetic makeup to her behaviors to the social, cultural, and environmental context in which genetic vulnerabilities and individual traits and behaviors are developed and expressed. Over the last 20 years, much has been learned about what the determinants of women's health are.

The committee found that many behavioral determinants (such as smoking, eating habits, and lack of physical activity) are risk factors for most of the conditions under consideration. Those behavioral factors, in turn, are shaped by cultural, social, and societal contexts. Marked differences in the prevalence of and mortality from various conditions in women who experience social disadvantage due to race and ethnicity, lack of education, low income, and other factors have been documented. The differences stem from a variety of social determinants, including differential exposure to stressors and violence, which are more common in more disadvantaged communities. Such exposures are related to wide-ranging outcomes, including injury and trauma, depression, arthritis, asthma, heart disease, human immunodeficiency virus/acquired immunodeficiency syndrome (HIV/AIDS), and other sexually transmitted infections.

The underlying determinants of health and their relative power may differ by sex and gender, and tailored interventions might be more effective than generic treatments. As discussed in Chapter 2, few studies have tested ways to modify behavioral determinants in women, and even less research has been conducted on the effects of social and community factors in specific groups of women.

IS WOMEN'S HEALTH RESEARCH FOCUSED ON THE MOST APPROPRIATE AND RELEVANT HEALTH CONDITIONS?

The committee discussed the research of a number of conditions as examples of conditions that greatly affect women. It categorized those conditions as having major, some, or little progress (see Table S-1).

Conditions on Which Research Has Contributed to Major Progress

The committee identified breast cancer, CVD, and cervical cancer as the conditions on which major progress has been made.

Mortality from breast cancer has decreased in the last 20 years. Consumer demand and involvement and increased funding have spurred breast-cancer research at the molecular, cellular, and animal levels as well as clinical trials and

TABLE S-1 Conditions Discussed by Committee, Categorized by Extent of Progress

Conditions on Which Research Has Contributed to Major Progress
Breast Cancer
Cardiovascular Disease
Cervical Cancer

Conditions on Which Research Has Contributed to Some Progress
Depression
HIV/AIDS
Osteoporosis

Conditions on Which There Has Been Little Progress
Unintended Pregnancy
Maternal Morbidity and Mortality
Autoimmune Diseases
Alcohol and Drug Addiction
Lung Cancer
Gynecological Cancers Other than Cervical Cancer
Non-Malignant Gynecological Disorders
Alzheimer's Disease

observational studies in women. That research has led to the development of more sensitive detection methods, biomarkers of risk and of more aggressive tumors, identification of risk factors, and treatment options that improve survival and posttreatment quality of life. The finding in the Women's Health Initiative (WHI) of increased risk of breast cancer from hormone therapy led to changes in practice, and a substantial drop in the incidence of breast cancer has been attributed to those changes in practice. Progress has not been seen to the same extent in all groups of women, however; for example, black women have higher mortality from breast cancer than white women despite a lower incidence.

CVD is the leading cause of death of both women and men. As in men, age-adjusted mortality from coronary heart disease was reduced by half in women from 1980 to 2000. About half the decline is attributable to changes in behavioral factors, including a drop in smoking; the other half is attributable to new clinical treatments that emerged from research. Studies led to recognition of CVD in women and, subsequently, extension of diagnosis and treatments for CVD to women. Awareness of CVD among women has increased, in part because of educational campaigns. However, the history of years of the study of CVD only in men has delayed greater progress.

Reductions in the incidence of and mortality from cervical cancer began as early as the 1960s and continued over the last 20 years as diagnosis and screening have improved further. In addition, during the last few years a vaccine that is effective in preventing infection by human papillomavirus, the virus that causes most cervical cancer, was developed. The vaccine was developed and brought into clinical practice through research on the basic biology of the virus and its relationship to cervical cancer in human cells and animals and through epidemiologic studies of cervical cancer's etiology. Although overall gains have been seen in mortality from cervical cancer, rates remain higher in black and Hispanic women than in white and Asian women.

Conditions on Which Research Has Contributed to Some Progress

The committee identified depression, HIV/AIDS, and osteoporosis as conditions on which some progress has been made as a result of women's health research.

The incidence and consequences (such as effects on educational attainment) of depression are higher in women than in men. Advances have been made in the treatment of depression in the last 20 years, although their impact has not been maximized, because of inadequate translation particularly in relation to primary providers. There have been rapid and major advances in the treatment of HIV/AIDS in the last 20 years, mostly through research in men. The rapid development of treatments has benefited women despite the focus of the research on men; however, the predominance of male-focused studies has limited some of the benefits for women. For example, issues with the toxicity of HIV/AIDS treatments in women (for example, increased risk of anemia and acute pancreatitis as compared to men) are only now being identified through women-based research. Over the last 20 years there have been advances in the knowledge of the basic science underlying osteoporosis and in the diagnosis and treatment of osteoporosis. That includes the identification of genes whose expression affects the risk of osteoporosis. Recent trends show a decrease in the incidence of hip factures. Osteoporosis remains, however, a condition that greatly impacts the quality of life of a large number of women, particularly as they age.

Conditions on Which Little Progress Has Been Made

The committee identified a number of conditions on which little progress has been made in reducing incidence or mortality, including unintended pregnancy[2] and autoimmune disease. The risk factors for unintended pregnancy are known, and effective contraceptives are available to prevent pregnancy. The fact that unintended pregnancies continue to occur at a high rate points to the need for research on the use of contraceptive regimens, the need for development of new contraceptives, including non-hormonal contraceptives, that are more acceptable to groups of women in which unintended pregnancies occur with greater frequency, and the need for social and community-level interventions to decrease unintended pregnancies. Autoimmune diseases constitute about 50 diseases, most of which are more common in women. As a group, they are the leading cause of morbidity in women, and they affect women's quality of life greatly. Despite their prevalence and morbidity, little progress has been made toward a better understanding of those conditions, identifying risk factors, or developing a cure.

Looking at the set of conditions on which little progress has been made—including unintended pregnancy; autoimmune disease; alcohol-addiction and drug-addiction disorders; lung, ovarian, endometrial, and colorectal cancer; non-malignant gynecologic disorders; and Alzheimer's disease—the committee tried to identify characteristics or explanations for the lack of progress. The committee could not determine specifically why progress was seen for some conditions and not others, but it considered a number of potential reasons, including degree of attention and subsequent research funding from government agencies, consumer advocacy groups, and Congress; availability of interested researchers trained in a given field; adequacy of understanding of the underlying pathophysiology of a condition; availability of sensitive and specific diagnostic tests and screening programs to identify persons who are at risk for or who have a condition; mor-

---

[2]The committee considered whether to discuss unintended pregnancy as a health outcome or a determinant of health. It decided to discuss it as an outcome, along with maternal mortality and morbidity, and also to discuss the determinants that increase the rate of unintended pregnancies in Chapter 2.

bidity, rather than mortality, as the outcome of a disease; and barriers associated with political or social concerns.

IS WOMEN'S HEALTH RESEARCH STUDYING THE MOST RELEVANT GROUPS OF WOMEN?

Many of the conditions that the committee reviewed are more common or have poorer outcomes in women who are socially disadvantaged than in women who are not. They include the three diseases on which there has been major progress—breast cancer, CVD, and cervical cancer. The fact that subgroups of women are not benefiting from the progress that has been made could indicate that the most relevant groups, the groups that have the greatest burden of disease, are not being adequately studied and research results are not being translated into practice and policies.

ARE THE MOST APPROPRIATE RESEARCH METHODS BEING USED TO STUDY WOMEN'S HEALTH?

The women's health research reviewed includes basic research (studies in animals and at the molecular and cellular levels), epidemiologic or clinical research (research conducted or observed in human subjects), and studies of health systems. All those study types have contributed to progress in women's health, and all yielded important findings on the conditions on which there has been major progress—breast cancer, CVD, and cervical cancer.

The committee identified a number of issues specific to the studies reviewed or to women's health. Large observational studies—such as the observational arm of the WHI, the Nurses' Health Study, and the Study of Women's Health Across the Nation (SWAN)—were coordinated among multiple research centers to accrue large and diverse samples and were especially useful for generating hypotheses for further testing. The postmenopausal hormone therapy and the calcium and vitamin D components of the WHI were randomized clinical trials that were based on the findings from such observational research. In addition, the observational studies led to animal and in vitro studies aimed at elucidating the pathophysiology of conditions and identifying potential treatments.

Different study types have different limits, and results from diverse study designs can combine to provide extremely useful information that is directly relevant to the health of women and some have led to clear improvements in women's health. The committee recognizes that there are drawbacks to different study types. For example, observational studies and clinical trials can be expensive, can have subject attrition, can be of long duration, and, in the case of observational studies, can have difficulty in finding appropriate comparison populations and in controlling for potential confounders. Large human studies, such as the WHI, are further hindered by complex study designs and associated pitfalls.

Despite those drawbacks, the committee concluded that information from large, complex observational and clinical studies could not be obtained with other study designs and are integral to progress in women's health. New study designs that yield similar levels of certainty would be valuable. Smaller studies, in contrast, provide different information and can often be better controlled, potentially faster (depending on the end points studied), and less expensive. Internal validity (for example, the ability to establish causal relationships) is generally stronger in such studies, but this may be at the cost of external validity (that is, generalizability). Smaller studies are important to provide information on which to base large studies and to test specific hypotheses.

Although women are now routinely included in clinical research, the initial design often is not optimal for obtaining data on women, including problems in the inclusion criteria and selection of end points that do not apply to women. Sample size and the ability to recruit adequate numbers of women in studies to allow appropriate analyses can be challenging. Sex- and gender-specific analyses must be published and used for drug development or clinical guidelines. Even when sex-specific analyses are conducted by researchers, the analyses are not always included in publications, because of page limitations or journal restrictions.

Studies often use incidence and 5-year survival rates as end points; fewer studies look at morbidity or quality of life after treatment and survival. Given that women tend to report worse overall health than do men and tend to emphasize quality of life when considering their health, the lack of assessment of quality of life in studies of women's health is problematic.

ARE THE RESEARCH FINDINGS BEING TRANSLATED IN A WAY THAT AFFECTS PRACTICE?

It can take 15–20 years for research findings to be incorporated into practice. Barriers to translation of findings on women's health include barriers that impede translation of science to practice more generally, such as the iterative nature of research in which inconsistent or contradictory results often are published before a clear picture emerges; social and cultural opposition to some new treatments or approaches; entrenched financial or other interests that favor the status quo or a specific approach; and lack of reimbursement for new treatments or practices. Patients themselves faced with a multitude of research findings and complex decisions can have difficulty in weighing new options for their health.

Other barriers, however, differentially affect the translation of research into better care for women. They are derived from the fragmentation of care that results when women see multiple providers for different health concerns, failure of performance measures to include many conditions that are specific to women, and failure to analyze sex-based differences in care, which undermines the use of incentives to implement research findings in women's health care.

ARE THE RESEARCH FINDINGS BEING
COMMUNICATED EFFECTIVELY TO WOMEN?

Complex and sometimes inconsistent or contradictory results present challenges to the communication of research findings, including those relevant to women. Often, the implications of a given finding are complex, so it is difficult to give a clear, concise message. The emergence of the Internet and the World Wide Web has increased the amount of and access to health-related information for the general public, but it has also added to the confusion about the findings and to concerns about the validity of the available information. Communication is complicated by competing forces, for example, when health messages compete with the marketing forces of industries.

GAPS IN WOMEN'S HEALTH RESEARCH

Relatively few studies have been published on a number of conditions important to women, including ovarian and endometrial cancer, pre-eclampsia (a major cause of maternal morbidity and mortality), and conditions that affect elderly women, including frailty. There is little information on many autoimmune diseases, such as lupus. Research on prevention of and treatment for Alzheimer's disease, obesity, and diabetes has rarely examined sex differences. Despite the prevalence of co-occurring conditions and the need to evaluate risk–benefit tradeoffs across multiple outcomes, such issues are rarely incorporated into studies of specific conditions. More information on how the physical and social environment affect health is needed, including an understanding of how they may result in health disparities in disadvantaged groups. In some cases, particularly reproductive health, strong data supporting the safety and efficacy of treatments may be insufficient to fuel their use if there is social or political opposition on nonmedical grounds. Advances in women's health may require attention to such obstacles in addition to those inherent in the research.

COMMITTEE'S KEY FINDINGS AND RECOMMENDATIONS

Substantial progress has been made since the expansion of investment in women's health research. Research findings have changed the practice of medicine and public-health recommendations in several prominent contexts, including changes in standards of care for women. There have also been decreases in mortality in women from breast cancer, heart disease, and cervical cancer. In other contexts, however, there has been less progress, including research on other conditions that affect women and identification of ways to reduce disparities among subpopulations of women.

Several barriers to further progress in improving the health status of women were identified. For example, there has been inadequate attention to the social and environmental factors that, along with biologic risk factors, influence health. There also has been inadequate enforcement of requirements that representative numbers of women be included in clinical trials and that women's results be reported. A lack of taking account of sex and gender differences in the design and analysis of studies, and a lack of reporting on sex and gender differences, has hindered identification of potentially important sex differences and slowed progress in women's health research and its translation to clinical practice. The committee recommends that all published scientific reports that receive federal funding and all medical product evaluations by the Food and Drug Administration present efficacy and safety data separately for men and women.

Poor communication of the results of women's health research has in many cases led to substantial confusion and may affect the care of women adversely. Research findings will have a greater impact if they are coupled with a well thought-out plan for communication and dissemination. Development of a plan for communication and dissemination should be a standard component of federally sponsored women's health research and the clinical recommendations that are made on the basis of that research.

The committee's specific findings and recommendations follow.

Finding 1

Investment in women's health research has afforded substantial progress and led to improvements in women's health with respect to such important conditions as some cancers and heart disease. Greater progress in women's health has occurred in conditions characterized by multipronged research involving molecular, animal, and cellular data; in observational studies to identify effects in the overall population; and in clinical trials or intervention studies from which evidence-based conclusions on treatment effectiveness can be drawn.

Recommendation 1

US government agencies and other relevant organizations should sustain and strengthen their focus on women's health, including the spectrum of research that includes genetic, behavioral, and social determinants of health and how they change during one's life. In addition to conducting women-only research as appropriate, a goal should be to integrate women's health research into all health research—that is, to mainstream women's health research—in such a way that differences between men and women and differences between subgroups of men and women are routinely assessed in all health research. Relevant US government agencies include the Department of Health and Human Services and its institutes and agencies—especially the National Institutes of Health, the Centers for Disease Control and Prevention, the Food and Drug Administration, the Agency for Healthcare Research and Quality, and the Substance Abuse and Mental Health Services Administration—and such others as the Department of Veterans Affairs, the Department of Defense, and the Environmental Protection Agency.

Finding 2

Women who experience social disadvantage as a result of race or ethnicity, low income, or low educational level suffer disproportionate disease burdens, adverse health outcomes, and barriers to care but have not been well represented in studies of behavior and health.

Recommendation 2

The National Institutes of Health, the Agency for Healthcare Research and Quality, and the Centers for Disease Control and Prevention should develop targeted initiatives to increase research on the populations of women that have the highest risks and burdens of disease.

Finding 3

The incidence, prevalence, morbidity, or mortality associated with a number of conditions—for example, unintended pregnancy, maternal mortality and morbidity, nonmalignant gynecologic disorders, alcohol- and drug-addiction disorders, autoimmune diseases, and lung, ovarian, and endometrial cancer—have not improved. Most of those conditions substantially affect the quality of life of those who experience them. The major focus of health research has been on reducing mortality; a singular focus on mortality, however, can divert attention from other health outcomes despite the high value that women place on quality of life.

Recommendation 3

Research should include the promotion of wellness and quality of life in women. Research on conditions that have high morbidity and affect quality of life should be increased. Research should include the development of better measures or metrics to compare effects of health conditions, interventions, and treatments on quality of life. The end points examined in studies should include quality-of-life outcomes (for example, functional status or functionality, mobility, and pain) in addition to mortality.

Finding 4

Social factors and health-related behaviors and their interactions with genetic and cellular factors contribute to the onset and progression of multiple diseases; they act as pathways that are common to multiple outcomes. Considerable progress has been made in understanding the behavioral determinants of women's health, but less is known about how to change them and about the broader determinants of women's health that involve social, community, and societal factors.

Recommendation 4

Cross-institute initiatives in the National Institutes of Health—such as those in the Division of Program Coordination, Planning, and Strategic Initiatives—should support research on common determinants and risk factors that underlie multiple diseases and on interventions on those determinants that will decrease the occurrence or progression of diseases in women. The National Institutes of Health's Office of Research on Women's Health should increase collaborations with the Office of Behavioral and Social Sciences Research to design and oversee such research initiatives.

Finding 5

Limitations in the design, analysis, and scientific reporting of health research have slowed progress in women's health. Inadequate enforcement of recruitment of women and of reporting data by sex has fostered suboptimal analysis and reporting of data on women from clinical trials and other research. That failure has limited possibilities for identifying potentially important sex or gender differences. New methods and approaches are needed to maximize advances in promoting women's health.

Recommendation 5

- Government and other funding agencies should ensure adequate participation of women, analysis of data by sex, and reporting of sex-stratified analyses in health research. One possible mechanism would be expansion of the role of data safety monitoring boards to monitor participation, efficacy, and adverse outcomes by sex.
- Given the practical limitations in the size of research studies, research designs and statistical techniques should be explored that facilitate analysis of data on sociodemographic subgroups without substantially increasing the overall size of a study population. Conferences or meetings with a specific goal of developing consensus guidelines or recommendations for such study methods (for example, the use of Bayesian statistics and the pooling of data across study groups) should be convened by the National Institutes of Health, other federal agencies, and relevant professional organizations.
- To gain knowledge from existing studies that individually do not have sufficient numbers of female subjects for separate analysis, the director of the Office of the National Coordinator for Health Information Technology in the Department of Health and Human Services should support the development and application of mechanisms for the pooling of patient

and subject data to answer research questions that are not definitively answered by single studies.

- For medical products (drugs, devices, and biologics) that are coming to market, the Food and Drug Administration should enforce compliance with the requirement for sex-stratified analyses of efficacy and safety and should take those analyses into account in regulatory decisions.
- The International Committee of Medical Journal Editors and other editors of relevant journals should adopt a guideline that all papers reporting the outcomes of clinical trials report on men and women separately unless a trial is of a sex-specific condition (such as endometrial or prostatic cancer). The National Institutes of Health should sponsor a meeting to facilitate establishment of the guidelines.

Finding 6

The translation of research findings into practice can be delayed or precluded by various barriers—the complexity of science and research and challenges in communicating understandable and actionable messages, social or political opposition to advances for nonmedical reasons, fragmentation of health-care delivery, health-care policies and reimbursement, consumer confusion and apprehension, and so on. Many of those barriers are seen in connection with translation of research in general, but some have aspects that are peculiar to women, and few studies have been conducted to examine how to increase the speed or extent of the translation of findings related specifically to women's health into clinical practice. Methods of translation that have been used and that warrant evaluation for translating research findings in women include clinical-practice guidelines, mandatory standards, reimbursement practices, laws (including public-health laws), health-professions school curricula, and continuing education.

Recommendation 6

Research should be conducted on how to translate research findings on women's health into clinical practice and public-health policies rapidly. Research findings should be incorporated at the practitioner level and at the overall public-health systems level through, for example, the use of education programs targeted to practitioners and the development of guidelines. As programs and guidelines are developed and implemented, they should be evaluated to ensure effectiveness.

Finding 7

The public is confused by conflicting findings and opposing recommendations that emerge from health research, including women's health research. Conflicting results and work to resolve disagreements are part of the scientific process, but that iterative aspect of scientific discovery is not clearly conveyed to, or understood by, the public. The resulting uncertainty and distrust of research may affect women's care adversely. Relevant knowledge from studies of communication often is not used by researchers, funders, providers, and public-health professionals to target health messages and information to women.

Recommendation 7

The Department of Health and Human Services should appoint a task force to develop evidence-based strategies to communicate and market health messages that are based on research results to women. In addition to content experts in relevant departments and agencies, the task force should include mass-media and targeted-messaging and marketing experts. The strategies should be designed to communicate to the diverse audience of women; to increase awareness of women's health issues and treatments, including preventive and intervention strategies; and to decrease confusion regarding complex and sometimes conflicting findings. The goals of the task force should be to facilitate and improve the communication of research findings by researchers to women. Strategies for the task force to consider or explore might include

- requiring a plan for the communication and dissemination of findings of federally funded studies to the public, providers, and policy makers; and
- establishing a national media advisory panel of experts in women's health that would be readily available to provide context to reporters, scientists, clinicians, and policy makers at the time of release of new research reports.

1

Introduction

BACKGROUND

Women make up just over half the US population (US Census Bureau, 2009) and should not be considered a special, minority population, but rather an equal gender whose health needs require equal research efforts as those for men. Historically, however, the health needs of women have lagged in medical research. In 1985, the Public Health Service Task Force on Women's Health Issues, formed in light of the changing role of women in society, highlighted the need for research in women's health and issued *Women's Health: Report of the Public Health Service Task Force on Women's Health Issues* (HHS, 1985). It concluded that the historical lack of research focus on women's health concerns has compromised the quality of health information available to women as well as the health care they receive.

Since the publication of that report, there has been a transformation in women's health research—including changes in government support of research, in policies, in regulations, and in organization—that has resulted in the generation of new scientific knowledge of women's health. Offices on women's health in the National Institutes of Health (NIH) and in the Substance Abuse and Mental Health Services Administration were mandated by law. Other offices focusing on women's health were established in the Department of Health and Human Services (HHS), in its Food and Drug Administration (FDA) and Health Resources and Services Administration, and in other government agencies, and are now codified under the Patient Protection and Affordable Care Act of 2010 (Public Law [PL] 111-148).

A number of nongovernment organizations have also provided leadership in research in women's health. Women as advocates, research subjects, researchers, clinicians, administrators, and US representatives and senators played a major role in building a women's health movement.

Government Activities

In 1986, NIH established a policy for the inclusion of women in clinical research;[1] guidelines for the implementation of the policy were included in its 1987 *Guide to Grants and Contracts*. A similar policy encouraging enrollment of minority-group members was issued in 1987 (ORWH, 2009). Before that, little clinical research on women's health was conducted, for reasons that included concern about ethical issues of possible fetal exposure to an experimental substance, the variability in hormonal status in women, comorbidities, the assumption that results of research on men could be extrapolated to women, and legal issues. Several developments led to a questioning of the exclusion of women from clinical trials: with the onset of the epidemic of the acquired immunodeficiency syndrome, clinical trials explicitly solicited only men, thereby denying to women the potential of a life-saving treatment; results of clinical trials in men were not being extrapolated to women, as seen in the initial unequal application of stents, beta blockers, and cholesterol-lowering drugs; and the male model did not always corresponds to health and disease status in women, especially with regard to cardiovascular disease (McCarthy, 1994; Merkatz and Junod, 1994). As a result of congressional inquiries, particularly from the bipartisan Congressional Caucus on Women's Issues (Carnes et al., 2008), in the early 1990s the General Accounting Office[2] (GAO) reviewed how well NIH had implemented its 1986 policy[3] to encourage the inclusion of women in research study populations (GAO, 1990). GAO found that the policy was not well communicated within NIH or the research community; there were inconsistencies in application of the policy in the grant-review process; the policy applied only to extramural research, and the smaller intramural research program had no policy; and NIH officials took little action to encourage researchers to analyze results by sex. GAO also concluded that there was "no readily accessible source of data on the demographics of NIH

---

[1]NIH definition of clinical research: "1. Patient-oriented research. Research conducted with human subjects (or on material of human origin such as tissues, specimens and cognitive phenomena) for which an investigator (or colleague) directly interacts with human subjects. Excluded from this definition are in vitro studies that utilize human tissues that cannot be linked to a living individual. Patient-oriented research includes: a. Mechanisms of human disease, b. Therapeutic interventions, c. Clinical trials, and d. Development of new technologies. 2. Epidemiologic and behavioral studies. 3. Outcomes research and health services research" (HHS, 2009).

[2]In 2004, the agency name was changed to Government Accountability Office.

[3]According to GAO (1990), "although the policy first was announced in October, 1986, guidance for implementation was not published until July, 1989, and the policy was not applied consistently before the 1990 grant review cycles."

study populations" and it was "impossible to determine the impact of the policy." The resulting public outrage and response by Congress led to many of the developments in the early 1990s discussed below (Carnes et al., 2008). Table 1-1 highlights some of the milestones in women's health research at the federal level.

The National Institutes of Health Revitalization Act of 1993 (PL 103-43, Subtitle B, "Clinical Research Equity Regarding Women and Minorities") required that NIH grantees include women and minority groups in human-subjects research and, for clinical trials, "ensure that the trial is designed and carried out in a manner sufficient to provide for a valid analysis of whether the variables being studied in the trial affect women or members of minority groups, as the case may be, differently than other subjects in the trial."[4] Cost was not allowed as an acceptable reason for exclusion. In addition, NIH developed a database to monitor compliance with the law. However, the law for clinical trials applied only to phase III trials.[5] The act also formalized the NIH Office of Research on Women's Health (ORWH), which was established in September 1990, and charged it with reporting on progress related to the law throughout NIH.[6] Inclusion guidelines for complying with the law were published in 1994 and effectively stated that "that NIH could not and would not fund any grant, cooperative agreement or contract or support any intramural project . . . which did not comply with this policy" (NIH Tracking/Inclusion Committee, 2009).

In 2000, a second analysis by GAO documented that NIH had made significant progress toward the goal of including women and minorities in research.

---

[4]The National Institutes of Health Revitalization Act of 1993 essentially reinforced the existing NIH policies but with four major differences: (1) that NIH ensure that women and minorities and their subpopulations be included in all clinical research, (2) that women and minorities and their subpopulations be included in phase III clinical trials in numbers adequate to allow valid analyses of differences in intervention effect, (3) that cost not be allowed as an acceptable reason for excluding these groups, and (4) that NIH initiate programs and support for outreach efforts to recruit and retain women and minorities and their subpopulations as participants in clinical studies (HHS, 2008).

[5]According to NIH (2008), phase I trials are "initial studies to determine the metabolism and pharmacologic actions of drugs in humans, the side effects associated with increasing doses, and to gain early evidence of effectiveness; may include healthy participants and/or patients"; phase II trials are "controlled clinical studies conducted to evaluate the effectiveness of the drug for a particular indication or indications in patients with the disease or condition under study and to determine the common short-term side effects and risks"; and phase III trials are "expanded controlled and uncontrolled trials after preliminary evidence suggesting effectiveness of the drug has been obtained, and are intended to gather additional information to evaluate the overall benefit-risk relationship of the drug and provide an adequate basis for physician labeling."

[6]ORWH, in collaboration with the Office of Extramural Research and the Office of Intramural Research, monitors efforts for compliance, including convening a "trans-NIH" Tracking and Inclusion Committee. Inclusion of women and minorities in NIH-supported clinical research is documented by fiscal year in a series of reports, which are available to the public at http://orwh.od.nih.gov/inclusion/inclreports.html (accessed June 17, 2010). ORWH has also helped to develop outreach documents for investigators and study staff of NIH-supported research that include guidance on inclusion, recruitment, and retention of women and minorities in clinical research (ORWH, 2009).

TABLE 1-1 Key Federal and Legislative Milestones in Women's Health
Research from 1977 to Present

Year	Event
1977	FDA restricts women of childbearing potential from participating in clinical research because of thalidomide and diethylstilbestrol tragedies
1985	*Women's Health: Report of the Public Health Service Task Force on Women's Health Issues* concludes that "the historical lack of research focus on women's health concerns had compromised the quality of health information available to women as well as the health care they receive"
1986	NIH establishes policy to increase women's health research
1987	NIH issues guidelines *urging* inclusion of women for first time in NIH Guide to Grants and Contracts
1989	Nurses' Health Study focus is expanded[a]
1990	Women's Health Equity Act is passed
	Breast and Cervical Cancer Mortality Prevention Act establishes the CDC's National Breast and Cervical Cancer Early Detection Program
	GAO review of inclusion of women in clinical research concludes that • NIH policy on inclusion of women in clinical trials was not well communicated or understood within NIH or research community, was applied inconsistently among institutes, and was applied only to extramural research • There was "no readily accessible source of data on the demographics of NIH study populations," so it was impossible to determine whether NIH was enforcing its own recommendations
1990	NIH Office of Research on Women's Health is established by NIH and requires inclusion of women in clinical research
1991	HHS establishes Office on Women's Health
	WHI, largest clinical study in women, is launched by NIH[b]
	NIH ORWH launches strategic planning process to define research priorities for women's health research in NIH
1992	GAO issues report on inclusion of women in clinical trials used by FDA in evaluating drugs for marketing approval. The report finds that • Although women were sometimes included in drug trials, they were significantly underrepresented • Even when women were included, data were not analyzed to determine whether women's responses to drugs differed from those of men The report recommends that FDA ensure that drug companies consistently include "sufficient numbers of women in drug testing to identify gender-related differences in drug response and that such sex differences are explored and studied"
	Mammography Quality Standard Act is signed into law. It links accreditation of mammography facilities to evidence that facilities met standards for personnel, equipment, quality-assurance procedures, clinical images, phantom images, and dose

TABLE 1-1 Continued

Year	Event
1993	NIH Revitalization Act is signed into law. It requires inclusion of women in all clinical research and analysis of results by sex for phase III clinical trials and formalizes NIH ORWH in law
1993	FDA reverses its 1977 guidelines barring women of childbearing potential from participating in clinical research and publishes new guideline, *Guideline for the Study and Evaluation of Gender Differences in the Clinical Evaluation of Drugs*. The new guideline • Encourages inclusion of women in phase I and II studies • Requires inclusion of women in efficacy studies • Requires analysis of data on sex differences • Encourages consideration of effects of menstrual cycle on drug effect, effects of exogenous hormone therapy on drug effect, and effect of drug on the effects of oral contraceptives, when feasible
1994	Offices of women's health are established in FDA and CDC
	SWAN, the first study on the natural history of menopause, is established[c]
	NIH guidelines on the inclusion of women and minority-group members as subjects in clinical research (first issued in 1990 and supported by 1993 NIH Revitalization Act) become effective on publication in *Federal Register* of March 28, 1994; guidelines state that NIH must: • "Ensure that women and members of minorities and their subpopulations are included in all human subject research; • For Phase III clinical trials, ensure that women and minorities and their subpopulations must be included such that valid analysis of differences in intervention effect can be accomplished; • Not allow cost as an acceptable reason for excluding these groups; and, • Initiate programs and support for outreach efforts to recruit these groups into clinical studies."[d]
1996	HHS OWH launches National Centers of Excellence in Women's Health; first six centers are established; program was later terminated
1998	NIH ORWH launches second strategic planning process to define research priorities for women's health research in NIH, and releases report, *Agenda for Research on Women's Health for the 21st Century*
	FDA publishes its final rule permitting agency to place clinical hold on investigational new drug application if men or women were excluded because of potential risk of reproductive or developmental toxicity
1999	AHRQ Centers for Education and Research of Therapeutics program begins. The Centers address a variety of topics over time including the following which were specific to women: hip fractures, irregular heart rhythms and the menstrual cycle, gaps in osteoporosis treatment, arthritis resources, prescription drug use by pregnant women, and hormone therapy

continued

TABLE 1-1 Continued

Year	Event
2000	GAO issues followup audit of NIH that concludes that although women are in clinical trials at rates proportional to their numbers in general population, "NIH has made less progress in implementing the requirement that certain clinical trials be designed and carried out to permit valid analysis by sex, which could reveal whether interventions affect women and men differently"
	NIH ORWH initiates Building Interdisciplinary Research Careers in Women's Health program to support research career development of junior faculty members, known as Interdisciplinary Women's Health Research scholars, who have recently completed clinical training or postdoctoral fellowships and are commencing basic research, translational research, clinical research, or health-services research relevant to women's health
2001	Interim report released in January on GAO audit of FDA records reveals that 8 of last 10 drugs withdrawn from market caused more adverse effects in women than in men; 4 of those drugs were more often prescribed to women than to men, so the higher number of adverse events in women was not unexpected; other 4 drugs were prescribed equally to men and women, but number of adverse events was higher in women, and this suggested a true sex difference in incidence of adverse effects
	GAO final report on audit of FDA records reveals that • 30% of study documents examined failed to fulfill requirements for presentation of outcome data by sex • Nearly 40% of study documents examined did not include required demographic information Auditors conclude that "FDA has not effectively overseen the presentation and analysis of data related to sex differences in drug development."
2003	Study by FDA's OWH found that nearly equal numbers of men and women were participating in clinical trials but noted that data were not being analyzed by sex
	NIH establishes Specialized Centers of Research on Sex and Gender Factors Affecting Women's Health program to develop innovative approaches to advancing research on role of sex and gender factors in health and disease AHRQ begins the annual release of National Healthcare Quality Report and the National Healthcare Disparities Report that address various health care issues, including the following that were specific to women: disparities among women, including race, ethnicity, and socio-economic status; disparities between men and women; and trends and variations over time
2008	HHS implements strategic plan for 2010 through 2015

TABLE 1-1 Continued

Year	Event
2009	NIH OWHR launches third strategic planning process to identify research priorities in women's health for NIH
2010	Patient Protection and Affordable Care Act (Public Law 111-148) formally codifies the Offices of Women's Health within HHS. It also formally establishes an Office of Women's Health in the director's office of AHRQ, CDC, FDA, HRSA, and SAMHSA. It formally establishes an HHS Coordinating Committee on Women's Health and the National Women's Health Information Center. Each agency is appropriated such sums as may be necessary for FY 2010 through 2014

[a]The Nurses' Health Studies are among the largest and longest-running observational investigations of factors that influence women's health. They were started in 1976 to investigate potential long-term consequences of use of oral contraceptives and expanded in 1989. Information provided by 238,000 nurse-participants has led to many insights into health and disease. Prevention of cancer is still the primary focus, but the studies have also produced landmark data on cardiovascular disease, diabetes, and many other conditions. Most important, these studies have shown that diet, physical activity, and other lifestyle factors can powerfully promote better health.

[b]WHI is major 15-year research study to address most common causes of death, disability, and poor quality of life in postmenopausal women: cardiovascular disease, cancer, and osteoporosis. One major goal was to assess the effect of hormone therapy on those clinical end points.

[c]SWAN is a multisite longitudinal epidemiologic study designed to examine health of women during their middle years, including the menopausal transition. Study examines physical, biologic, psychologic, and social changes during this transitional period. The goal of SWAN's research is to help scientists, health-care providers, and women to learn how midlife experiences affect health and quality of life during aging.

[d]NIH defines a phase III clinical trial as "a broadly based . . . clinical investigation usually involving several hundred or more research subjects, for the purpose of evaluating an experimental intervention in comparison with a standard or control intervention or comparing two or more existing treatments."

ABBREVIATIONS: AHRQ, Agency for Healthcare Research and Quality; CDC, Centers for Disease Control and Prevention; FDA, Food and Drug Administration; FY, fiscal year; GAO, Government Accountability Office (formerly General Accounting Office); HHS, Department of Health and Human Services; HRSA, Health Resources and Services Administration; NIH, National Institutes of Health; ORWH, Office of Research on Women's Health; OWH, Office of Women's Health; SAMHSA, Substance Abuse and Mental Health Services Administration; SWAN, Study of Women's Health Across the Nation; WHI, Women's Health Initiative.

However, for the policy to have its intended effect, GAO emphasized that NIH needed to expand its focus beyond simple inclusion to ensure that, when it is scientifically appropriate, clinical trials be designed and carried out to allow for analysis by sex (GAO, 2000). NIH concurred with GAO's recommendations and stated they would make efforts to improve tracking of statistical analysis of data on women in clinical trials (GAO, 2000).

In addition to the activities related to NIH discussed above, there have been several activities related to FDA. One of FDA's primary regulatory responsibilities is to review applications for new drugs, biologics, and medical devices before they are marketed to the public. As part of that responsibility, the agency provides guidance for manufacturers that are conducting clinical trials and evaluating the safety and efficacy of new medical products. In 1977 guidance to manufacturers, FDA precluded women of childbearing potential from participating in phase I and early phase II trials (FDA, 1977) to avoid the possibility of exposing a fetus to a drug that had not satisfied preliminary safety and efficacy testing. Women of childbearing potential were permitted to participate in clinical trials that were conducted after evidence of a drug's effectiveness in humans was obtained (that is, in late phase II and phase III trials) and after data from animal reproductive studies were examined to see whether the drug caused birth defects; but in practice, women were underrepresented in the later phases as well (GAO, 1992). However, there were concerns that if FDA approved drugs on the basis of clinical trials in which women were underrepresented, their effectiveness and safety in women would not be known (GAO, 1992; Haseltine and Jacobson, 1997). For example, a drug dose established in small early-phase clinical trials that used mostly men might be too high for women, especially because men typically weigh more than women.

Concerns led to a GAO review (1992) that found that although women were included in phase III clinical trials for all the drugs surveyed, they were generally underrepresented, especially in trials of cardiovascular drugs (GAO, 1992). The report recommended that FDA ensure that drug companies consistently include "sufficient numbers of women in drug testing to identify gender-related differences in drug response and that such sex differences are explored and studied." In 1993, FDA issued a *Federal Register* (FR) notice (58 FR 39406), "Guideline for the Study and Evaluation of Gender Differences in Clinical Evaluation of Drugs," which reversed the 1977 guidance and recommended inclusion of women in early-phase clinical trials. FDA also amended its regulations to require efficacy and safety data on sex, age, and racial subgroups (21 Code of Federal Regulation [CFR] Parts 312 and 314, February 11, 1998. Final Rule: Investigational New Drug Applications and New Drug Applications). The final published rule permits the agency to place a clinical hold[7] on one or more studies that is the subject of an investigational new drug application if men or women with reproductive

---

[7]A clinical hold is an order issued by FDA to the sponsor of an investigational new drug to delay or to suspend a clinical investigation.

potential are excluded from participation only because of the risk or potential risk of reproductive or developmental toxicity associated with use of the investigational drug (21 CFR 312, June 1, 2000. Final Rule: Investigational New Drug Applications: Amendment to Clinical Hold Regulations for Product Intended for Life Threatening Disease).

In 2001, GAO again reviewed the inclusion of women in clinical drug trials submitted to FDA and found that women made up a majority (52%) of the trial participants in the new drug applications (NDAs) examined and that every NDA included enough women in the pivotal studies to make it possible to determine statistically whether the drugs were effective in women (GAO, 2000, 2001).[8] However, GAO had three concerns (GAO, 2001):

1. There was a relatively small proportion of women in early small-scale safety studies, which provide important information on a drug's toxicity and safe dosages for later stages of clinical development.
2. Although "most of the NDAs included analyses to detect differences between men and women, fewer of the NDAs explicitly included descriptions of both safety and efficacy analyses that compared women taking the drug with a comparison group of women taking a placebo or an alternative treatment," and "NDA sponsors did not recommend different dosage levels for men and women based on the sex differences they detected." Furthermore, GAO found "no evidence that any of the sex differences reported in any NDA on any dimension—safety, efficacy, or pharmacokinetics—even when statistically significant, were judged to be clinically relevant by either the NDA sponsors or the FDA reviewers, and no dose adjustments based on sex were recommended" (because NDA summary documents are not required to include analyses of sex differences, many of them do not, and FDA reviewers do not consistently request that information).
3. FDA lacks appropriate management systems to document the number of women in clinical trials, to comply with regulations for presenting outcomes data by sex, and to confirm that its reviewers have adequately addressed sex-related issues in their reviews.

---

[8]In addition, in 2002, the FDA Office on Women's Health funded an internal review of participation of women in clinical trials and sex analysis of data on biologics (such as vaccines, blood and blood components, allergenics, somatic cells, gene therapy, tissues, and recombinant therapeutic proteins) for which a new product or biologic license application was approved by the Center for Biologics Evaluation and Research during calendar years 1995–1999. The review found that nearly equal numbers of men and women were participating in the trials. However, analysis of data by sex occurred for only a small number of the studies reviewed (FDA, 2009).

Previous Institute of Medicine Report—*Does Sex Matter?*

In 2001, the Institute of Medicine (IOM) published *Exploring the Biological Contributions to Human Health: Does Sex Matter?* The committee that prepared the report focused on the basic differences between males and females that appear to have primarily biologic origins (that is, sex differences). Although it acknowledged the importance of social factors (such as female role expectations and socialization—that is, gender differences), it did not review data on those factors as health determinants. It also did not discuss the influence of reproductive factors (such as pregnancy, parity, and parenthood) on health (IOM, 2001), believing that these deserve a separate evaluation.

After a review of the evidence and discussions with scientific experts, that committee came to the following three overarching conclusions and the recommendations in Box 1-1 (IOM, 2001):

1. **Sex matters.** Being male or female is an important basic human variable and should be considered in designing and analyzing studies in all areas and at all levels of biomedical and health-related research.

BOX 1-1
Recommendations from *Exploring the Biological Contributions to Human Health: Does Sex Matter?*

Recommendations for Research
- Promote research on sex at the cellular level.
- Study sex differences from womb to tomb.
- Mine cross-species information.
- Investigate natural variations.
- Expand research on sex differences in brain organization and function.
- Monitor sex differences and similarities for all human diseases that affect both sexes.

Recommendations for Addressing Barriers to Progress
- Clarify use of the terms *sex* and *gender.*
- Support and conduct additional research on sex differences.
- Make sex-specific data more readily available.
- Determine and disclose the sex of origin of biological research materials.
- Longitudinal studies should be conducted and should be constructed so that their results can by analyzed by sex.
- Identify the endocrine status of research subjects.
- Encourage and support interdisciplinary research on sex differences.
- Reduce the potential for discrimination based on identified sex differences.

---

2. **The study of sex differences is evolving into a mature science.** There is sufficient knowledge of the biologic basis of sex differences to validate their scientific study and to allow the generation of hypotheses.
3. **Barriers to the advancement of knowledge about sex differences in health and illness exist and must be eliminated.** Scientists conducting research on sex differences are confronted with barriers to progress, including ethical, financial, sociologic, and scientific factors.

Since that report, a large amount of research on women's health has been conducted with a variety of research approaches, methods, and studies.

CHARGE TO THE COMMITTEE

Given the differences that have been identified between men and women with regard to health and given the transformation in approaching women's health and the increase in women's health research conducted over the last 2 decades, in the Consolidated Appropriations Act of 2008 (PL 110-161) Congress provided the HHS Office on Women's Health (OWH) with funds for the IOM "to conduct a comprehensive review of the status of women's health research, summarize what has been learned about how diseases specifically affect women, and report to the Congress on suggestions for the direction of future research." In response to that congressional language, the HHS OWH requested that the IOM conduct a study of women's health research; the charge to the committee for the project is presented in Box 1-2.

In response to that request, the IOM convened a committee of 18 members who have a wide variety of expertise, including expertise in biomedical research, research translation, research communication, disabilities, epidemiology, healthcare services, behavioral and social determinants of health, health disparities, nutrition, public health, women's health, clinical decision making, and such other medical specialties as cardiovascular disease, mental health, endocrinology, geriatrics, and immunology.

BOX 1-2
Charge to the Committee

An Institute of Medicine committee will examine what the research on women's health has revealed; how that research has been communicated to providers, women, the public and others; and identify gaps in those areas. The committee will identify examples of successful dissemination of findings paying particular attention to how the communication has influenced women's use of care and preventive services. The committee will make recommendations where appropriate.

This consensus report is the result of the committee's research and deliberations.

THE COMMITTEE'S APPROACH TO ITS CHARGE

In light of the expansive nature of its charge, the broad expertise of the committee, and the audience for this report, the committee recognized the need to focus its information gathering, the need to ensure that terms are defined and used consistently, and the need to have an organizational framework. The committee's information gathering approach, definitions, and framework are described below.

Definitions Used by the Committee

In Box 1-3 the committee defines a number of terms that will be used throughout this report. In 1946, the World Health Organization defined health as

---

BOX 1-3
Key Definitions

Women's Health Research
Women's health research is confined for this report to the scientific study of health conditions that are specific to women, are more common or more serious in women, or have distinct causes, manifestations, outcomes, or treatments in women; it includes the study of factors that are determinants of health (biologic, psychologic, environmental, and sociocultural), especially factors that might affect women disproportionately or uniquely.

Sex
"The classification of living things, generally as male or female according to their reproductive organs and functions assigned by chromosomal complement." (IOM, 2001)

Gender
"A person's self-representation as male or female, or how that person is responded to by social institutions on the basis of the individual's gender presentation. Gender is shaped by environment and experience." (IOM, 2001)

Research Translation
The application of the knowledge and findings from research (such as basic experimental research, observational and clinical studies, and research on health-care services) to health-care practices and public-health policies.

Health Communication
The dissemination of research findings to the public.

"a state of complete physical, mental and social well-being and not merely the absence of disease or infirmity" (WHO, 1946). The committee agrees that health is not merely the absence of disease and disability. The committee approached women's health as a concept that has expanded beyond a narrow focus on the female reproductive system to encompass other conditions that create a significant burden in women's lives. It confines its discussion of women's health research to the scientific study of health conditions that are specific to women, are more common or more serious in women, have distinct causes or manifestations in women, or have different outcomes or treatments in women; and it includes the study of factors that are determinants of health (biologic, psychologic, environmental, and sociocultural factors), especially factors that might affect women disproportionately or uniquely.

Being a man or a woman has a substantial influence on health as a result of biologic and sociocultural differences. It is important to distinguish sex-based differences and gender-based differences. The committee uses those terms as they were defined in the IOM report *Exploring the Biological Contributions to Human Health: Does Sex Matter?* (IOM, 2001). That report defined *sex* as "the classification of living things, generally as male or female according to their reproductive organs and functions assigned by chromosomal complement." *Gender* is defined as "a person's self-representation as male or female, or how that person is responded to by social institutions on the basis of the individual's gender presentation. Gender is shaped by environment and experience."

The committee is charged not only with highlighting what has been learned from women's health research but with providing conclusions and recommendations related to the translation and communication of those research findings. For the purposes of this report, the committee defines research translation as the application or implementation of the findings of research studies in changes in health-care practice and public-health policies, and it defines health-research communication as the dissemination of the findings of research studies related to women's health to the general public. As discussed in *Healthy People 2010* (HHS ODPHP, 2009):

> Health communication encompasses the study and use of communication strategies to inform and influence individual and community decisions that enhance health. It links the domains of communication and health and is increasingly recognized as a necessary element of efforts to improve personal and public health [Jackson and Duffy, 1998; NCI, 1989; Piotrow et al., 1997]. Health communication can contribute to all aspects of disease prevention and health promotion and is relevant in a number of contexts, including (1) health professional-patient relations, (2) individuals' exposure to, search for, and use of health information, (3) individuals' adherence to clinical recommendations and regimens, (4) the construction of public health messages and campaigns, (5) the dissemination of individual and population health risk information, that is, risk communication, (6) images of health in the mass media and the culture at large, (7) the educa-

tion of consumers about how to gain access to the public health and health care systems, and (8) the development of telehealth applications [Atkin and Wallack, 1990; Backer et al., 1992; Eng and Gustafson, 1999; Freimuth et al., 1989; Harris, 1995; Jackson and Duffy, 1998; Maibach and Parrott, 1995; Northouse and Northouse, 1998; Ray and Donohew, 1990].

Information Gathering

The committee met six times, including two open information-gathering sessions at which the members heard from stakeholders and researchers. Appendix A presents the agendas of those public meetings. During that time, the NIH ORWH held a series of scientific workshops and public hearings involving a variety of stakeholders (health-care providers, public-policy experts, advocates, and the general public) to gather information to update its women's health research agenda. Committee members or IOM staff attended portions of those meetings so that they could be aware of ORWH research–priority development and hear further stakeholder input on research priorities in women's health.

The committee conducted extensive literature searches related to women's health research and on the translation and communication of research findings in numerous databases, including PubMed and Embase. The committee focused on research published in the last 15–20 years, which is roughly the period during which policies were implemented to promote women's health research. The committee's evaluation included research on biologically determined sex differences in health and research on the influence of social, behavioral, and environmental factors on women's health. Searches were conducted both on studies of women's health research in general and on specific diseases, conditions, and determinants of health. Because of the large number of published articles, summaries and review articles were used when possible. Data from a broad spectrum of research were reviewed, including clinical trials, observational studies, basic research (spanning human, animal, and cellular studies), and research on health-care services, such as women's use of and access to high-quality health care. The committee focused on research relevant to the health of US women and to differential effects in groups of women.

In light of the breadth of the topic and the enormous base of published scientific articles, reviews, and summaries, the committee does not provide a comprehensive summary of findings of research related to women's health but instead identifies selected conditions in which there has been progress. In addition, health issues in which progress has been lacking or narrowly limited and in which additional research is needed are mentioned; the committee focuses on a few examples that make it possible to identify overarching lessons and recommendations.

Focus of Charge

Given the breadth of its charge, the committee developed a series of questions to focus deliberations and ensure appropriate response to the charge. Although not officially outlined in the statement of task, the questions provided more specific tasks for the committee to use in addressing its overall charge. The questions are presented in Box 1-4. The committee refers to those questions in this report to link the information in the various chapters to its charge.

Framework for the Committee's Work

Women's health research (like health research in general) traditionally has been conducted with an organ- or disease-based approach. With advancing knowledge, however, it has become apparent that a woman's health encompasses more than the sum of the absence or presence of discrete disease states and is much more complex. Moreover, health and disease are influenced by a number of factors and the interplay among them, including genetics; physiologic, psychologic, social, and environmental forces; and growth, development, and aging. Health research has expanded to be interdisciplinary and collaborative among specialties (for example, a clinical trial might be developed and conducted jointly by internists, oncologists, cardiologists, epidemiologists, psychologists, and nutritionists). The present committee was faced with a decision of whether to work with a disease-based framework, in keeping with the conduct and funding of most of the research reviewed, or to take an interdisciplinary approach by incorporating multiple determinants of health and considering health outcomes in addition to disease. The committee used both approaches. In Chapter 2, health determinants are discussed in the context of an ecologic framework that distinguishes

---

BOX 1-4
Committee Questions to Focus Deliberations

1. Is women's health research studying the most appropriate and relevant determinants of health?
2. Is women's health research focused on the most appropriate and relevant conditions and end points?
3. Is women's health research studying the most relevant groups of women? For example, are women with sociodemographic characteristics that place them at higher risk adequately studied?
4. Are the most appropriate research methods being used to study women's health?
5. Are the research findings being translated in a way that affects practice?
6. Are the research findings being communicated effectively to women?

individual-level determinants of health (such as biologic and physiologic factors and health behaviors) from broader determinants of health (such as environmental and social determinants) (see, for example, Dahlgren and Whitehead, 1991; Evans and Stoddart, 1990; IOM, 2000). Such an approach is better suited to understanding not only the pathophysiology of a health outcome but also preventive measures that can help to ensure optimal health. When summarizing advances in the understanding of the biology and pathology related to women's health in Chapter 3, however, the committee organized findings by health outcome in light of the nature of the literature reviewed.

The committee did not conduct a comprehensive review of all research on all diseases, disorders, and conditions that are women's health issues. It reviewed data on the status of women's health in terms of morbidity and mortality, and it assessed improvements in those respects in the context of research that has been conducted on the various diseases and health issues. The overall leading causes of death in women from 1989 through 2006 are presented in Appendix B. The committee focused its review in Chapter 3 on progress that has been made in reducing mortality or morbidity associated with specific conditions. The committee also highlights a few conditions or diseases in which little progress has been made so that it can identify lessons learned and future needs.

Because the incidence and prevalence of conditions and the leading causes of mortality in women vary with age, it is important to remember that the main causes of death in women overall do not necessarily reflect the main health concerns and issues at different points in a women's life cycle and that events that occur in one stage can affect health later in life. Furthermore, women have a longer life expectancy than men so many diseases of aging are of a greater concern for women than men.

The population of women in the United Sates is diverse and growing more so. As can be seen in Appendix B, demographic groups vary in the prevalence, incidence, and severity of conditions and their determinants. The committee has reviewed the data on disparities to determine whether research is being conducted on appropriate populations of women. The committee recognizes that different groups of women (such as lesbians,[9] military and veterans, prisoners, and disabled women) can have different health needs or benefit from different means of meeting their health needs. The committee has not compiled a comprehensive list of such populations but discusses the needs of particular groups as appropriate when data are available. Finally, in addition to health conditions, the committee considered such emerging issues as genetics and the effect of health information technology.

---

[9]The IOM is currently preparing a report on lesbian, gay, bisexual, and transgender health issues as well as research gaps and opportunities.

ORGANIZATION OF THIS REPORT

The remainder of this report is organized in five chapters and three appendixes. Chapter 2 focuses on findings over the last 2 decades related to the determinants of health outcomes and diseases in women. Chapter 3 provides an overview of some of the major research advances of the last 1–2 decades in understanding the biology of women's health, including the biology of conditions relevant to women and diagnosing and treating those health conditions. Those two chapters present the evidence that supports the committee's conclusions regarding questions 1, 2, and 3 in Box 1-4, that is, whether women's health research is focused on the most appropriate and relevant determinants of health, the most appropriate and relevant health conditions, and the most relevant groups of women. In Chapter 4, the committee looks at the methods that have been used in women's health research on pathology and health determinants and draws conclusions related to question 4 in Box 1-4, that is, whether the most appropriate research methods are being used to study women's health? The committee addresses questions 5 and 6, about how well research findings in women's health have been translated into practice and communicated to women, in Chapter 5. The committee's findings are synthesized in Chapter 6, which presents the committee's responses to its six questions, a summary of the basis for its responses, and its overall conclusions and recommendations on women's health research.

The report includes three appendixes. Appendix A presents the agendas of the open sessions held by the committee. Appendix B summarizes data on the overall causes of morbidity or causes of mortality in women. The committee used the latter information to focus its review of research on women's health on issues that have the greatest impact on women. A number of large research studies or trials have been conducted in women in recent years, such as the Nurses' Health Study and the Women's Health Initiative. The findings of those studies are discussed in almost all the chapters in this report. To facilitate the discussions and avoid repetition of the descriptions of the study designs, Appendix C, which is included on the enclosed compact disk, describes those large trials.

REFERENCES

Atkin, C. K., and L. M. Wallack. 1990. *Mass Communication and Public Health: Complexities and Conflicts.* Edited by Anonymous, Sage focus editions. Newbury Park, CA: Sage Publications.

Backer, T. E., E. M. Rogers, and S. Pradeep. 1992. *Designing Health Communication Campaigns: What Works?* Newberry Park, CA: Sage Publications.

Carnes, M., C. Morrissey, and S. E. Geller. 2008. Women's health and women's leadership in academic medicine: Hitting the same glass ceiling? *Journal of Women's Health* 17(9):1453–1462.

Dahlgren, G., and M. Whitehead. 1991. *Policies and Strategies to Promote Social Equity in Health.* Stockholm, Sweden: Institute for the Futures Studies.

Eng, T. R., and D. H. Gustafson, eds. 1999. *Wired for Health and Well-being: The Emergence of Interactive Health Communication.* Washington, DC: Office of Disease Prevention and Health Promotion.

Evans, R. G., and G. L. Stoddart. 1990. Producing health, consuming health care. *Social Science & Medicine* 31(12):1347–1363.

FDA (US Food and Drug Administration). 1977. *General Considerations for the Clinical Evaluation of Drugs.* Rockville, MD: US Department of Health, Education, and Welfare, Public Health Service, FDA.

————. 2009. *Participation of Females in Clinical Trials and Gender Analysis of Data in Biologic Product Applications.* http://www.fda.gov/BiologicsBloodVaccines/DevelopmentApproval Process/InvestigationalNewDrugINDorDeviceExemptionIDEProcess/ucm094300.htm (accessed July 14, 2009).

Freimuth, V. S., J. A. Stein, and T. J. Kean. 1989. *Searching for Health Information: The Cancer Information Service Model.* Philadelphia: University of Pennsylvania Press.

GAO (US General Accounting Office). 1990. *National Institutes of Health: Problems in Implementing Policy on Women in Study Population: Statement of Mark V. Nadel, Associate Director, National and Public Health Issues, Human Resources Division, Before the Subcommittee on Health and the Environment, Committee on Energy and Commerce, House of Representatives.* Washington, DC: GAO.

————. 1992. *Women's Health: FDA Needs to Ensure More Study of Gender Differences in Prescription Drug Testing: Report to Congressional Requesters.* Washington, DC: GAO.

————. 2000. *Women's Health: NIH Has Increased Its Efforts to Include Women in Research: Report to Congressional Requesters.* Washington, DC: GAO.

————. 2001. *Women's Health: Women Sufficiently Represented in New Drug Testing, but FDA Oversight Needs Improvement.* Washington, DC: GAO.

Harris, L. M., ed. 1995. *Health and the New Media: Technologies Transforming Personal and Public Health, Lea's Communication Series.* Mahwah, NJ: Erlbaum.

Haseltine, F. P., and B. G. Jacobson, eds. 1997. *Women's Health Research: A Medical and Policy Primer.* Washington, DC: American Psychiatric Publishing, Inc.

HHS (US Department of Health and Human Services). 1985. Women's health. Report of the Public Health Service Task Force on Women's Health Issues. *Public Health Reports* 100(1):73–106.

————. 2008. *Monitoring Adherence to the NIH Policy on Inclusion of Women and Minorities as Subjects of Clinical Research.* http://orwh.od.nih.gov/inclusion/FinalAnnualReport2007.pdf (accessed July 15, 2009).

————. 2009. *Application for a Public Health Service Grant–PHS 398.* http://grants1.nih. gov/grants/ funding/phs398/phs398.doc (August 3, 2010).

HHS ODPHP (US Department of Health and Human Services, Office of Disease Prevention and Health Promotion). 2009. *Healthy People 2010: Health Communication.* http://www.healthypeople. gov/document/HTML/Volume1/11HealthCom.htm (accessed July 15, 2009).

IOM (Institute of Medicine). 2000. *Promoting Health: Intervention Strategies from Social and Behavioral Research.* Washington, DC: National Academy Press.

————. 2001. *Exploring the Biological Contributions to Human Health: Does Sex Matter?* Washington, DC: National Academy Press.

Jackson, L. D., and B. K. Duffy, eds. 1998. *Health Communication Research: A Guide to Developments and Directions.* Westport, CT: Greenwood.

Maibach, E., and R. Parrott. 1995. *Designing Health Messages: Approaches from Communication Theory and Public Health Practice.* Thousand Oaks, CA: Sage Publications.

McCarthy, C. R. 1994. Historical background of clinical trials involving women and minorities. *Academic Medicine* 69(9):695–698.

Merkatz, R. B., and S. W. Junod. 1994. Historical background of changes in FDA policy on the study and evaluation of drugs in women. *Academic Medicine* 69(9):703–707.

NCI (National Cancer Institute). 1989. *Making Health Communications Work.* Pub. No. NIH 89-1493. Department of Health and Human Services.

NIH (National Insitutes of Health). 2008. *Glossary of Clinical Trial Terms.* http://clinicaltrials.gov/ct2/info/glossary#phasel (accessed January 22, 2010).

NIH Tracking/Inclusion Committee. 2009. *Monitoring Adherence to the NIH Policy on the Inclusion of Women and Minorities as Subjects in Clinical Research: Comprehensive Report: Tracking of Human Subjects Research as Reported in Fiscal Year 2007 and Fiscal Year 2008.* Washington, DC: HHS and NIH.

Northouse, L. L., and P. G. Northouse. 1998. *Health Communication: Strategies for Health Professionals.* 3rd ed. Stamford, CT: Appleton & Lange.

ORWH (Office of Research on Women's Health). 2009. *Inclusion of Women in Clinical Research.* http://orwh.od.nih.gov/inclusion/inclintro.html (accessed July 15, 2009).

Piotrow, P. T., D. L. Kincaid, J. G. Rimon II, and W. Reinhardt. 1997. *Health Communication: Lessons from Family Planning and Reproductive Health.* Westport, CT: Praeger.

Ray, E. B., and L. Donohew, eds. 1990. *Communication and Health: Systems and Applications, Communication Textbook Series; Applied Communication.* Hillsdale, NJ: L. Erlbaum Associates.

US Census Bureau. 2009. *Population Estimates.* http://www.census.gov/popest/national/asrh/NC-EST2007-srh.html (accessed April 29, 2009).

WHO (World Health Organization). 1946. *Preamble to the Constitution of the World Health Organization as Adopted by the International Health Conference, New York, 19–22 June, 1946; Signed on 22 July 1946 by the Representatives of 61 States (Official Records of the World Health Organization, no. 2, p. 100) and Entered into Force on 7 April 1948.* http://www.who.int/about/definition/en/print.html (accessed July 14, 2009).

2

Research on Determinants
of Women's Health

Improvements in women's health require an understanding of the determinants of disease, functioning, and well-being and the capacity to intervene in connection with the determinants. Intervention can occur at any level from cells to communities. Some determinants are linked to specific disorders; others have broad effects. Addressing common determinants of multiple diseases increases the potential for a greater overall influence on women's health.

Several models have been developed to illustrate determinants of population health. Although they are not specific to women, they are useful for describing the variety of factors in women's health. Models of determinants of health have generally distinguished individual-level characteristics (such as biologic and physiologic factors and health-related behaviors) from the broader determinants (such as environmental and social determinants) in which the individual-level characteristics develop and are expressed. There is some variability among models with regard to labeling determinants of health and the organizing frameworks for determinants (Dahlgren and Whitehead, 1991; Evans and Stoddart, 1990; IOM, 2000a), but in general, biologic and physiologic, or "downstream," determinants of health are identified as modifiable through complex pathways by proximal determinants (such as drugs, surgical interventions, and health behaviors) and "upstream" determinants (such as social and economic policies).

To organize its review of research on the determinants of women's health, the committee adopted a model of health determinants similar to that described in *The Future of the Public's Health in the 21st Century* (IOM, 2002a). Adapted from Dahlgren and Whitehead (1991), the model (see Figure 2-1) is consistent with this committee's approach that determinants of health encompass biologic, behavioral, and social factors. In addition this model acknowledges the interac-

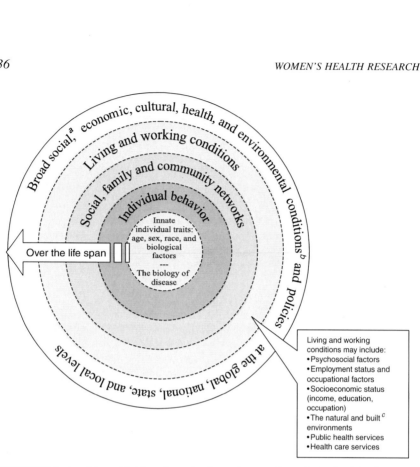

FIGURE 2-1 A guide to thinking about the determinants of population health. The model was originally adapted from Dahlgren and Whitehead (1991). The dotted lines between levels of the model denote interaction effects between and among the various levels of health determinants.

[a]Social conditions include economic inequality, urbanization, mobility, cultural values, and attitudes and policies related to discrimination and intolerance on the basis of race, sex, and other differences. Although race is an individual characteristic, its influence on health is strongly influenced by the social context of race.

[b]Other conditions at the national level might include major sociopolitical shifts, such as recession, war, and government collapse.

[c]The built environment includes transportation, water and sanitation, housing, and other dimensions of urban planning.

SOURCE: IOM (2002a).

tion between and among the various levels of health determinants. The organizing framework includes the following determinants of health:

- innate traits and characteristics;
- individual behavior;

- social, family, and community relationships and networks;
- living and working conditions; and
- societal, economic, cultural, and environmental policies and conditions.

Some determinants may operate at more than one level, and most health outcomes will be related to determinants from more than one level of the model. The model is consistent with the committee's belief that quality of life is a particularly important component of women's health. The determinant-based framework has advantages over a strictly disease-based framework in that it more readily allows consideration of functioning, wellness, and quality of life in addition to the understanding, detecting, and treating of diseases. It also allows discussion of interventions that can occur at the individual, community, and population levels, and how determinants are related to health across a woman's life span.

This chapter presents evidence of the impact of a number of behavioral factors (smoking, eating habits and physical activity, sexual risk behavior, and alcohol use), social and community factors (violence against girls and women, social connections and stress, and social disadvantage), and societal factors (cultural factors and health care) that affect women's health. Those factors are discussed as examples of factors that affect women's health and should not be considered a comprehensive list of determinants of women's health. Biologic determinants are discussed in Chapter 3 in the context of their roles in specific diseases.

BEHAVIORAL FACTORS

In the last 20 years, there has been substantial progress in understanding how behavior affects people's health, including the health of women and girls. Research has identified modifiable risk factors for a variety of health outcomes and has led to a better understanding of the level at which behavior leads to improvements in or deterioration of health. Human behavior is one of the biggest contributors to death and disease (McGinnis and Foege, 1993; McGinnis et al., 2002). With respect to US women, for example, substantial numbers of deaths have been attributed to smoking, physical inactivity, and dietary factors, which are preventable (Figure 2-2). As discussed in the Institute of Medicine (IOM) report *Health and Behavior: The Interplay of Biological, Behavioral, and Societal Influences*, the extent to which a given behavior affects health varies during the course of life (IOM, 2001a), and life span and stage of development are important to consider. Several IOM reports have also discussed strategies for modifying behavioral norms to improve the health of specific populations (IOM, 2000b, 2005a,b, 2010). This section discusses research on behavioral factors that are major contributors to morbidity and mortality among women: smoking, eating habits and physical activity, sexual risk behavior, and alcohol use.

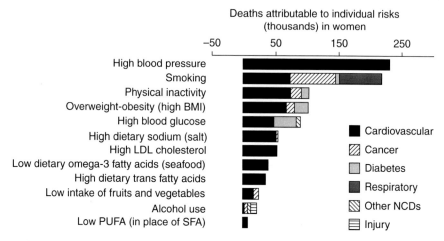

FIGURE 2-2 Deaths in women attributable to total effects of individual risk factors, by disease. Data are for all women and do not reflect differences across racial, ethnic, and socioeconomic groups.
ABBREVIATIONS: BMI, body-mass index; LDL, low-density lipoproteins; NCD, non-communicable disease; PUFA, polyunsaturated fatty acid; SFA, saturated fatty acid.
SOURCE: Danaei et al. (2009).

Smoking

The US surgeon general issued reports outlining the state of the evidence on the health consequences of smoking and progress in understanding the factors that influence smoking by women and girls in 1980 (HHS, 1980) and 2001 (HHS, 2001). Hundreds of observational studies conducted since the 2001 surgeon general's report have been published and have added substantially to the knowledge base on smoking by women and girls and have helped to improve women's health. In 2007, about one-fifth of US women 18 years old or older were current smokers[1] (CDC, 2008a). Smoking has been declining in both women and men in recent decades, but the rate of decline has been slower in women. Similarly, declines in lung-cancer deaths have been slower in women than in men.

Vulnerable Populations

Smoking is strongly associated with socioeconomic status (Dube et al., 2009). The prevalence of smoking is over 3 times as high in women who have 9–11 years of education (33.6%) as in women who have an undergraduate degree

---

[1]Defined as "those who smoked more than 100 cigarettes in their lifetime and now smoke every day or some days" (CDC, 2008a).

(9.7%). The difference by education is even greater in pregnant women: 25.5% in pregnant women who have 9–11 years of education vs 2.2% in college graduates. Similarly, smoking is higher in women who live below the poverty level (31.7%) than in those living at or above the poverty level (17.0%). American Indian or Alaskan native women are more likely to smoke (22.4%) than women who are white (20.6%), black (17.8%), or Hispanic (10.7%); Asian American or Pacific Islanders (4.7%) are the least likely to do so (Dube et al., 2009).

Health Consequences of Smoking

Research has painted an increasingly bleak picture of the health consequences of smoking in women and girls. As is true for the US population as a whole, tobacco use is the leading cause of preventable death in women. Smoking substantially increases women's risk of a number of cardiovascular outcomes, including coronary heart disease and stroke (Bermudez et al., 2002; Kawachi et al., 1993; Stampfer et al., 2000). In women who smoke and use oral contraceptives, the risk of heart attack is even greater; the risk of heart attack is increased by as much as a factor of 30 and the risk of stroke by a factor of 3 compared with the risk in nonsmokers who use oral contraceptives (Burkman et al., 2004). Smoking is the major cause of lung cancer in women, with about 80% of lung cancers in women attributable to smoking. In 1987 lung cancer surpassed breast cancer to become the leading cause of cancer deaths in women (HHS, 2004; RWJF, 2009). Observational studies have established that smoking also increases the risk of cancers of the larynx, oral cavity and esophagus, stomach, bladder, kidneys, and pancreas (HHS, 1980, 2001, 2004). For women specifically, smoking results in increased risk of cancers of the cervix and vulva and of such gynecologic and reproductive complications as menstrual problems, reduced fertility, and premature menopause (Gold et al., 2001; Laurent et al., 1992; Luborsky et al., 2003). Postmenopausal women who smoke experience accelerated loss of bone mass, which may put them at increased risk for osteoporosis and hip fracture (HHS, 2001, 2004; Law and Hackshaw, 1997).[2] Smoking during pregnancy can result in placental abruption and previa (CDC, 2007a; HHS, 2001; RWJF, 2009).

Research on Smoking Initiation, Prevention, and Interventions

Since the late 1960s the tobacco industry has targeted women and girls by using specific cigarette brands and marketing techniques (RWJF, 2009).[3] The US surgeon general's reports on women and smoking and more recent reports by the

---

[2]For a fuller list of the health consequences of smoking for women and girls, see HHS (2001, 2004).

[3]In 1968, Philip Morris introduced Virginia Slims, the first female-specific brand of cigarette (RWJF, 2009).

National Cancer Institute, the Robert Wood Johnson Foundation, and others have described tobacco companies' use of themes of associations between smoking and social desirability, independence, and weight control to target adolescent girls, who are at an impressionable age (HHS, 1980, 2001; NCI, 2008; RWJF, 2009). Such targeted marketing has been identified as a reason that lung cancer–death rates initially increased and then have been slower to decline in women than in men in recent years (Jemal et al., 2008; RWJF, 2009).

The large majority of women who smoke, as with men, began doing so during adolescence; this is cause for concern because risks of many of the health consequences of smoking are a function of the duration (years smoked), in addition to intensity (cigarettes per day) of use (Flanders et al., 2003; Hegmann et al., 1993; Terry and Rohan, 2002). Most interventions to prevent smoking initiation, therefore, have targeted adolescents. Interventions have included school-based or health-care–based educational and informational programs, environmental and policy change interventions that restrict tobacco advertising and youth access to tobacco products, smoking bans, and taxation of tobacco products (IOM, 2009a). Several interventions have been found to reduce youth smoking but, as discussed in a report of the surgeon general in 2001, little systematic effort has been focused on developing and evaluating prevention interventions specifically in girls (HHS, 2001), and more research on differences in smoking cessation for girls and boys is needed (Thorner et al., 2007).

The Department of Health and Human Services report *Treating Tobacco Use and Dependence: 2008 Update* concluded that women benefit from the same interventions as men but that the data are mixed as to whether they benefit by the same magnitude. The smoking quit ratio—proportion of ever smokers who are now former smokers—has increased in both men and women, but women have consistently had lower quit ratios (Gritz et al., 1996). Several factors are associated with poorer cessation outcomes in women and girls: being less ready to stop smoking; being more addicted to cigarettes, as indicated by the smoking of more cigarettes per day; having less confidence in resisting temptation; having less social support; and socioeconomic disadvantages (being unemployed and having less education and lower employment) (HHS, 2001). Psychosocial interventions—including telephone counseling, individually tailored followup, and advice to quit geared toward children's health—are effective in women smokers (HHS, 2008a). Weight gain is associated with smoking cessation (Caan et al., 1996; Flegal et al., 1995), and is often of concern to women (Copeland et al., 2006). There is some evidence that exercise is effective in reducing weight gain after smoking cessation in women, but the findings are not consistent (HHS, 2008a).

Several pharmacologic aids have been developed in the last 25 years to help smokers quit and to help prevent relapse by reducing cigarette cravings and withdrawal symptoms. A few trials have compared the benefit of the aids in women and men. In the overall population, nicotine-replacement therapies (NRTs), such as the nicotine patch and chewing gum, double the odds of quitting smoking relative to placebo (Silagy et al., 2004). Although NRTs appear to lead to higher cessation rates in women than placebo especially when combined with cessation counseling (Reynoso et al., 2005), there is some evidence that NRTs are more efficacious in men than in women. In part because of concerns about exposure of the fetus to NRTs, few studies have tested NRTs in pregnant women (see for example, HHS, 2008a; Schnoll et al., 2007).

Pregnancy appears to be a time of high motivation for many women to quit smoking, but relapse often occurs after birth (Reichert et al., 2004). In the health-care setting, multipronged psychosocial interventions (for example, a combination of pregnancy-specific self-help materials and counseling with a health educator) have been found to be significantly effective in getting women to quit smoking during pregnancy. Psychosocial interventions for postpartum abstinence from smoking had positive but nonsignificant effects (HHS, 2008a). Spousal support for quitting, including the spouse's own change in smoking, is particularly helpful (HHS, 2004). Partner smoking is associated with continued smoking by women during pregnancy; this suggests the need for partner-focused interventions along with interventions for pregnant women themselves (DiClemente et al., 2000).

Eating Habits and Physical Activity

The prevalence of obesity, defined as a body-mass index (BMI) of 30 or more, in the United States has more than doubled in the last 3 decades, with increases seen in women, men, and children (Flegal et al., 2002; Mokdad et al., 1999; Ogden et al., 2006; Sturm, 2003). More than one-third of US adults were obese and more than two-thirds of adults were either obese or overweight (BMI 25–29.9) in 2007–2008 (Flegal et al., 2010). Class 3 or extreme obesity, which has been defined as a BMI of 40 or more, is associated with an increased risk of all-cause mortality and comorbidities. The prevalence of Class 3 obesity more than doubled in women between the early 1990s and 2000, and in 2000 was 2.8%, which was about twice as high as in men. The prevalence was highest in black women (6%) and those without a high-school education (Freedman, 2002). Recent data from the National Health and Nutrition Examination Survey (NHANES) provide some evidence that the rate of increase in obesity is slowing, particularly in women. Unlike the increases seen between 1976–1980 and 1988–1994, and between 1988–1994 and 1999–2000, "the prevalence of obesity showed no statistically significant changes over the 10-year period from 1999 through 2008" (Flegal et al., 2010).

Eating habits and physical activity are the primary drivers of weight; overconsumption of calories and insufficient physical activity are fueling high rates of people who are overweight or obese (Patrick et al., 2004; Weinsier et al., 1998). Calorie consumption has increased over the past 4 decades, in part from larger portion sizes, increased consumption of high-sugar and high-fat foods, increased consumption of high-calorie and low-nutrient food and beverages (for example, sodas), and increased eating out (Levi et al., 2009). Over the past 5 decades, physical activity has decreased with Americans walking less, having less time to exercise in part from longer working hours and longer commutes, and reduced physical demands of work, household management, and travel (Levi et al., 2009). In addition, the built environment[4] can "facilitate or constrain physical activity" (NRC, 2005), and many people live in areas that facilitate driving rather than walking, or in areas where parks and recreational facilities are not considered safe (Levi et al., 2009).

Substantial headway has been made over the last 20 years in understanding how eating habits and physical activity affect the health of women. Whereas prior evidence came largely from studies of men, several large US cohort studies of women—such as the Nurses' Health Study, the Women's Health Initiative (see Box 2-1 for a brief description), the Women's Health Study, and the Black Women's Health Study—have resulted in a vast literature on the roles of eating habits and physical activity in women's health (Hu et al., 2001; Martinez et al., 1997). That research has informed the design of interventions to increase physical activity and improve eating habits in women and girls.

Much more is known about determinants of being overweight and obese, but there is still a lack of effective interventions. Although the rate of increase in obesity has decreased, the prevalence of obesity doubled in the last 2 decades (Flegal et al., 2002; Mokdad et al., 1999; Sturm, 2003); in 2001–2004, more than one-third of US adults were obese (BMI, over 30), and two-thirds were overweight or obese (BMI, 25–29.9) (Ogden et al., 2006).

According to a self-report survey of adults conducted in 2007, 40% of US women did not meet the *2008 Physical Activity Guidelines for Americans* for adequate physical activity (CDC, 2008b),[5] despite the documented health benefits of physical activity. The eating habits of women in the United States are also far from optimal. For example, less than one-third of women in 2005 met recommendations to eat five or more servings of fruits and vegetables per day (CDC, 2007b). It is a reflection of the poor diets and lack of physical activity of most

---

[4]The built environment is "defined broadly to include land use patterns, the transportation system, and design features that together provide opportunities for travel and physical activity. *Land use patterns* refer to the spatial distribution of human activities. The *transportation system* refers to the physical infrastructure and services that provide the spatial links or connectivity among activities. *Design* refers to the aesthetic, physical, and functional qualities of the built environment, such as the design of buildings and streetscapes, and relates to both land use patterns and the transportation system" (NRC, 2005).

[5]According to the guidelines, the minimum recommended aerobic physical activity required to produce substantial health benefits in adults is 150 minutes of moderate-intensity activity, or 75 minutes of vigorous-intense activity, or an equivalent combination of moderate- and vigorous-intensity physical activity per week (CDC, 2008b).

BOX 2-1
General Description of Women's Health Initiative

The Women's Health Initiative (WHI) was a multi-million-dollar, large prospective clinical study coordinated by the National Heart Lung and Blood Institute. Enrollment of 68,132 postmenopausal women ages 50 to 79 ran from 1993 to 1998. To address some research questions, women were randomized to various studies: (1) a dietary modification arm, which assigned 48,835 women to follow a 20% low-fat eating plan or self-selected diet; (2) a hormone therapy arm consisting of conjugated equine estrogen-plus-progestin or placebo for 16,608 women with uterus; or (3) another hormone therapy arm consisting of conjugated equine estrogen-only or placebo for 10,739 women with a hysterectomy. Other WHI studies included 8,050 women who followed both the dietary modification and a hormone therapy, and a calcium and vitamin D study that started 1 year later and included 36,282 of the women. In addition, 93,676 women from the same population agreed to be in an observational study (Prentice and Anderson, 2008).

---

women that over 60% of women 20 years old and older are overweight or obese (Ogden et al., 2006).[6] This can have serious effects on subsequent generations as studies have shown that a child with an obese parent is 60% as likely to become an obese adult (IOM, 2005b; Whitaker et al., 1997).

A greater proportion of women than men are obese; the difference is greatest among some racial and ethnic populations (see Figure 2-3) (CDC, 2009a). Non-Hispanic black women (about 53%) and Mexican-American women (about 42%) are more likely to be obese than non-Hispanic white women (about 32%). The percent of obese non-Hispanic Black women is higher (about 61%) in women 60 years old and older (Pan et al., 2009).

Physical Activity

With some consistency, studies have shown that women engage in less physical activity than do men and that activity declines with age and is lower in nonwhite women (Biddle and Mutrie, 2008). Both girls and women have been found to engage in leisure-time physical activity,[7] such as sports and recreational

---

[6]On the basis of data from the NHANES for the period 2003–2006. Definitions: healthy weight = BMI ≥ 18.5 to < 25; overweight = BMI ≥ 25 to < 30; obesity = BMI ≥ 30; and extreme obesity = BMI ≥ 40.

[7]Leisure-time physical activity has been measured and defined differently among studies but generally does not include activity in working, in performing household tasks, or in transportation-related activity, such as walking to work.

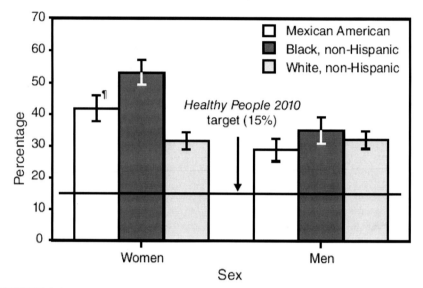

FIGURE 2-3 Prevalence of obesity, defined as a body-mass index (weight [kg]/height [m^2]) ≥ 30, in the United States. Prevalence estimates are age-adjusted to the 2000 US standard population. Age-adjusted percentage of adults 20 years old or older who were obese during 2003–2006 varied by race or ethnicity in women and ranged from 53.3% of non-Hispanic black women to 41.8% of Mexican American women and 31.6% of non-Hispanic white women. Obesity levels were more similar among Mexican American men (28.8%), non-Hispanic black men (35.0%), and non-Hispanic white men (32.0%). None of the groups had met the *Healthy People 2010* target of 15% (objective 19-02). Non-Hispanic black and non-Hispanic white include persons who reported only one race and exclude persons of Hispanic ethnicity. Persons of Mexican American ethnicity might be of any race.

¶95% confidence interval.

SOURCE: CDC (2009a).

activities, less often than their male counterparts, and there is a substantial decrease in activity in girls during adolescence (Kimm et al., 2002; Sallis et al., 2000; Trost et al., 2002).[8] There is some evidence that girls become less active during adolescence because of shifting self-perceptions associated with pubertal development, heightened awareness of peers, and changes in self-esteem (Kimm et al., 2001; Murdey et al., 2004).

Findings depend on the type of physical activity assessed. For instance, although older women engage in fewer sports and less planned exercise than men,

---

[8]In a 10-year longitudinal study of youth assessed at ages 9–19 years, rates of habitual physical activity among girls (including sports and leisure activities) declined by 83% from year 1 (ages 9–10 years) to year 10 (18–19 years) (Kimm et al., 2002).

reported activity levels may increase when household and caregiving activities are considered (Sternfeld et al., 2000). White women and those with more education and income, who generally have more resources and flexibility, are more likely to engage in leisure activities, whereas other groups of women are more likely to be classified as physically active when occupational activity, household activity, and walking for transportation are considered as physical activities (Brownson et al., 2000; Eyler et al., 2002; Sternfeld et al., 1999; Young and Cochrane, 2004).

Childbearing and motherhood, especially the early years of raising children, have been identified as common barriers to regular physical activity in women 25–35 years old (Cramp and Brawley, 2006). Whereas in the past it was recommended that pregnant women limit strenuous exercise or stop altogether (ACOG, 1985), today, moderate exercise has been established as safe for healthy women and has been shown to reduce gestational diabetes and pre-eclampsia and to help in preventing excess maternal weight gain (Clapp and Little, 1995; Dempsey et al., 2004a; Saftlas et al., 2004; Sorensen et al., 2003). Because of a lack of dissemination of that evidence, however, some women may remain uncertain about the safety of exercise during pregnancy (Mudd et al., 2009). Indeed, evidence from both retrospective and prospective studies shows that intensity and duration of leisure-time physical activity are lower during pregnancy than before it and lower in the third trimester than in the first (Poudevigne and O'Connor, 2006). There appear to be smaller decreases in household and caregiving activities during pregnancy (Mottola and Campbell, 2003; Schmidt et al., 2006; Taber-Chasan et al., 2007). One of the strongest determinants of whether a woman will be active during pregnancy is her level of activity during the year before pregnancy; inactivity during pregnancy is more common among multiparous women, especially those who are economically disadvantaged or who have less education (Ning et al., 2003; Poudevigne and O'Connor, 2006).

In recent years, there has been wide use of ecologic models that emphasize social and environmental influences on physical activity in addition to individual-level influences (Biddle and Mutrie, 2008; King et al., 2002; Spence and Lee, 2003). Evidence from mostly cross-sectional studies shows that attributes of the neighborhood environment—such as availability of recreational facilities and parks, low crime rates, seeing others exercise, less traffic, sidewalks, and street lighting—are associated with more physical activity (Duncan et al., 2005; Humpel et al., 2004; Owen et al., 2004). A recent dissertation on the effect of elementary school policies on physical activity and obesity in children found that the presence of a gymnasium in a school is associated with more time in physical education class and that children from disadvantaged backgrounds are less likely to have a gymnasium, but it did not find a significant correlation between presence of a school gymnasium and rates of being overweight or obese (Fernandes, 2010). Having the recommended time for recess and physical education was associated with a decrease in BMI for boys, but not for girls (Fernandes, 2010).

Eating Habits

Having a high quality diet means taking in adequate amounts of healthy foods, including fruits and vegetables,[9] and limiting intake of unhealthy foods, such as fats and sugar (HHS and USDA, 2005). Ingestion of energy (or calories) via consumption of carbohydrates, proteins, and fats in the diet is necessary to maintain body functions such as respiration, circulation, physical activity, and protein synthesis (IOM, 2005c). Women eat more fruits and vegetables than men[10] and are more aware of recommendations for fruit and vegetable intake and of the links between fruit and vegetable consumption and disease prevention (Baker and Wardle, 2003; Wardle et al., 2004). Sex differences in fruit and vegetable consumption in adolescents have been less clear, although where differences have been noted, consumption has been higher in girls (Cooke and Wardle, 2005; Rasmussen et al., 2006). Other determinants positively associated with fruit and vegetable consumption in adults include higher socioeconomic status (SES), being married, and having good local availability (Kamphuis et al., 2006). Among the determinants consistently found to influence fruit and vegetable intake in children and adolescents are SES, preferences, parental eating habits, and home availability and accessibility (Rasmussen et al., 2006). Availability of fruits and vegetables in schools has the potential to increase consumption in youth, but only about one-fifth of US middle and high schools offer fruit and vegetables as competitive foods (CDC, 2009b).

Minorities, including minority-group women and girls, on the average have diets that are lower in quality and nutrient intake than non-minorities (Neumark-Sztainer et al., 1998; Xie et al., 2003). Neighborhood SES may play a role, as indicated by findings that residents of lower-SES neighborhoods have poorer fruit and vegetable availability and an overabundance of fast and convenience food (Bodor et al., 2008; Morland et al., 2002).[11] Relative costs of healthy and unhealthy foods and cultural differences in food choices and methods of food preparation may also play some role in differences in diet quality in populations of women. Research involving Latina women has found that acculturation into mainstream culture in the United States is associated with a degradation of diet

---

[9]Consumption of fruits and vegetables is associated with lower risk of numerous chronic diseases, including some cancers and cardiovascular disease. When eaten as part of a reduced-energy diet, fruits and vegetables are also beneficial in weight management because of their low energy density (AICR, 2007; Liu et al., 2000; Rolls et al., 2004).

[10]In an analysis of data on over 1.2 million adults who participated in the Behavioral Risk Factor Surveillance System, researchers found that several groups of women had significant increases in fruit and vegetable consumption during 1994–2005: women 25–34 years (+3.65 percentage points, $P < 0.001$), non-Hispanic black women (+4.08 percentage points, $P = 0.0002$), and women who were nonsmokers (+1.43 percentage points, $P = 0.004$) (Blanck et al., 2008).

[11]There is a large body of evidence that diet quality follows a socioeconomic gradient, with higher-SES groups more likely to consume whole grains, lean meats, fish, low-fat dairy products, and fresh fruits and vegetables than groups of lower-SES groups (Darmon and Drewnowski, 2008).

quality, including lower intake of fruits and vegetables and higher consumption of fats and drinks that contain refined sugar, an effect often modified by SES (Perez-Escamilla and Putnik, 2007).

Family-level factors are among the strongest influences on food choices and eating behavior in children, including girls. Much research has documented similarities between parents and their children in food acceptance and preferences for foods, such as fruits and vegetables (Patrick and Nicklas, 2005), as well as in physical activity and other factors that decrease the risk of weight-related problems (Neumark-Sztainer, 2005). During adolescence, peers can be especially influential in adolescent eating behavior, particularly in girls, who, in general, have more body-image and weight concerns than their male peers. Lieberman et al. (2001) found that adolescent girls' eating behavior was strongly predicted by peer pressure even after controlling for other interpersonal variables. There is also evidence that public policies, such as taxing unhealthful food and beverages, such as pizza and soda, could help improve eating habits (Duffey et al., 2010).

Health Consequences Related to Eating Habits and Physical Activity

Findings of hundreds of studies on the protective and detrimental effects of dietary exposures have added to the knowledge base on how eating habits affect women's health, including the increasingly common problem of obesity. *Trans* fatty acids and saturated fats, high-glycemic-index foods, red meat, and a Western dietary pattern, to name a few examples, have been found to increase the incidence of coronary heart disease in studies involving women, whereas such foods as fruits and vegetables, nuts, and omega-3 fatty acids have been shown to reduce the risk of coronary heart disease (Mente et al., 2009). Excess body fat is probably the most important determinant of type 2 diabetes in women and men (Hu et al., 2001); however, there is some evidence from large observational studies of women that, even after controlling for BMI, women who consume a high-fiber, low-glycemic-index diet are less likely to develop type 2 diabetes (Hu et al., 2001; Liu et al., 2000; Salmeron et al., 1997).

Physical activity has been shown to reduce the incidence of cardiovascular conditions in women, including coronary heart disease and stroke (Ellekjaer et al., 2000; Hu et al., 2000, 2004; Li et al., 2006; Manson et al., 1999; Oguma and Shinoda-Tagawa, 2004; Stevens et al., 2002; Weinstein et al., 2008; Wessel et al., 2004). For example, the Nurses Health Study showed the health benefits of brisk walking, including an association between walking briskly for 3 or more hours per week and a reduced risk of coronary heart disease (Manson et al., 1999). Several publications on physical activity and type 2 diabetes in women have reported significant inverse associations between physical activity and incident diabetes (Folsom et al., 2000; Hsia et al., 2005; Hu et al., 1999, 2003; Jeon et al., 2007; Weinstein et al., 2004). Moreover, evidence is mounting that physical activity before and during pregnancy can reduce the chances that a woman will develop gestational diabetes mellitus during pregnancy (Dempsey et al., 2004b; Oken et al., 2006; Zhang et al., 2006). In addition to reducing colon cancer (Chao et al., 2004; Martinez et al., 1997; Wolin et al., 2007), physical activity may help to reduce risk of premenopausal and postmenopausal breast cancer and endometrial cancer in women (AICR, 2007; Maruti et al., 2008). Studies have also demonstrated less cognitive decline in women with higher physical activity (Weuve et al., 2004; Yaffe et al., 2001). Inactivity or a sedentary lifestyle increases women's risks of several chronic conditions and is linked with weight gain, overweight, and obesity, which themselves are linked to detrimental health outcomes independent of physical activity.[12] An inverse dose–response relationship of physical activity with health outcomes is frequently observed: benefits are conferred by moderate activities, such as walking, and even more by vigorous activity. Reduction in the risk of cardiovascular disease and type 2 diabetes in women has been found with as little as 15 or 30 minutes of physical activity per day (Brown et al., 2007).

Besides cardiovascular outcomes, cancers, and type 2 diabetes, research has looked at other health outcomes in women as well. For instance, physical activity and dietary exposures, such as to calcium and vitamin D, have been studied in relation to women's bone health as possible risk modifiers for conditions, such as osteoporosis and hip fracture, that are more likely to occur in older women (Feskanich et al., 2003; Jackson et al., 2006). The findings on calcium and vitamin D remain less certain, but it appears that girls and young women who are regularly active achieve a greater peak bone mass—a factor that decreases risk of osteoporosis—than those who do not and that older women can prevent bone loss with regular activity (NIAMS, 2009).

A relatively small but growing field of research is focused on how physical activity and eating habits may influence how well women who are living with chronic conditions, or who have experienced a health-related event, fare and recover. For women who have early-stage breast cancer, for instance, there is some evidence that physical activity is favorably associated with quality of life and improved survival (Bicego et al., 2009; Holmes et al., 2005; McNeely et al., 2006; Pierce et al., 2007).

In girls and women, increments in adipose tissue (fat) tend to be distributed in both upper (abdominal) and lower (hips) body compartments (Kissebah et al., 1983). Accumulation of fat in either may reduce the image and esteem of a girl or woman in her own mind as well as among her peers: this situation may occur in girls and women more than boys and men (Crocker, 1999; Wing et al.,

---

[12]For example, overweight and obesity are clearly associated with an increased risk of many cancers, including cancers of the breast in postmenopausal women, colon cancer, endometrial cancer, adenocarcinoma of the esophagus, and renal cancer. Evidence is highly suggestive that obesity also increases the risk of cancers of the pancreas, gallbladder, thyroid, ovary, and cervix, and of multiple myeloma and Hodgkin lymphoma (Kushi et al., 2006).

1991). Trends in fat accumulation that may begin in childhood and accelerate during adolescence are increasingly consequential during young adulthood and middle age. The sex differences in patterns of fat buildup become clearer: men add weight (especially fat) in a central, upper-body, waist-expanding fashion (sometimes termed the android pattern), and women classically selectively increase fat deposits in a more peripheral, lower-body, hip- and thigh-expanding distribution (the gynoid pattern) (Ley et al., 1992). The health implications of that gender difference are profound and evident in the waist:hip ratio, which is lower in many women than in men (Ley et al., 1992). A high waist:hip ratio correlates with measures of insulin insensitivity and the metabolic syndrome (Björntorp, 1997; Goodpaster et al., 2005), high blood pressure (Kalkhoff et al., 1983), dyslipidemia (increased low-density lipoprotein and decreased high-density lipoprotein) (Björntorp, 1997), thrombosis (Walker et al., 1996), type 2 diabetes (Barker et al., 1993; Stern and Haffner, 1986), and cardiovascular disease (Stern and Haffner, 1986). High waist circumference, an indicator of visceral fat, also correlates with adverse health outcomes (Li et al., 2007), including an increased risk of myocardial infarction (Yusuf et al., 2005), type 2 diabetes (Wang et al., 2005), and all-cause mortality (Bigaard et al., 2005).

Research on Interventions

Evidence of the effectiveness of interventions to increase physical activity and improve eating habits in women and girls comes largely from studies that have targeted these behaviors, often in concert, as a means of reducing or managing weight or reducing the risk of diabetes, cardiovascular disease, and other health outcomes (Bayne-Smith et al., 2004; Pate et al., 2005). The antecedents of changes in behavior (such as changes in knowledge about risks and self-efficacy, that is, their belief in their ability to change their behavior) and physical activity and dietary change themselves have been used as measures of intervention effectiveness (Edmundson et al., 1996; Emmons et al., 1999; Saksvig et al., 2005). Some studies have used biomarkers—such as weight or BMI change, serum cholesterol, and blood pressure—as measures of effectiveness (Andersen et al., 1999; Elmer et al., 2006; Moreau et al., 2001; Stefanick et al., 1998).

Many interventions that have targeted children and adolescents have been school-based and have targeted boys and girls together. The Task Force on Community Preventive Services found insufficient evidence to determine the effectiveness of school-based interventions in increasing fruit and vegetable intake or in decreasing fat and saturated-fat intake. Although generally positive, the effects of individual interventions are modest and based on self-reports (Guide to Community Preventive Services, 2004).

With respect to physical activity, it appears that modified curricula that increase the length or intensity of activity in schools' physical-education classes are effective in increasing physical activity and improving fitness in girls and boys among diverse racial, ethnic, and socioeconomic groups (Guide to Community Preventive Services, 2004). A more recent review, however, concluded that the evidence does not support the effectiveness of school-based physical-activity interventions in general in increasing the percentage of children and adolescents who are physically active during leisure time or in reducing BMI (Dobbins et al., 2009). Where increases in activity have been documented, they have tended to be modest and of short duration, and have not generalized to nonschool settings. Moreover, maintenance of physical-activity increases has been poor or, because of short followup, not assessed (Marcus et al., 2006).

Low income is associated with low fruit and vegetable consumption in part because of poorer access (Steptoe et al., 2003). On the basis of the socioecologic model, some efforts to improve access to fruits and vegetables, such as food vouchers for farmers' markets and supermarkets, have been successful in increasing fruit and vegetable intake in low-income women. In a study of Women, Infants, and Children participants, women who received food vouchers increased their consumption of fruits and vegetables significantly and sustained the increase 6 months after the intervention was terminated (model-adjusted R2 0.13; P < 0.001) (Herman et al., 2008).

Clinical settings offer a way to reach women to increase physical activity and improve eating habits. A review of 32 studies of nutrition-counseling and physical-activity interventions to reduce the risk of cardiovascular disease in women found that, overall, interventions administered in health-care settings tended to produce modest but statistically significant effects on physical activity or exercise, dietary fat, weight loss, blood pressure, and serum cholesterol (Wilcox et al., 2001). Diet-only and combined interventions were equally effective in reducing dietary fat, and physical-activity-only and combined interventions were about equally effective in increasing physical activity. Effects were observed even after modest interventions, such as brief behavioral counseling by a health-care provider and printed educational materials. The length of followup varied among studies. With respect to physical activity in particular, interventions with less than 6 months of followup had greater effects, indicating a problem with sustaining the activity. Studies that were tailored to ethnic group and stage or readiness for change had larger effects, but the authors indicated that more research was needed to confirm their findings (Wilcox et al., 2001).

Little research has been carried out on strategies for encouraging physical activity during or after pregnancy (Cramp and Brawley, 2006). In a review of weight-management interventions for pregnant and postpartum women, Kuhlmann et al. (2008) concluded that interventions that addressed modifications in eating habits and exercise and included individual or group counseling sessions, combined with written and telephone correspondence or food and exercise diaries, resulted in significantly better outcomes on weight measures than other interventions, although refusal and attrition rates were high.

The Centers for Disease Control and Prevention's (CDC's) VERB campaign—

which encouraged daily physical activity in children aged 9–13 years old through paid advertisements, school and community promotions, and Internet activities— had some success. After 1 year of the program, a significant positive relationship was detected between the level of awareness of VERB and weekly median sessions of free-time physical activity in the total population. Significant overall effects were observed in girls exposed to the campaign compared with girls unaware of the campaign (Huhman et al., 2005). Studies of mass-media campaigns that deliver messages on a local or regional level via television, newspaper, and radio, however, can be successful in producing recall of campaign messages but show mixed results as to attitude and behavioral change in targeted populations (Marcus et al., 2006).

Although interventions that promote healthy eating have the potential to improve health, short-term "diets" may be more harmful than helpful. A careful review of research on dieting found in long-term followup (4–7 years) that one-third to two-thirds of dieters gain more weight than they lost on their diets (Mann et al., 2007).

Sexual Risk Behaviors

Sexual risk behaviors increase the chances of adverse outcomes associated with sexual contact, including sexually transmitted infections (STIs) and unintended pregnancy. In the research literature, sexual risk behaviors have commonly included nonuse and incorrect and inconsistent use of condoms and other birth control methods, sex with multiple partners, sex with high-risk or casual partners, and use of drugs or alcohol (which can impair judgment and decision making) before or during sex (Blake et al., 2003; LaBrie et al., 2007; Pulerwitz et al., 2002; Santelli et al., 1998). Although those behaviors put women at risk for both unintended pregnancy and STIs, the research has tended to look at these separately in a reflection of differences in funding streams and service delivery. Unintended pregnancy and its health consequences and prevention are discussed further in Chapter 3. The rates of many STIs have decreased in recent years, but in 2008 it was estimated that one-fourth of females 14–19 years old had one of the most common STIs—human papillomavirus (HPV) infection, chlamydiosis, herpes simplex, or trichomoniasis (Forhan et al., 2008). Chlamydiosis has not decreased, but this may be because there have been more screening and more sensitive tests. About half of pregnancies are unintended (Finer and Henshaw, 2006).

Vulnerable Populations

In 2008, the overall rate of chlamydial infection in the United States in women (584 cases per 100,000 women) was almost 3 times the rate for men (CDC, 2009c). Of females, those 15–19 and 20–24 years old have the highest rates of chlamydial infection (CDC, 2009c). Poorer women and girls, and those who are members of racial and ethnic minorities are disproportionately affected by STIs and their sequelae, and by unintended pregnancy (Finer and Henshaw, 2006; Guttmacher Institute, 2006). The prevalence of chlamydial infection is greater in economically disadvantaged women than among those who are more advantaged (Harrison et al., 1983; Jolly et al., 1995). Gonorrhea rates in men and women are generally similar and have remained fairly stable over the last 12 years (CDC, 2009d). In 2008, 15- to 19-year-old black women had the highest gonorrhea rates of any group, followed closely by 20- to 24-year-old black women (CDC, 2009d).

Syphilis declined from 1992 to 2003 but increased from 0.8 case per 100,000 women in 2004 to 1.5 cases per 100,000 in 2008 (CDC, 2009e). Syphilis is a greater problem in the South and in urban areas in other regions of the country and is more prevalent in some minority groups. Similar patterns emerge across STIs: rates are highest in blacks, followed by Hispanics and American Indians and Alaskan Natives; they are lowest in Asian Americans and Pacific Islanders; and they are intermediate in whites (CDC, 2009e).

Health Consequences

Women are at higher risk than men for most STIs and at higher risk of adverse complications. For instance, bacterial STIs in women that are left untreated can lead to pelvic inflammatory disease (PID), which can cause infertility, ectopic pregnancy when pregnant, and chronic pelvic pain. About 1 million US women experience an episode of acute PID each year.[13] Symptoms of bacterial STIs (such as chlamydiosis and gonorrhea) are often subtle or "silent," especially in females, and this can delay testing and treatment. HPV increases men's risks of some cancers, but it contributes to twice as many cancers in women as in men, primarily HPV-associated cervical cancers. There were 104,097 cases of HPV-associated invasive carcinoma in women during 1998–2003 compared with 45,410 in men (Watson et al., 2008).

The consequences, biology, and diagnosis of and treatment for those conditions are discussed in Chapter 3.

Research on Sexual Risk Behavior and Protective Factors

Rates of STIs and unintended pregnancy in those who are sexually active are highest in adolescence and young adults in their early 20s (Finer and Henshaw, 2006). In addition to social and psychologic factors, biologic vulnerabilities may play a role. For example, the cervix of adolescent girls is more susceptible to STIs than those in older women (IOM, 1997; Lee et al., 2006). A review of US studies

---

[13]Recent data from CDC indicate that 10–40% of untreated chlamydia cases in women lead to PID and that as many as 20% of women with PID will develop infertility (Hillis and Wasserheit, 1996).

published in 1990–2007 (Kirby, 2007) found that multiple factors act to increase or decrease the chances that adolescent girls will engage in sexual risk behavior. They include individual biology (such as pubertal timing); factors in adolescents' lives and environments (such as physical and emotional abuse and exposure to drugs and alcohol); sexual values, attitudes, norms, and modeled behavior (of teens themselves and their parents, friends, and romantic partners); and connections with parents, other adults, and organizations (such as school and places of worship) that discourage sex, unprotected sex, and early childbearing.[14]

Several gender-related differences and findings specific to girls have been recognized. Having an older romantic partner is a stronger factor in risky sex in girls than in boys. When teen girls have sex at an early age with much older partners, the chances are greater that their first sexual experiences will be involuntary or unwanted and that they will become pregnant (Kirby, 2007; Manlove et al., 2006). The different decision-making roles and power of male and female partners in a relationship affect decisions about contraceptive use, particularly coitus-dependent methods, such as condoms (Pulerwitz et al., 2000, 2002). Greater communication with parents about sex appears to be protective in both sexes, but the effects on behavior are greater in girls. For teen girls, but not teen boys, participation in sports results in delayed initiation of sex, less frequent sex, greater use of contraception, and lower pregnancy rates (Kirby et al., 2007).[15] Multiple studies, including prospective studies that followed victims of abuse over time, have shown that adolescent girls who have a history of sexual abuse engage in more risky sexual behavior and are more likely to become pregnant (Logan et al., 2007).

Research on Interventions

Many curriculum-based interventions to affect adolescent sexual behavior have been developed and evaluated. Most have been implemented in schools, and most have used a comprehensive approach that addresses avoidance of pregnancy and STIs through abstinence and through the use of condoms and other forms of contraception. Although some interventions are ineffective, studies have indicated strongly that well-designed comprehensive interventions generally reduce sexual risk behaviors and do not increase sexual activity (Kirby, 2007). According to self-reporting, interventions appear about equally effective in girls and boys in reducing the number of sexual partners, increasing the use of condoms, increasing the use of other contraceptives, and reducing the overall frequency of unprotected sex (Coyle et al., 2001; Kirby, 2007; Shrier et al., 2001). Even though girls have

---

[14]For a more detailed list of risk and protective factors, see Hillis and Wasserheit (1996).

[15]The finding regarding pregnancy is less clear, because girls who are athletes are more likely than nonathletes to be young, better educated, and to be non-Hispanic white—characteristics that reduce the risk of becoming pregnant (Kirby, 2007).

less control over condom use than boys do, after some interventions girls are more likely to report that male sex partners used condoms (Coyle et al., 2001; Kirby et al., 2007; Shrier et al., 2001). At their most effective, the curriculum-based interventions appear to reduce adolescent sexual risk-taking (Kirby et al., 2007). Virtually all studies use risk-behavior change as the outcome rather than rates of pregnancies and STIs because obtaining an adequate number of end points to test for the effect of an intervention requires large samples and long followup.

A number of abstinence-only interventions for adolescents have been developed and evaluated in recent years because of requirements for funding introduced in 1996. Systematic reviews of the programs have suggested that their effects on behavior vary, but that overall they had a minimal impact on risky behavior (Bennett and Assefi, 2005; Kirby, 2007; Kohler et al., 2008; Trenholm et al., 2007).

Non–curriculum-based interventions have also been developed and tested, but there is not yet enough evidence to support conclusions about their effectiveness. Examples include human immunodeficiency virus (HIV) and STI educational programs that facilitate discussion between adolescent girls and their parents (Dancy et al., 2006; DiIorio et al., 2006; Nicholson and Postrado, 1991) and video- and computer-based programs for girls (Downs et al., 2004). Many communitywide STI–HIV and pregnancy-prevention initiatives to improve teenage girls' performance in school, plans for the future life, and connections to family, school, and faith institutions have been found to result in reduced community-level pregnancy and birth rates (Kirby et al., 2007).

Research to evaluate school-based clinics and condom-availability programs finds that teens use those sources to obtain condoms and other contraceptives. School policies that accept condom dissemination have been shown not to increase sexual activity in youth who are not sexually active while increasing condom use by those who are sexually active (Blake et al., 2003). Publicly funded family-planning services overall increase use of contraceptives by women and girls and avert an estimated 1.4 million unintended pregnancies and 600,000 abortions each year (Frost et al., 2008).

Cultural values that promote and emphasize the role of women as mothers and the value of children and that accept adolescent pregnancy can contribute to increased rates of unplanned pregnancy. Promotion of traditional gender roles wherein girls and women are expected to be more naïve and less active in sexual decision making may also contribute to unplanned sexual behavior and to higher rates of STIs and pregnancy in subpopulations of women and girls (Gomez and Van Oss Marin, 1996; Shearer et al., 2005; Weiss et al., 2000).

Most interventions for STIs and unplanned pregnancy have focused on girls or women, and very few have targeted boys and men, who are the ones who *use* condoms (Amaro, 1995). Intervention approaches studied include involving partners and family members in the intervention; implementation of interventions in churches, community centers, and other locations where people may congregate along cultural lines; communitywide interventions that aim to change broad per-spectives about roles of women and girls; and skill-based interventions to help women and girls in negotiating condom use with their partners (Orr et al., 1996; Roye et al., 2007; Scholes et al., 2003). On the basis of risk-factor research, such organizations as the National Campaign to Prevent Teen and Unplanned Preg-nancy have produced evidence-based materials outlining how programs to reduce sexual risk behaviors can better reach high-risk populations, such as black and Hispanic individuals and communities (The National Campaign to Prevent Teen Pregnancy, 2010).[16]

Alcohol Use

Alcohol use is more complicated than other risk factors; studies have shown both beneficial and harmful effects. The use of alcohol and the use of other sub-stances, if excessive, constitute serious health conditions of their own; and mod-erate use can affect the risk of other diseases. Chapter 3 deals specifically with alcohol and drug addiction as a disease, including sex- and gender-differences in its biology and treatment; here, the committee considers the use of alcohol as a more general determinant of women's health.

Although men are more likely than women to drink alcohol and to drink in large amounts, differences in body structure and chemistry cause women to take longer to break alcohol down and remove it from their bodies. In addition, women, particularly elderly women, typically have lower body weights than men. On drinking equal amounts, women have higher blood alcohol concentrations than men, and the immediate effects occur more quickly and last longer (CDC, 2008c). Furthermore, although women generally begin using alcohol later than men do, they move more quickly (telescoping) to dependence and manifestation of associated adverse health effects (Diehl et al., 2007; Greenfield, 2002). Alcohol use in women appears to have some unique features, including more concur-rent psychological and medical problems, which may be more pronounced than in men (Ashley et al., 1977; CDC, 2008c; Chatham et al., 1999; Conner et al., 2007).

Alcohol is a widely used substance with complex relationships to health. Moderate consumption of alcohol is associated with decreased risk of heart disease in women (Hvidtfeldt et al., 2010; Mente et al., 2009). However, as little as one alcoholic beverage per day can increase the chances that a woman will develop breast cancer, particularly if she is postmenopausal or has a family history of breast cancer (AICR, 2007; NIAAA, 2008). Women appear to have greater susceptibility than men to alcohol-related hepatic and cardiac disease, even though on the average women drink less (NIAAA, 2008). Heavy alcohol use has been linked with an increased risk of colorectal cancer in both women and

---

[16]See http://www.thenationalcampaign.org/resources/reports.aspx#hisp (accessed May 2, 2010)

men (AICR, 2007). Because of the acute toxic effects of alcohol, including impairment of psychomotor function and judgment, alcohol intoxication increases the risk of injury (for example, in motor-vehicle crashes). Especially for women, heavy drinking increases the chances of being a victim of violence or sexual assault (NIAAA, 2008).

SOCIAL AND COMMUNITY FACTORS

In addition to the individual biologic determinants (discussed in Chapter 3) and behavioral determinants that affect women's health, social and community factors affect health as well, and they modify responses to other determinants. This section discusses some of those factors—exposure to violence, stress and social connections, social disadvantage, and environmental factors.

Exposure to Violence

Violence against women and children, including sexual assault and rape, has attracted national and international attention as a serious public-health concern (WHO, 2005).[17] About one-fourth of US women (26.4%) report a lifetime occurrence of intimate-partner violence[18] victimization vs 15.9% of men (HHS, 2008b). Women are more likely than men to be injured during an assault, and the risk is highest when they are victimized by current or former partners (Tjaden and Thoennes, 2000). It is estimated that women and men suffer 2 million and 600,000 injuries, respectively, and 1,200 deaths a year of women from intimate-partner violence (HHS, 2008b).

Vulnerable Populations

Women who are "multiracial, non-Hispanic" and "American Indian or Alaska Native" report higher rates of exposure to violence than do white women (HHS, 2008b). Those groups are overrepresented in communities characterized by poverty, in which community violence is more common. Urban vs rural residence, however, has not been found to be related to violence exposure (Breiding et al., 2009). Violence against women is not limited to those in heterosexual relationships. A national survey of lesbian women found that 32% and 11.4% of lesbian women reported experiencing rape and intimate-partner violence, respectively;

---

[17]Violence against women is defined as "any act . . . that results in, or is likely to result in, physical, sexual or psychological harm or suffering to women, including threats of such acts, coercion or arbitrary deprivation of liberty, whether occurring in public or in private life" (United Nations, 1993).

[18]Intimate-partner violence includes violence between two people in a close relationship, including current and former spouses and dating partners.

black lesbians are more likely than their Latina or white counterparts to report being raped (Descamps et al., 2000).

Health Consequences

Violence against women within intimate relationships and within the community and violence against girls have direct health effects through injury and trauma and contribute to the development of later health problems (Tjaden and Thoennes, 1998). Women who experience violence have higher rates of later arthritis, asthma, heart disease, gynecological problems, and risk factors for HIV or sexually transmitted diseases and have lower self-rated health than those who do not experience violence (Campbell et al., 2002; HHS, 2008b). Women who experience psychologic intimate-partner violence, even in the absence of physical violence, are at greater risk for a number of adverse health outcomes, including a disability that prevents work, arthritis, chronic pain, migraine and other frequent headaches, STIs, chronic pelvic pain, gastric ulcers, spastic colon, and frequent indigestion, diarrhea, or constipation (Coker et al., 2000). Women of reproductive age who experience violence are at increased risk for unintended pregnancy (O'Donnell et al., 2009; Pallitto et al., 2005; Silverman et al., 2007), miscarriage (Silverman et al., 2007) and low–birth-weight babies (Campbell et al., 2002; Coker et al., 2002; Ellsberg et al., 2008). Intimate-partner violence is associated with psychologic disorders, including eating disorders, drug and alcohol abuse, and depression (McCauley et al., 1995). In a study of self-identified Latina or Hispanic urban women, those reporting intimate-partner violence were 3 times more likely to meet the criteria of posttraumatic stress disorder (PTSD) than those not reporting it (Fedovskiy et al., 2008).

Intimate-partner violence is also linked to STIs, including HIV infection. In a clinic-based sample of black and Latina women, those who experienced partner violence were more likely to report having multiple partners, a history of STIs, and inconsistent condom use (Wu et al., 2003), which are risk factors for HIV transmission (Silverman et al., 2004). Negotiating condom use in abusive relationships is particularly difficult (Campbell et al., 2002; Wingood and DiClemente, 1997).

Exposure to community violence has been associated with greater anxiety, depression, and PTSD and with adjustment or behavioral problems in school, particularly in urban populations (Gorman-Smith and Tolan, 1998; Ozer and Weinstein, 2004; Schwab-Stone and Ayers, 1995). Young men are more likely than their female counterparts to be exposed to community violence (Cooley-Quille et al., 2001; Malik et al., 1997; Ozer and Weinstein, 2004; Schwab-Stone and Ayers, 1995). One study indicated that girls are more likely than boys to demonstrate internalizing behavior (such as withdrawal and anxiety) after community-violence victimization (Cooley-Quille et al., 2001). However, another study that looked at depression and PTSD in urban adolescents did not demonstrate gender differences (Ozer and Weinstein, 2004).

Research on Prevention

Research on community violence has identified social conditions that foster violence victimization and perpetration. Previously conflated in the literature, violence victimization and the witnessing of community violence are now considered separate phenomena (O'Donnell et al., 2002). Less obvious forms of abuse at the hands of intimate partners have been identified; qualitative studies have described coercive tactics used by male partners to influence women's reproductive lives (for example, intentionally breaking condoms, preventing a partner from accessing birth control, and using threats to influence decisions about pregnancy and abortion) (Hathaway et al., 2005; Miller et al., 2007a). Those forms of abuse are not currently captured in standard clinical assessments of intimate-partner violence. Such assessments might also miss women and girls who are the victims of trafficking associated with being brought to the United States for domestic labor, sex work, or adoption (Miller et al., 2007b; US Department of State, 2009). There has been little research on differences in mechanisms of exposure to violence between racial and ethnic groups, social classes, sexual orientations, and cultures.

Research is starting to identify factors that may buffer girls and women from some of the sequelae of exposure to violence. A study of young adolescents found that support from parents and teachers was a protective factor against adverse outcomes after community-violence victimization, but that peer support was not related (Ozer and Weinstein, 2004). Although gang involvement can increase risky behavior, such as early sexual initiation and substance use (Cepeda and Valdez, 2003), good mother–daughter relationships were protective against alcohol and substance use regardless of gang involvement (Valdez et al., 2006).

Research on Interventions

The prevention of violence involves educating the general population (primary prevention) and identifying at-risk populations in which targeted prevention (secondary prevention) and intervention programs may be effective. Primary prevention programs are often school-based (Mytton et al., 2002) and focus on violence related to dating. For example, "Safe Dates" is a program tested in rural public schools to prevent adolescent dating violence and to stop victimization from continuing in abusive relationships (Foshee et al., 1998). It uses peer education to change gender norms that supported violence in dating relationships (Foshee et al., 1998, 2005) and significantly reduced a number of measures of victimization in boys and girls (Foshee et al., 2005).

In the clinical arena, effective HIV-prevention programs that include attention to how intimate-partner violence and dating violence affect HIV risk are emerging. An intervention conducted among black adolescent girls who were seeking care at community-based clinics used health and peer educators to discuss gender norms and resulted in a significant increase in consistency of condom use and a decrease in partner-related barriers to safe sex among those who had experienced dating violence (Wingood et al., 2006). Another promising intervention, conducted in abused adult women who had co-occurring mental-health and substance-use disorders, incorporated group trauma treatment focused on knowledge about personal safety, empowerment, coping skills, HIV-prevention education, and risk-reduction skills (Amaro et al., 2007). Women who did not receive the intervention were more likely than those who did to report unprotected sex 6 months and 12 months after the intervention.

Stress and Social Connections

Stress

A substantial body of research links stress and disease. Stress is the state that occurs when people are faced with a threat that they feel unable to counteract (McEwen and Stellar, 1993). Much of the research has examined short-term effects of acute stress on biologic processes—such as blood pressure, heart rate, cortisol, and proinflammatory cytokines—whereas more recent research is examining the health effects of chronic exposure to stress (Burkman, 1988; Dreher, 2004; Fleury et al., 2000; McEwen, 2004; Vitaliano et al., 2002). The occurrence of a threatening situation in itself does not engender stress; it occurs only when a person does not have adequate resources to deal with it. Facing threats that can be controlled or eliminated is generally experienced as a challenge rather than as a threat and has a different physiologic response. Challenge responses are characterized by increased cardiac performance, greater excretion of epinephrine, and greater vasodilation (Blascovich and Mendes, 2000; Blascovich et al., 1996). In contrast, threat responses engage the hypothalamic–pituitary–adrenal (HPA) axis and are accompanied by greater excretion of cortisol and norepinepherine and greater vasoconstriction. Accumulating data suggest that chronic stress accelerates the aging process and shortens life expectancy (Hawkley and Cacioppo, 2004).

In the last 20 years, more has been learned about the effects of repeated exposure to stress and specifically to the chronic stress associated with social disadvantage (McEwen and Gianaros, 2010; Seeman et al., 2009). There have also been advances in the understanding of differences in how men and women respond to stress, which have implications for health. For example, one hypothesis is that women are more likely than men to respond to threats not with the "flight or fight" response and but with a "tend and befriend" response that involves oxytocin, sex hormones, and endogenous opiods, and that increases the parasympathetic response while reducing sympathoadrenal and HPA activity. The "tend and befriend" response may buffer women from some of the adverse effects of stress (Taylor et al., 2000). Because the predominant model of stress response has been the male model, women's counterregulatory processes have had less attention, and there are fewer data on the extent to which they operate.

Women's roles subject them to different types and degrees of stressors than men generally experience. Women often experience stress associated with caregiving, which can take a toll on the body. For example, caregivers showed a significantly weaker antibody response in the months after receipt of a vaccination for pneumonia than did those who had never been caregivers and those who had been caregivers but no longer were (Glaser et al., 2000). Stress associated with caregiving can be seen even at the cellular level as reflected in telomere length. Telomeres cap the end of chromosomes and generally shorten with age. Telomere length is predictive of development of cardiovascular and other diseases and of death (Blackburn, 1991). Epel and colleagues (2004) compared telomere length in cells drawn from blood samples of middle-aged women who were caring for a child with a serious health problem and those who were caring for healthy children. The mothers of ill children who showed psychologic distress had significantly shorter telomeres than the other women; the difference was equivalent to 9 years of aging. The length of the women's telomeres was significantly related to the number of years in which they had been in a caretaking role. The finding was replicated in a sample of male and female caregivers for patients who had dementia of the Alzheimer's type. Caregivers had shorter telomeres (the equivalent of 4–8 years of aging), greater depression, higher concentrations of cytokines, and fewer lymphocytes than age- and sex-matched non-caregiving controls (Damjanovic et al., 2007; Epel et al., 2004).

Social Connections

Social connections are an important resource for buffering stress. Humans are social animals, and our links to one another can be a source of comfort as well as of conflict (as described in the section "Exposure to Violence"). A substantial literature shows that socially isolated people are at increased risk for death from multiple causes (Berkman and Syme, 1979; Friedmann et al., 2006) and that those who are more engaged in social relationships are generally healthier (Berkman and Glass, 2000).

Researchers have made much progress in delineating social processes that can affect health. For example, they have differentiated social support, social integration, and negative interactions, each of which shows associations with health (Cohen, 2004). Social integration reflects the variety of social roles in which a person is engaged. In general, occupying more social roles is linked to better health. For example, Cohen and colleagues (1997) used an experimental protocol in which healthy volunteers were exposed to a standard rhinovirus. Those who occupied more social roles were less likely to develop a clinical cold than were those with fewer; the effect was especially strong in those who were most isolated.

Marriage is an important social role that can be a source of both support and conflict. Being married is consistently linked to better health in men but less so in women. For example, in analyses of the Framingham Offspring Study, Eaker and colleagues (2007) found that married men (mean age at study onset, 48.8 years) are half as likely to die during the 10 years of followup compared with unmarried men, but found no benefit of marriage for women. They also demonstrated that marital quality and the ways in which women responded to marital conflicts predicted that mortality.

As more women have moved into the workplace, there has been increasing research on possible conflicts of work and home roles. Working women may experience work–home conflicts, but they also appear to benefit from the additional social roles afforded them by their work status (Barnett, 2004; Barnett and Hyde, 2001; Ruderman et al., 2002). The benefits of working depend on the characteristics of the work environment, including exposure to physical or chemical hazards and to psychosocial factors, such as the balance of effort and reward and decision latitude. Although a great deal is known about the health effects of work environments, relatively little work has compared the impact of work conditions on women's health with that on men's health (Theorell, 2000).

Social networks also affect health through their influence on health-promoting or -damaging behaviors. They provide health-relevant information and influence behavior through social norms. Data from Alameda County, California, showed a link between social integration and health risks, including smoking, sedentary lifestyle, and obesity. The probability of engaging in high-risk behaviors decreased monotonically as social connections increased (Berkman and Glass, 2000). Recent studies of the Framingham study data found that obesity spread through social networks—one's likelihood of obesity increased if others in one's network were obese (Christakis and Fowler, 2007).

Important gaps in the understanding of the effects of social connections on women's health remain. There has been relatively little work on sex differences in the impact of social ties (other than marriage) on health.

Research on Interventions

The adverse effects of stress on health can be reduced by reducing exposure to stressors and by modifying the people's psychologic and physiologic responses to it. Interventions to address the former include programs to help people to anticipate and manage stress (Taylor, 1990); those addressing the latter include training in coping skills that enable people to reframe situations that they encounter so that they do not elicit a stress response. Exercise and such techniques as meditation have been shown to buffer the impact of stress on the body (Carlson et al., 2003; McComb et al., 2004; Rejeski et al., 1992; Sandlund and Norlander,

2000; Speca et al., 2000) and form the basis of new interventions. Although there is substantial documentation of the association between greater social connection and health, no successful interventions have been developed to improve health by strengthening social ties.

Social Disadvantage

There are multiple reasons why groups are relegated to more disadvantaged positions in society, and those positions have health consequences. In addition to social limitations imposed by gender, some of the most common bases of social disadvantage are race, ethnicity, and SES. Social epidemiology studies over the past 20 years demonstrate that health inequities exist and change with societal conditions and policies (Beckfield and Krieger, 2009). Social conditions linked with low SES have been termed the fundamental determinants of health (Link and Phelan, 1995) because they affect almost all the more proximal determinants of health and illness. SES encompasses a person's income and wealth, educational attainment, and occupational position (Braveman et al., 2005; Kaplan and Keil, 1993; Link and Phelan, 1995). Each of those domains provides both material and social resources and shapes the environments in which people live and work.

The meaning and measurement of SES in women is not always equivalent to those in men. For many years, women were classified according to their husbands' socioeconomic characteristics (Zaher, 2002). Data on women's occupational status has been harder to capture because more women than men are voluntarily out of the workforce for long periods. Income can be measured in terms of a person's individual or household income. If the latter is used, one needs to take into account household size. Some women lack control over funds, and household income may have different implications for their expenditures and experiences (Phipps and Burton, 1998).

Differences in health associated with SES can be seen from birth and occur throughout the course of life. Premature birth, low birth weight, and birth defects are all more common in babies whose mothers have less money or education. In childhood, rates of asthma, ear diseases, injuries, and limiting chronic conditions decrease as SES increases (Chen et al., 2002). Moreover, childhood disadvantage has residual effects on adult health; a recent study, for example, showed independent associations of socioeconomic disadvantage, abuse, and social isolation experienced in childhood with levels of depression and with biomarkers of metabolic risk and inflammation in adulthood (Danese et al., 2009).

In adulthood, rates of many diseases—including cardiovascular disease, diabetes, such infectious diseases as HIV/acquired immunodeficiency syndrom (AIDS), respiratory illnesses, and mental illness—are higher in low-SES populations. The relative risk of dying before the age of 65 years is 3 times as great as those whose family annual incomes are under $10,000 (based on 1999 dollars) than in those whose incomes are above $100,000 (Adler et al., 2007). The gaps between high- and low-SES groups in morbidity and mortality diminish after the age of 65 years, although they can still be seen (Robert and Li, 2001).

In recent years, research on the joint effects of gender, race and ethnicity, and SES has provided increased evidence that many of the health effects of disadvantage are mediated by SES. Differences in life expectancy between the poorest and the wealthiest groups are twice as great as differences between whites and blacks (Lin et al., 2003); within every racial or ethnic group, the affluent have substantially better health than the poorest. For many diseases, racial and ethnic differences are substantially reduced or even disappear when SES is controlled for. The exception is birth outcomes, in which there is a substantial difference between black and white women at every SES level; in contrast with other outcomes, in which differences between the groups are smaller at higher levels of SES (Williams, 1999), the gap in birth outcomes is greater among higher-SES women than among those with less education or lower income (Cramer, 1995; Kallan, 1993). SES, however, does not explain all effects of race and ethnicity; at every level of SES blacks have higher mortality than whites (Lin et al., 2003).

At the same time, cultural factors may moderate the effects of SES. For example, although Latinos as a group have less education and are more likely to be poor, they have better outcomes on some health measures than similarly disadvantaged groups and better outcomes than some more advantaged groups, including non-Hispanic whites (Hayes-Bautista et al., 1994). Cultural factors may affect men and women differently; for example, US-born Mexican Americans have much higher rates of substance abuse than Mexican-born Mexican Americans and the differences are greater in women than in men (Lara et al., 2005; Vega et al., 1998).

In the last 2 decades, there have been substantial advances in research on SES and health. Initial studies established that the association was not due simply to the poorer health of the most disadvantaged but that health is monotonically related to SES; each step up the SES ladder is associated with better health (Adams et al., 2003; Adler and Stewart, 2010; Smith, 2004). That is the case with income in both men and women; those at the bottom have by far the greatest burden of disease and show the greatest gain in health with higher income, and those in the middle suffer poorer health than the most affluent. About one-fourth of deaths before the age of 65 years occur in the poorest 8% of the population (Santiago et al., 2009; Smith, 2004).

The picture is more complicated for education. White men get health returns for each additional educational milestone passed, from high-school graduation to earning a postcollege degree. The data on white women, however, are mixed. Women's health improves with high-school and college graduation, but postcollege education does not seem to provide health benefits, and some studies even find slightly poorer health associated with graduate degrees (Krishnan et al., 2010; Lantz et al., 1998). The pattern is similarly complicated for black men and women (Krishnan et al., 2010; Williams and Collins, 2001).

After studies established the strong graded association between SES and health, researchers turned to studies that could uncover the mechanisms by which socioeconomic factors operated to influence health. It is clear that there is no single pathway; the major mechanisms are discussed below.

SES is linked to exposure to health hazards including carcinogens and pathogens that directly affect disease risk. For example, people who live in poorer neighborhoods are subjected to deteriorated housing and have greater exposure to lead (Pirkle et al., 1998). Rates of high-blood-lead concentrations are substantially greater in residents of low-income neighborhoods, and the risk is especially high in poor blacks (Brody et al., 1994; Lanphear et al., 1998). SES-related features of communities can encourage or constrain health behaviors. For example, poorer neighborhoods have less access to supermarkets that provide more choice and lower prices of healthy foods, such as fruits and vegetables (Moore and Diez Roux, 2006). Such neighborhoods also have fewer recreational facilities and may not be conducive to walking or jogging (Macintyre, 2000; Sallis and Glanz, 2009). Most behavioral risk factors for disease are more common in low-SES populations. For example, rates of smoking differ dramatically with educational level: less than 10% of college graduates smoke, but over 30% of those who never graduated from high school are smokers (CDC, 2004).

People's social environments also differ by SES. Low-SES neighborhoods and work settings are generally more unpredictable, allowing less control, and have more conflict and threat. As a result, at work and at home, those who have less education, lower income, and jobs with less prestige and power encounter more stressors and have fewer resources for dealing with them (Fleury et al., 2000; Hallman et al., 2001).

Neighborhood effects appear to be greater in women than in men (Diez Roux et al., 1997; Winkleby et al., 2007). For example, women's engagement in exercise was more affected by the proximity of recreational facilities than men's (Diez Roux et al., 2007), and women's but not men's BMI was associated with proximity of supermarkets and convenience stores (Wang et al., 2007). Those findings are consistent with research that showed a stronger association of SES with cardiovascular disease in women than in men (Diez Roux et al., 2007).

SES has a major influence on health-care access and quality of care. People who have fewer economic resources and are employed in lower-SES occupations are less likely to have health insurance or access to care. Lower-SES people are likely to encounter problems as a result of poorer health literacy (IOM, 2004a). Issues of health care are discussed in more detail later in this chapter and in Chapter 5.

Interventions that modify income, education, or occupation are not within the purview of the health-care sector but fall into other domains. A few programs have been evaluated and found to have health effects. Most promising are new programs, largely in Latin American countries, in which conditional cash transfers are linked to performance of behaviors that have health consequences. The model program is Progresa/Oportunidades, in Mexico, which was tested using a randomized design with rigorous evaluation. Results are still emerging, but show that the program has favorable effects, such as increased contraceptive use by 20- to 24-year-olds and beneficial effects on children's growth (Fernald et al., 2009; Molyneux, 2006). In the United States, the Moving to Opportunity is a program of the Department of Housing and Urban Development in which families living in high-poverty public housing receive housing vouchers to move to a privately owned rental property in a low-poverty area. Among those who moved, the women showed significant gains in mental-health outcomes (Katz et al., 2001; Leventhal and Brooks-Gunn, 2003).

Many more interventions are addressing the pathways by which SES affects health, including community-level interventions to address the physical or social environment. Increased knowledge of the effects of SES on health behaviors may also allow for the development of more effective interventions that address the context in which these behaviors are established and maintained in women of different socioeconomic backgrounds.

Environmental Factors

Environmental factors can play a role in health, including women's health. Environmental exposures, such as exposure to chemicals, combine with genetic and other factors to determine health. As is the case with genetic contributions, very few diseases are determined solely by environmental factors (Davey Smith and Ebrahim, 2003; Jirtle and Skinner, 2007). Even in the face of relatively dominant hereditary input (such as *BRCA1*), it appears that enabling environmental and hereditary (non-*BRCA1*) contributions are at play (Chia, 2008; Laden and Hunter, 1998; Wolff et al., 1996). Similar gene–environment interactions determine a woman's health and risk-seeking behavior, not to mention the proclivity to smoking, drug abuse, and obesity (Gammon et al., 1998; Hamajima et al., 2002; Russo, 2002; Wolff et al., 1996). Although some environmental exposures, such as to drugs of abuse and smoking, are due to individual behaviors, others are the result of community factors.

SOCIETAL FACTORS

Societal factors, such as cultural norms and health care, can have a large impact on women's health. Those factors are discussed in this section.

Cultural Factors

Transmitted from generation to generation, culture is defined in many ways, but is generally considered a distinguishing set of characteristics of a population group. It consists of a group's shared values, norms, practices, systems of meaning, ways of life, and other social regularities (Kreuter et al., 2003). Culture can be a powerful influence on health, health behavior, and experiences in the health care system. Influencing perceptions and interpretations of symptoms, culture shapes help seeking, expectations of the sick role, and the level and nature of communication between patient and provider. In particular, cultural differences in language and SES between patient and provider may present barriers to appropriate diagnosis and treatment (Perez-Stable et al., 1997).

Lifestyle behaviors are influenced by culture as evidenced in food preferences and dietary practices. Cultural traditions associated with the consumption of high-fat, high-salt, and high-sugar foods among African Americans contribute to an increased risk for hypertension, diabetes, and heart disease (Airhihenbuwa et al., 1996). On the other hand, several studies of Hispanic diets show a greater consumption of carbohydrates, protein, and fiber and less saturated fats than whites, although the use of traditional foods among Mexican American women appear to decrease with increased acculturation to mainstream society (Guendelman and Abrams, 1995). For both African American and Latino women, cultural factors influence a greater acceptance of being overweight and body image satisfaction than among white women (Fitzgibbon and Beech, 2009; Phelan, 2009).

While cultural factors in some instances may contribute to risks for poor health, aspects of culture may also bring positive protective influences. A study by Nasim and colleagues (2007) found that cultural factors associated with religious beliefs and family values served as protective factors against tobacco and marijuana smoking among African American female college students at a predominantly white university. In another example, Wasserman and colleagues (2006) report how promotoras (lay health advisors) facilitated cervical cancer screening among Latina immigrant women.

Providing parameters for women's gender roles, culture prescribes acceptable norms in the family and community for behavior associated with being male or female. Cultural norms may determine whether women engage in employment outside the home, the circumstances under which caregiving is undertaken, how women respond to domestic violence, and the nature and type of social support given and received. Cultural norms also affect health decisions from prevention to treatments and may influence choices regarding sexual risk behaviors, contraception, and the acceptability of the HPV vaccine.

Culture appears to mediate the effect of poverty on depression rates in minorities. The recent Collaborative Psychiatric Epidemiology Survey program, which used common core questions and unified sampling weights, found that Hispanic Americans (except those from Puerto Rico), Asian Americans, and black Americans have fewer common mental disorders, such as depression, than do white Americans, even though many of these cultural groups are more likely to be impoverished than their white counterparts (Alegría et al., 2008; Breslau et al.,

2007; Himle et al., 2009; Jackson et al., 2007; Suarez et al., 2009; Takeuchi et al., 2007a,b; Williams et al., 2007). Similarly, American Indians have lower risk of depression than a representative sample of the US population. For Mexican, African, and Caribbean immigrants, the risk of depression is particularly low but increases with time spent in the United States (Alegría et al., 2007; Cutrona et al., 2000; Escobar et al., 2000; Laden and Hunter, 1998; Morales et al., 2002).

However, Page (2005) points out that culture is not static but is viewed as a process. This is seen in the changing gender roles of women, as well as the acculturation of immigrant groups. In addition, data from NHANES shows that foreign-born Hispanics obtained more energy from food groups such as legumes, fruits, and low-fat/high-fiber breads than US-born Hispanics (Duffey et al., 2008). While considerable research has focused on the health of women of various ethnic groups, cultural factors are not consistently examined. Given the increasing ethnic diversity in the US population, understanding cultural factors and their relationship to specific health outcomes remains an ongoing challenge.

Health Care

Prior IOM reports have summarized the adverse health consequences of poor health care, and these are not reiterated here (IOM, 2001b, 2002b,c, 2003, 2004b, 2009b). The present committee accepted the premise that a lack of health care or high-quality health care adversely affects a woman's health. A large body of research has examined the factors that affect people's use of health care. Women use more health services than men (HRSA, 2008; Salganicoff et al., 2005), but there is inadequate understanding of the factors that influence health-care use by men and women and of the extent to which these factors reflect issues related to gender or differential treatment by the health-care system.

Health-Care Access and Quality for Women

Health policies, both private and public, shape our delivery system and influence access and quality of care, especially insofar as they affect health insurance coverage and affordability.

Women and Health-Insurance Coverage   In the United States, women are covered by patchwork of private insurance and public coverage programs and by direct financing programs that provide services primarily to low-income or uninsured women. Eligibility for those programs and benefits is determined primarily by a person's work status, age, household income, and state of residence (DeNavas-Walt et al., 2009). The Patient Protection and Affordability Act of 2010 (Public Law 111-148) will make major changes in health coverage, but most of those changes will not be implemented until 2014.

Most US adults under age 65 years old are covered by an employment-based health insurance plan (DeNavas-Walt et al., 2009). Because women are less likely than men to work full-time, access to the system can be tenuous. Women with employer-based insurance are almost twice as likely as men to be covered as dependents, and this makes them vulnerable to losing their insurance if they become widowed or divorced or if their husbands or partners lose their jobs (Kaiser Family Foundation, 2009). Women are increasingly obtaining coverage in their own names as the share of women in the full-time workforce grows (Glied et al., 2008).

Nationally, about 6% of women purchase coverage through the individual insurance market in which insurers can deny coverage if an applicant has a "pre-existing condition," such as pregnancy, mental illness, or a chronic health condition. In 38 states, insurers can charge women who purchase individual insurance more than men for the same coverage even if they do not cover maternity care (Codispoti et al., 2008; Pollitz et al., 2007). That practice has been banned under the new health reform law, but will not be fully implemented until 2014.

One-tenth of women are covered by Medicaid (Kaiser Family Foundation, 2007). Women are more likely than men to qualify for Medicaid because women on the average have lower incomes and are more likely to fall into one of the program's eligibility categories (that is, she is pregnant, the parent of a dependent child, over 65 years old, or disabled). Women make up over two-thirds of adult beneficiaries of Medicaid (Kaiser Family Foundation, 2007). Medicaid covers many services that are important to women, paying for two-fifths of births in the United States, nearly two-thirds of all publicly funded family-planning services, a wide array of preventive screening services without copayments, and long-term care (Kaiser Family Foundation, 2007). On a number of primary and preventive indicators, women on Medicaid have access that is on a par with that of women with private insurance (Almeida et al., 2001; Salganicoff et al., 2005).

Women who are 65 years old and older or who are permanently disabled are covered by Medicare, but it has sizable gaps in coverage, notably for vision, dental, and hearing care and, most important for women, long-term care. Sizable out-of-pocket costs associated with the program can pose a major problem for older women, who have lower average Social Security and pension benefits than men (Congressional Research Service, 2008; Salganicoff et al., 2009).

Finally, almost 17 million women—17% of nonelderly women—are uninsured (Kaiser Family Foundation, 2009). Many working women lack access to employer-based coverage because they work part-time or in firms or industries that do not offer insurance. Poor and low-income women, young women, and

Latina and American Indian women are uninsured or underinsured at higher rates than other groups (Kaiser Family Foundation, 2009).[19]

Coverage, Out-of-Pocket Costs, and the Use of Health-Care Services   The literature on women's access to and use of care has been comprehensively summarized by Brittle and Bird (2007). Women who have health insurance have higher rates of use of a broad array of services than those who are uninsured (Almeida et al., 2001; Taylor et al., 2006). Uninsured women obtain fewer recommended preventive services, such as mammography and Papanicolaou (Pap) tests (Salganicoff et al., 2005); are less likely to have a usual source of care (RWJF, 2002); are less likely to get timely prenatal care (Braveman et al., 2003); and have lower rates of use of prescription drugs (Ranji et al., 2007).

Costs of care are a major concern for women, and reproductive and gender-specific conditions place a heavy burden on women's health-care out-of-pocket spending throughout their lives (Bertakis et al., 2000; Kjerulff et al., 2007; Salganicoff et al., 2005). The impact of such costs may be particularly burdensome for women, who are disproportionately in a low-income bracket (Glied et al., 2008; Rustgi et al., 2009; Salganicoff et al., 2005). For example, a larger share of women than of men have a usual source of care, which is linked to timely receipt of preventive services (DeVoe et al., 2003), but among those without a usual source of care, women were more likely than men to report that the cost was the major reason that they did not have one (AHRQ, 2009a). Higher levels of cost sharing result in lower use of services, particularly in low-income populations, including fewer visits to doctors, lower use of prescription medicines and mental-health treatment, and fewer dental visits (Hudman and O'Malley, 2003). Medicaid historically has either prohibited cost sharing or kept it to nominal levels. States that have raised cost-sharing levels have sometimes seen declines in service use thereafter (Artiga and O'Malley, 2005).[20]

Unlike Medicaid, Medicare has relatively high cost-sharing requirements, which affects level of use by beneficiaries, particularly those who have low incomes (Fitzpatrick et al., 2004). Increased cost sharing tends to reduce the appropriate use of prescription drugs through a number of means, including skipping doses, halting medication use, and not filling prescriptions (Rice and Matsuoka, 2004). Cost sharing was also found to be associated with substantial decreases in mammography rates among female Medicare beneficiaries who were enrolled in managed-care plans that instituted even small copayments (Trivedi et al., 2008).

---

[19]This is the group of women which is most likely to be assisted by the passage of the Patient Protection and Affordable Care Act of 2010 (Public Law 111-148).

[20]For example, in 2003 under a Medicaid waiver, Oregon increased premiums for poor adults on Medicaid to $6–20, depending on income. Of those who had unmet needs, 35% could not get needed care because of cost, 24% reported that they did not have the copayment, and 17% reported that they did not get care because they owed the physician money (Artiga and O'Malley, 2005).

Quality of Care

The quality of care received in the US health-care system is problematic (IOM, 2001b, 2002c, 2003) and, although quality has improved, the gains have been modest (AHRQ, 2009b). Substantial research efforts have focused on the development and application of quality measures. In the case of women's health, measures have historically focused on a narrow band of process indicators, typically limited to receipt of early prenatal care, mammography, and Pap tests. Although there is increasing attention to expanding the measures that started in the 1990s, cost challenges and concerns about administrative burdens have slowed progress. Furthermore, despite clear evidence that there are differences in how women are treated for such conditions as stroke, cardiovascular disease, and diabetes (Brittle and Bird, 2007), most of the quality measures collected by hospitals, plans, and government agencies are not disaggregated by sex. Failure to report by sex hinders evaluation of the quality of care received by men and women and slows progress in improving quality (McGlynn et al., 1999; McKinley et al., 2002; Weisman, 2000).

The National Healthcare Quality Report and the National Healthcare Disparities Report, both issued annually by the Agency for Healthcare Research and Quality (AHRQ, 2009a,b), provide national- and state-level data on a wide array of process, intermediate, and outcome quality measures in different health settings, including outpatient, inpatient, and nursing-home care. Although women are designated as a high-priority population in the reports, there are few indicators for women's health-care quality. Data are presented for women-specific conditions, including two dimensions of treatment for breast cancer[21] and receipt of first-trimester prenatal care. In addition, a subset of sex-specific data is presented for a few indicators that are relevant to both sexes. Such indicators include exercise counseling for obese patients (obese women are more likely to be counseled than obese men), mortality from myocardial infarction (women have significantly higher mortality rate than men), new AIDS cases, and having a usual source of care. Results on those measures are stratified by age and race or ethnicity. They are the only measures, however, that receive such analysis in either report.

The Health Plan Employer Data and Information Set (HEDIS) provides health-quality indicators that are used by commercial managed-care plans and by Medicaid and Medicare managed-care organizations (NCQA, 2010). It contains indicators that measure plan performance on conditions specific to women (for example, screening for breast and cervical cancer and chlamydiosis, and testing for and management of osteoporosis in women who have had a fracture) and on prenatal care (NCQA, 2010). HEDIS also collects other indicators that are

---

[21]Breast-cancer treatment measures include administration of radiation therapy within 1 year of diagnosis in women under 70 years old who are receiving breast-conserving surgery and axillary-node dissection or sentinel lymph-node biopsy at the time of surgery (lumpectomy or mastectomy) in women who have stage I-IIb breast cancer (AHRQ, 2009c).

important to women, such as weight, colorectal-cancer screening, persistence of beta-blocker treatment after a heart attack, comprehensive diabetes care, antidepressant-medication management, fall-risk management, aspirin use and discussion, and medical assistance with smoking and tobacco use. Those measures, however, are not reported by patient sex; this limits information on whether plans differ in their quality of care on indicators that are not sex specific. The same is true for differences by race and ethnicity.

Recent efforts to broaden the number of HEDIS measures to focus on women's health conditions have been met with limited success. Some important indicators have been added to the HEDIS data set, including osteoporosis screening and treatment and chlamydiosis testing in women. However, barriers to the collection of data on other relevant conditions, such as unintended pregnancy, remain; the barriers include difficulty in collecting information, cost and administrative burdens, and low frequency (Bird et al., 2003; McKinley et al., 2002; Weisman, 2000).

There are substantial gaps in knowledge of how quality of care affects women's health in relation to conditions that affect both men and women and conditions that affect women exclusively. Those issues are similar to challenges that have plagued clinical research, including a lack of sex-stratified analysis and measures that capture the broad array of sex-specific conditions (Correa-de-Araujo and Clancy, 2006; Kosiak et al., 2006). Improving quality requires improving data and analysis and is salient in relation to prevention of unintended pregnancy and to elements of maternity and older women's health care (Kelleher et al., 1997; Rehle et al., 2004; Sakala and Corry, 2007; Wilcox, 1999).

CONCLUSIONS

- There is substantial evidence of the role of individual behavior (for example, smoking, eating habits and physical activity, sexual risk behaviors, and alcohol use) in the prevention of disease and improvement of health. Many behavioral determinants act as common pathways to multiple conditions.
- Recent years have seen increased attention to factors beyond the individual that affect health and health behavior—such as social, cultural, family, and community determinants; living and working conditions (for example, environmental exposures); and societal factors—but more work is needed on these broader determinants of women's health.
- Although research has led to a greater understanding of the determinants of women's health, more is needed to develop effective interventions and prevention strategies to improve women's health by influencing the determinants.

- Although research has documented disparities in determinants across racial and ethnic groups, the efficacy of interventions has not been adequately evaluated in minority-group women, and this limits the generalizability of findings to subgroups of women.

REFERENCES

ACOG (American Congress of Obstetricians and Gynecologists). 1985. Exercise during pregnancy and the postnatal period. In *ACOG Technical Bulletin: Women and Exercise*. Washington, DC: ACOG.

Adams, P., M. D. Hurd, D. McFadden, A. Merrill, and T. Ribeiro. 2003. Healthy, wealthy, and wise? Tests for direct causal paths between health and socioeconomic status. *Journal of Econometrics* 112(1):3–56.

Adler, N., and J. Stewart. 2010. Health disparities across the lifespan: Meaning, methods, and mechanisms. *Annals of the New York Academy of Sciences* 1186:5–23.

Adler, N., J. Stewart, S. Cohen, M. W. Cullen, A. Diez Roux, W. Dow, G. Evans, I. Kawachi, M. Marmot, K. Matthews, B. McEwan, J. Schwartz, T. Seeman, and D. William. 2007. *Reaching for a Healthier Life: Facts on Socioeconomic Status and Health in the U. S.* San Francisco, CA: MacArthur Foundation.

AHRQ (Agency for Healthcare Research and Quality). 2009a. *National Healthcare Quality Report, 2008*. US Department of Health and Human Services.

———. 2009b. *National Healthcare Disparities Report, 2008*. Rockville, MD: US Department of Health and Human Services.

———. 2009c. *Measuring Healthcare Quality*. http://www.ahrq.gov/qual/measurix.htm (accessed September 10, 2009).

AICR (American Institute for Cancer Research). 2007. *Food, Nutrition, Physical Activity, and the Prevention of Cancer: A Global Perspective*. Washington, DC:AICR.

Airhihenbuwa, C. O., S. Kumanyika, T. D. Agurs, A. Lowe, D. Saunders, and C. B. Morssink. 1996. Cultural aspects of African american eating patterns. *Ethnicity and Health* 1(3):245–260.

Alegría, M., W. Sribney, M. Woo, M. Torres, and P. Guarnaccia. 2007. Looking beyond nativity: The relation of age of immigration, length of residence, and birth cohorts to the risk of onset of psychiatric disorders for Latinos. *Research in Human Development* 4(1):19–47.

Alegría, M., G. Canino, P. E. Shrout, M. Woo, N. Duan, D. Vila, M. Torres, C. N. Chen, and X. L. Meng. 2008. Prevalence of mental illness in immigrant and non-immigrant U. S. Latino groups. *American Journal of Psychiatry* 165(3):359–369.

Almeida, R. A., L. C. Dubay, and G. Ko. 2001. Access to care and use of health services by low-income women. *Health Care Financial Review* 22(4):27–47.

Amaro, H. 1995. Love, sex and power: Considering women's realities in HIV prevention. *American Psychologist* 50(6):437–447.

Amaro, H., M. J. Larson, A. Zhang, A. Acevedo, J. Dai, and A. Matsumoto. 2007. Effects of trauma intervention on HIV sexual risk behaviors among women with co-occurring disorders in substance abuse treatment. *Journal of Community Psychology* 35(7):895–908.

Andersen, K., L. J. Launer, M. E. Dewey, L. Letenneur, A. Ott, J. R. Copeland, J. F. Dartigues, P. Kragh-Sorensen, M. Baldereschi, C. Brayne, A. Lobo, J. M. Martinez-Lage, T. Stijnen, and A. Hofman. 1999. Gender differences in the incidence of ad and vascular dementia: The Eurodem studies. Eurodem Incidence Research Group. *Neurology* 53(9):1992–1997.

Artiga, S., and M. O'Malley. 2005. *Kaiser Commission on Medicaid and the Uninsured Issue Paper. Increasing Premiums and Cost Sharing in Medicaid and SCHIP: Recent State Experiences*. Menlo Park, CA: Kaiser Family Foundation.

Ashley, M. J., J. S. Olin, W. H. le Riche, A. Kornaczewski, W. Schmidt, and J. G. Rankin. 1977. Morbidity in alcoholics. Evidence for accelerated development of physical disease in women. *Archives of Internal Medicine* 137(7):883–887.

Baker, A. H., and J. Wardle. 2003. Sex differences in fruit and vegetable intake in older adults. *Appetite* 40(3):269–275.

Barker, D. J. P., C. N. Hales, C. H. D. Fall, C. Osmond, K. Phipps, and P. M. S. Clark. 1993. Type 2 (non-insulin-dependent) diabetes mellitus, hypertension and hyperlipidaemia (syndrome x): Relation to reduced fetal growth. *Diabetologia* 36(1):62–67.

Barnett, R. C. 2004. Women and multiple roles: Myths and reality. *Harvard Review of Psychiatry* 12(3):158–164.

Barnett, R. C., and J. S. Hyde. 2001. Women, men, work, family. *American Psychologist* 56(10): 781–796.

Bayne-Smith, M., P. S. Fardy, A. Azzollini, J. Magel, K. H. Schmitz, and D. Agin. 2004. Improvements in heart health behaviors and reduction in coronary artery disease risk factors in urban teenaged girls through a school-based intervention: The path program. *American Journal of Public Health* 94(9):1538–1543.

Beckfield, J., and N. Krieger. 2009. Epi + demos + cracy: Linking political systems and priorities to the magnitude of health inequities—evidence, gaps, and a research agenda. *Epidemiologic Review* 31:152–177.

Bennett, S. E., and N. P. Assefi. 2005. School-based teenage pregnancy prevention programs: A systematic review of randomized controlled trials. *Journal of Adolescent Health* 36(1):72–81.

Berkman, L. F., and T. Glass. 2000. Social cohesion, social capital, and health. In *Social epidemiology*, edited by L. F. Berkman and K. Ichiro. New York: Oxford University Press.

Berkman, L. F., and S. L. Syme. 1979. Social networks, host resistance, and mortality: A nine-year follow-up study of Alamedia County residents. *American Journal of Epidemiology* 109(2): 186–204.

Bermudez, E. A., N. Rifai, J. E. Buring, J. E. Manson, and P. M. Ridker. 2002. Relation between markers of systemic vascular inflammation and smoking in women. *American Journal of Cardiology* 89(9):1117–1119.

Bertakis, K. D., R. Azari, J. Helms, E. J. Callahan, and J. A. Robbins. 2000. Gender differences in the utilization of health care services. *Journal of Family Practice* 49(2):147–152.

Bicego, D., K. Brown, M. Ruddick, D. Storey, C. Wong, and S. R. Harris. 2009. Effects of exercise on quality of life in women living with breast cancer: A systematic review. *Breast Journal* 15:45–51.

Biddle, S., and N. Mutrie. 2008. *Psychology of Physical Activity: Determinants, Well-being, and Interventions.* 2nd ed. New York: Routledge.

Bigaard, J., K. Frederiksen, A. Tjonneland, B. L. Thomsen, K. Overvad, B. L. Heitmann, and T. I. Sorensen. 2005. Waist circumference and body composition in relation to all-cause mortality in middle-aged men and women. *International Journal of Obesity* 29(7):778–784.

Bird, C. E., A. Fremont, S. Wickstrom, A. S. Bierman, and E. McGlynn. 2003. Improving women's quality of care for cardiovascular disease and diabetes: The feasibility and desirability of stratified reporting of objective performance measures. *Women's Health Issues* 13(4):150–157.

Björntorp, P. 1997. Body fat distribution, insulin resistance, and metabolic diseases. *Nutrition* 13(9): 795–803.

Blackburn, E. H. 1991. Structure and function of telomeres. *Nature* 350(6319):569–573.

Blake, S. M., R. Ledsky, C. Goodenow, R. Sawyer, D. Lohrmann, and R. Windsor. 2003. Condom availability programs in Massachusetts high schools: Relationships with condom use and sexual behavior. *American Journal of Public Health* 93(6):955–962.

Blanck, H. M., C. Gillespie, J. E. Kimmons, J. D. Seymour, and M. K. Serdula. 2008. Trends in fruit and vegetable consumption among US men and women, 1994–2005. *Preventing Chronic Disease* 5(2):A35.

Blascovich, J., and W. B. Mendes. 2000. Consequences require antecedents: Toward a process model of emotion elicitation. In *Feeling and Thinking: The Role of Affect in Social Cognition, Studies in Emotion and Social Interaction*; second series, edited by J. P. Forgas. New York: Cambridge University Press.

Blascovich, J., J. Tomaka, and P. Z. Mark. 1996. The biopsychosocial model of arousal regulation. *Advances in Experimental Social Psychology* 28:1–51.

Bodor, J. N., D. Rose, T. A. Farley, C. Swalm, and S. K. Scott. 2008. Neighbourhood fruit and vegetable availability and consumption: The role of small food stores in an urban environment. *Public Health Nutrition* 11(4):413–420.

Braveman, P., K. Marchi, R. Sarnoff, S. Egerter, D. R. Rittenhouse, and A. Salganicoff. 2003. *Promoting Access to Prenatal Care: Lessons from the California Experience.* Menlo Park, CA: Kaiser Family Foundation.

Braveman, P. A., C. Cubbin, S. Egerter, S. Chideya, K. S. Marchi, M. Metzler, and S. Posner. 2005. Socioeconomic status in health research: One size does not fit all. *Journal of the American Medical Association* 294(22):2879–2888.

Breiding, M. J., J. S. Ziembroski, and M. C. Black. 2009. Prevalence of rural intimate partner violence in 16 US states, 2005. *Journal of Rural Health* 25(3):240–246.

Breslau, J., S. Aguilar-Gaxiola, G. Borges, K. S. Kendler, M. Su, and R. C. Kessler. 2007. Risk for psychiatric disorder among immigrants and their US-born descendants: Evidence from the National Comorbidity Survey Replication. *Journal of Nervous and Mental Disease* 195(3): 189–195.

Brittle, C., and C. E. Bird. 2007. *Literature Review on Effective Sex- and Gender-Based Systems/Models of Care.* Arlington, VA: Uncommon Insights.

Brody, D. J., J. L. Pirkle, R. A. Kramer, K. M. Flegal, T. D. Matte, E. W. Gunter, and D. C. Paschal. 1994. Blood lead levels in the US population: Phase 1 of the Third National Health and Nutrition Examination Survey (NHANES III, 1988 to 1991). *Journal of the American Medical Association* 272(4):277–283.

Brown, W. J., N. W. Burton, and P. J. Rowan. 2007. Updating the evidence on physical activity and health in women. *American Journal of Preventive Medicine* 33(5):404–411.

Brownson, R., A. Eyler, A. King, D. Brown, Y. Shyu, and J. Sallis. 2000. Patterns and correlates of physical activity among US women 40 years and older. *American Journal of Public Health* 90(2):264–270.

Burkman, R. 1988. Obesity, stress, and smoking: Their role as cardiovascular risk factors in women. *American Journal of Obstetrics and Gynecology* 158(6 Pt. 2):1592–1597.

Burkman, R., J. J. Schlesselman, and M. Zieman. 2004. Safety concerns and health benefits associated with oral contraception. *American Journal of Obstetrics & Gynecology* 190(4 Suppl.): S5–S22.

Caan, B., A. Coates, C. Schaefer, L. Finkler, B. Sternfeld, and K. Corbett. 1996. Women gain weight 1 year after smoking cessation while dietary intake temporarily increases. *Journal of the American Dietetic Association* 96(11):1150–1155.

Campbell, J., A. S. Jones, J. Dienemann, J. Kub, J. Schollenberger, P. O'Campo, A. C. Gielen, and C. Wynne. 2002. Intimate partner violence and physical health consequences. *Archives of Internal Medicine* 162(10):1157–1163.

Carlson, L. E., M. Speca, K. D. Patel, and E. Goodey. 2003. Mindfulness-based stress reduction in relation to quality of life, mood, symptoms of stress, and immune parameters in breast and prostate cancer outpatients. *Psychosomatic Medicine* 65(4):571–581.

CDC (Centers for Disease Control and Prevention). 2004. *Health, United States, 2004: With Chartbook on Trends in the Health of Americans.* Department of Health and Human Services, Centers for Disease Control and Prevention, National Center for Health Statistics. http://www.cdc. gov/nchs/hus.htm (accessed June 18, 2009).

————. 2007a. *Preventing Smoking and Exposure to Secondhand Smoke Before, During, and After Pregnancy.* http://www.cdc.gov/NCCdphp/publications/factsheets/Prevention/pdf/smoking.pdf (accessed September 10, 2009).

————. 2007b. *Average Fruit and Vegetable Consumption per Day. Nationwide—2007.* http://apps.nccd.cdc.gov/5ADaySurveillance/ (accessed June 18, 2009).

————. 2008a. *Current Smoking.* http://www.cdc.gov/nchs/data/nhis/earlyrelease/200812_08.pdf (accessed August 17, 2009).

————. 2008b. Prevalence of self-reported physically active adults—United States, 2007. *Morbidity and Mortality Weekly Report* 57(48):1297–1300.

————. 2008c. *Public Health: Excessive Alcohol Use and Risks to Women's Health.* http://www.cdc.gov/Alcohol/quickstats/womens_health.htm (accessed June 18, 2009).

————. 2009a. *Prevaence of Obesity Among Adults Aged ≥ 20 Years, by Race/Ethnicity and Sex—National Health and Nutrition Examination Survey, United States, 2003–2006.* hhttp://www.cdc.gov/mmwr/preview/mmwhrtml/mm5838a6.htm (accessed March 30, 2010).

————. 2009b. *State Indicator Report on Fruits and Vegetables, 2009.* http://www.fruitsandveggies matter.gov/health_professionals/statereport.html#Policy (accessed September 29, 2009).

————. 2009c. *Sexually Transmitted Diseases Surveillance, 2008: Chlamydia.* http://www.cdc.gov/std/stats08/chlamydia.htm (accessed March 16, 2010).

————. 2009d. *Sexually Transmitted Diseases Surveillance, 2008: Gonorrhea.* http://www.cdc.gov/std/stats08/gonorrhea.htm (accessed March 30, 2010).

————. 2009e. *Sexually Transmitted Diseases Surveillance, 2008: Syphilis.* http://www.cdc.gov/std/stats08/syphilis.htm (accessed March 30, 2010).

Cepeda, A., and A. Valdez. 2003. Risk behaviors among young Mexican American gang-associated females: Sexual relations, partying, substance use, and crime. *Journal of Adolescent Research* 18(1):90–106.

Chao, A., C. J. Connell, E. J. Jacobs, M. L. McCullough, A. V. Patel, E. E. Calle, V. E. Cokkinides, and M. J. Thun. 2004. Amount, type, and timing of recreational physical activity in relation to colon and rectal cancer in older adults: The Cancer Prevention Study II Nutrition Cohort. *Cancer Epidemiology, Biomarkers & Prevention* 13(12):2187–2195.

Chatham, L. R., M. L. Hiller, G. A. Rowan-Szal, G. W. Joe, and D. D. Simpson. 1999. Gender differences at admission and follow-up in a sample of methadone maintenance clients. *Substance Use & Misuse* 34(8):1137–1165.

Chen, E., K. A. Matthews, and W. T. Boyce. 2002. Socioeconomic differences in children's health: How and why do these relationships change with age? *Psychological Bulletin* 128(2):295–329.

Chia, K. S. 2008. Gene-environment interactions in breast cancer. *Novartis Foundation Symposium* 293:143–150; discussion 150–155, 181–183.

Christakis, N. A., and J. H. Fowler. 2007. The spread of obesity in a large social network over 32 years. *New England Journal of Medicine* 357(4):370–379.

Clapp, J. F., and K. D. Little. 1995. Effect of recreational exercise on pregnancy weight gain and subcutaneous fat deposition. *Medicine & Science in Sports & Exercise* 27(2):170–177.

Codispoti, L., B. Courtot, and J. Swedish. 2008. *Nowhere to Turn: How the Individual Health Insurance Market Fails Women.* Washington, DC: National Women's Law Center.

Cohen, S. 2004. Social relationships and health. *American Psychologist* 59(8):676–684.

Cohen, S., W. J. Doyle, D. P. Skoner, B. S. Rabin, and J. M. Gwaltney, Jr. 1997. Social ties and susceptibility to the common cold. *Journal of the American Medical Association* 277(24):1940–1944.

Coker, A. L., P. H. Smith, L. Bethea, M. R. King, and R. E. McKeown. 2000. Physical health consequences of physical and psychological intimate partner violence. *Archives of Family Medicine* 9(5):451–457.

Coker, A. L., K. E. Davis, I. Arias, S. Desai, M. Sanderson, H. M. Brandt, and P. H. Smith. 2002. Physical and mental health effects of intimate partner violence for men and women. *American Journal of Preventive Medicine* 23(4):260–268.

Congressional Research Service. 2008. *Income and Poverty Among Older Americans in 2007*. Washington, DC: Congressional Research Service.

Conner, K. R., V. M. Hesselbrock, S. C. Meldrum, M. A. Schuckit, K. K. Bucholz, S. A. Gamble, J. D. Wines, and J. Kramer. 2007. Transitions to, and correlates of, suicidal ideation, plans, and unplanned and planned suicide attempts among 3,729 men and women with alcohol dependence. *Journal of Studies on Alcohol and Drugs* 68(5):654–662.

Cooke, L. J., and J. Wardle. 2005. Age and gender difference in children's food preferences. *British Journal of Nutrition* 93(5):741–746.

Cooley-Quille, M., R. C. Boyd, E. Frantz, and J. Walsh. 2001. Emotional and behavioral impact of exposure to community violence in inner-city adolescents. *Journal of Clinical Child Psychology* 30(2):199–206.

Copeland, A. L., P. D. Martin, P. J. Geiselman, C. J. Rash, and D. E. Kendzor. 2006. Predictors of pretreatment attrition from smoking cessation among pre- and postmenopausal, weight-concerned women. *Eating Behaviors* 7(3):243–251.

Correa-de-Araujo, R., and C. M. Clancy. 2006. Catalyzing quality of care improvements for women. *Women's Health Issues* 16(2):41–43.

Coyle, K., K. Basen-Engquist, D. Kirby, G. Parcel, S. Banspach, J. Collins, E. Baumler, S. Carvajal, and R. Harrist. 2001. Safer choices: Reducing teen pregnancy, HIV, and STDs. *Public Health Reports* 116(1):82–93.

Cramer, J. C. 1995. Racial and ethnic differences in birthweight: The role of income and financial assistance. *Demography* 32(2):231–247.

Cramp, A. G., and L. R. Brawley. 2006. Moms in motion: A group-mediated cognitive-behavioral physical activity intervention. *International Journal of Behavioral Nutrition and Physical Activity* 3:23.

Crocker, J. 1999. Social stigma and self-esteem: Situational construction of self-worth. *Journal of Experimental Social Psychology* 35(1):89–107.

Cutrona, C. E., D. W. Russell, R. M. Hessling, P. A. Brown, and V. Murry. 2000. Direct and moderating effects of community context on the psychological well-being of African American women. *Journal of Personality and Social Psychology* 79(6):1088–1101.

Dahlgren, G., and M. Whitehead. 1991. *Policies and Strategies to Promote Social Equity in Health*. Stockholm, Sweden: Institute for the Futures Studies.

Damjanovic, A. K., Y. H. Yang, R. Glaser, J. K. Kiecolt-Glaser, H. Nguyen, B. Laskowski, Y. X. Zou, D. Q. Beversdorf, and N. P. Weng. 2007. Accelerated telomere erosion is associated with a declining immune function of caregivers of Alzheimer's disease patients. *Journal of Immunology* 179(6):4249–4254.

Danaei, G., E. L. Ding, D. Mozaffarian, B. Taylor, J. Rehm, C. J. Murray, and M. Ezzati. 2009. The preventable causes of death in the United States: Comparative risk assessment of dietary, lifestyle, and metabolic risk factors. *PLoS Medicine* 6(4):e1000058.

Dancy, B. L., K. S. Crittenden, and M. L. Talashek. 2006. Mothers' effectiveness as HIV risk reduction educators for adolescent daughters. *Journal of Health Care for the Poor and Underserved* 17(1):218–239.

Danese, A., T. E. Moffitt, H. Harrington, B. J. Milne, G. Polanczyk, C. M. Pariante, R. Poulton, and A. Caspi. 2009. Adverse childhood experiences and adult risk factors for age-related disease: Depression, inflammation, and clustering of metabolic risk markers. *Archives of Pediatrics & Adolescent Medicine* 163(12):1135–1143.

Darmon, N., and A. Drewnowski. 2008. Does social class predict diet quality? *American Journal of Clinical Nutrition* 87(5):1107–1117.

Davey Smith, G., and S. Ebrahim. 2003. "Mendelian randomization": Can genetic epidemiology contribute to understanding environmental determinants of disease? *International Journal of Epidemiology* 32(1):1–22.

Dempsey, J. C., C. L. Butler, T. K. Sorensen, I. M. Lee, M. L. Thompson, R. S. Miller, I. O. Frederick, and M. A. Williams. 2004a. A case–control study of maternal recreational physical activity and risk of gestational diabetes mellitus. *Diabetes Research and Clinical Practice* 66(2):203–215.

Dempsey, J. C., T. K. Sorensen, M. A. Williams, I. M. Lee, R. S. Miller, E. E. Dashow, and D. A. Luthy. 2004b. Prospective study of gestational diabetes mellitus risk in relation to maternal recreational physical activity before and during pregnancy. *American Journal of Epidemiology* 159(7):663–670.

DeNavas-Walt, C., B. Proctor, and J. D. Smith. 2009. *Income, Poverty, and Health Insurance Coverage in the United States: 2008.* Washington, DC: US Census Bureau.

Descamps, M. J., E. Rothblum, J. Bradford, and C. Ryan. 2000. Mental health impact of child sexual abuse, rape, intimate partner violence, and hate crimes in the National Lesbian Health Care Survey. *Journal of Gay & Lesbian Social Services* 11(1):27–56.

DeVoe, J. E., G. E. Fryer, R. Phillips, and L. Green. 2003. Receipt of preventive care among adults: Insurance status and usual source of care. *American Journal of Public Health* 93(5):786–791.

DiClemente, C. C., P. Dolan-Mullen, and R. A. Windsor. 2000. The process of pregnancy smoking cessation: Implications for intervention. *Tobacco Control* 9(3):19–21.

Diehl, A., B. Croissant, A. Batra, G. Mundle, H. Nakovics, and K. Mann. 2007. Alcoholism in women: Is it different in onset and outcome compared to men? *European Archives of Psychiatry and Clinical Neuroscience* 257(6):344–351.

Diez Roux, A. V., F. J. Nieto, C. Muntaner, H. A. Tyroler, G. W. Comstock, E. Shahar, L. S. Cooper, R. L. Watson, and M. Szklo. 1997. Neighborhood environments and coronary heart disease: A multilevel analysis. *American Journal of Epidemiology* 146(1):48–63.

Diez Roux, A. V., K. R. Evenson, A. P. McGinn, D. G. Brown, L. Moore, S. Brines, and D. R. Jacobs, Jr. 2007. Availability of recreational resources and physical activity in adults. *American Journal of Public Health* 97(3):493–499.

DiIorio, C., K. Resnicow, F. McCarty, A. K. De, W. N. Dudley, D. T. Wang, and P. Denzmore. 2006. Keepin' it R.E.A.L.: Results of a mother-adolescent HIV prevention program. *Nursing Research* 55(1):43–51.

Dobbins, M., K. DeCorby, P. Robeson, H. Husson, and D. Tirilis. 2009. School-based physical activity programs for promoting physical activity and fitness in children and adolescents aged 6–18. *Cochrane Database of Systematic Reviews* (1), http://www.mrw.interscience.wiley.com/cochrane/clsysrev/articles/CD007651/frame.html (accessed August 15, 2009).

Downs, J. S., P. J. Murray, W. Bruine de Bruin, J. Penrose, C. Palmgren, and B. Fischhoff. 2004. Interactive video behavioral intervention to reduce adolescent females' STD risk: A randomized controlled trial. *Social Science & Medicine* 59(8):1561–1572.

Dreher, H. 2004. Psychosocial factors in heart disease: A process model. *Advances in Mind-Body Medicine* 20(3):20–31.

Dube, S. R., K. Asman, A. Malarcher, and R. Carabollo. 2009. Cigarette smoking among adults and trends in smoking cessation—United States, 2008. *Morbidity and Mortality Weekly Report* 58(44):1227–1232.

Duffey, K. J., P. Gordon-Larsen, G. X. Ayala, and B. M. Popkin. 2008. Birthplace is associated with more adverse dietary profiles for US-born than for foreign-born Latino adults. *Journal of Nutrition* 138(12):2428–2435.

Duffey, K. J., P. Gordon-Larsen, J. M. Shikany, D. Guilkey, D. R. Jacobs, Jr., and B. M. Popkin. 2010. Food price and diet and health outcomes: 20 years of the CARDIA Study. *Archives of Internal Medicine* 170(5):420–426.

Duncan, M. J., J. C. Spence, and W. K. Mummery. 2005. Perceived environment and physical activity: A meta-analysis of selected environmental characteristics. *International Journal of Behavioral Nutrition and Physical Activity* 2:11.

Eaker, E. D., L. M. Sullivan, M. Kelly-Hayes, R. B. D'Agostino, Sr., and E. J. Benjamin. 2007. Marital status, marital strain, and risk of coronary heart disease or total mortality: The Framingham Offspring Study. *Psychosomatic Medicine* 69(6):509–513.

Edmundson, E., G. S. Parcel, H. A. Feldman, J. Elder, C. L. Perry, C. C. Johnson, B. J. Williston, E. J. Stone, M. Yang, L. Lytle, and L. Webber. 1996. The effects of the child and adolescent trial for cardiovascular health upon psychosocial determinants of diet and physical activity behavior. *Preventive Medicine* 25(4):442–454.

Ellekjaer, H., J. Holmen, E. Ellekjaer, and L. Vatten. 2000. Physical activity and stroke mortality in women. Ten-year follow-up of the Nord-Trondelag Health Survey, 1984–1986. *Stroke* 31(1):14–18.

Ellsberg, M., H. A. Jansen, L. Heise, C. H. Watts, and C. Garcia-Moreno; WHO Multi-country Study on Women's Health and Domestic Violence Against Women Study Team. 2008. Intimate partner violence and women's physical and mental health in the who multi-country study on women's health and domestic violence: An observational study. *Lancet* 371(9619):1165–1172.

Elmer, P. J., E. Obarzanek, W. M. Vollmer, D. Simons-Morton, V. J. Stevens, D. R. Young, P. H. Lin, C. Champagne, D. W. Harsha, L. P. Svetkey, J. Ard, P. J. Brantley, M. A. Proschan, T. P. Erlinger, and L. J. Appel. 2006. Effects of comprehensive lifestyle modification on diet, weight, physical fitness, and blood pressure control: 18-month results of a randomized trial. *Annals of Internal Medicine* 144(7):485–495.

Emmons, K. M., L. A. Linnan, W. G. Shadel, B. Marcus, and D. B. Abrams. 1999. The working healthy project: A worksite health-promotion trial targeting physical activity, diet, and smoking. *Journal of Occupational and Environmental Medicine* 41(7):545–555.

Epel, E. S., E. H. Blackburn, J. Lin, F. S. Dhabhar, N. E. Adler, J. D. Morrow, and R. M. Cawthon. 2004. Accelerated telomere shortening in response to life stress. *Proceedings of the National Academy of Sciences of the United States of America* 101(49):17312–17315.

Escobar, J. I., C. H. Nervi, and M. A. Gara. 2000. Immigration and mental health: Mexican Americans in the United States. *Harvard Review of Psychiatry* 8(2):64–72.

Evans, R. G., and G. L. Stoddart. 1990. Producing health, consuming health care. *Social Science & Medicine* 31(12):1347–1363.

Eyler, A. E., S. Wilcox, D. Matson-Koffman, K. R. Evenson, B. Sanderson, J. Thompson, J. Wilbur, and D. Rohm-Young. 2002. Correlates of physical activity among women from diverse racial/ethnic groups. *Journal of Women's Health and Gender-Based Medicine* 11(3):239–253.

Fedovskiy, K., S. Higgins, and A. Paranjape. 2008. Intimate partner violence: How does it impact major depressive disorder and post traumatic stress disorder among immigrant Latinas? *Journal of Immigrant and Minority Health* 10(1):45–51.

Fernald, L. C., P. J. Gertler, and L. M. Neufeld. 2009. 10-year effect of Oportunidades, Mexico's conditional cash transfer programme, on child growth, cognition, language, and behaviour: A longitudinal follow-up study. *Lancet* 374(9706):1997–2005.

Fernandes, M. M. 2010. *Evaluating the Impacts of School Nutrition and Physical Activity Policies on Child Health*. Dissertation, Pardee RAND Graduate School, Santa Monica, CA.

Feskanich, D., W. C. Willett, and G. A. Colditz. 2003. Calcium, vitamin D, milk consumption, and hip fractures: A prospective study among postmenopausal women. *American Journal of Clinical Nutrition* 77(2):504–511.

Finer, L. B., and S. K. Henshaw. 2006. Disparities in rates of unintended pregnancy in the United States, 1994 and 2001. *Perspectives on Sexual and Reproductive Health* 38(2):90–96.

Fitzgibbon, M. L., and B. M. Beech. 2009. The role of culture in the context of school-based BMI screening. *Pediatrics* 124 (Suppl. 1):S50–S62.

Fitzpatrick, A. L., N. R. Powe, L. S. Cooper, D. G. Ives, and J. A. Robbins. 2004. Barriers to health care access among the elderly and who perceives them. *American Journal of Public Health* 94(10):1788–1794.

Flanders, W. D., C. A. Lally, B. P. Zhu, S. J. Henley, and M. J. Thun. 2003. Lung cancer mortality in relation to age, duration of smoking, and daily cigarette consumption: Results from Cancer Prevention Study II. *Cancer Research* 63(19):6556–6562.

Flegal, K. M., R. P. Troiano, E. R. Pamuk, R. J. Kuczmarski, and S. M. Campbell. 1995. The influence of smoking cessation on the prevalence of overweight in the United States. *New England Journal of Medicine* 333(18):1165–1170.

Flegal, K. M., M. D. Carroll, C. L. Ogden, and C. L. Johnson. 2002. Prevalence and trends in obesity among US adults, 1999–2000. *Journal of the American Medical Association* 288(14):1723–1727.

Flegal, K. M., M. D. Carroll, C. L. Ogden, and L. R. Curtin. 2010. Prevalence and trends in obesity among US adults, 1999–2008. *Journal of the American Medical Association* 303(3):235–241.

Fleury, J., C. Keller, and C. Murdaugh. 2000. Social and contextual etiology of coronary heart disease in women. *Journal of Women's Health & Gender-Based Medicine* 9(9):967–978.

Folsom, A. R., L. H. Kushi, and C. P. Hong. 2000. Physical activity and incident diabetes mellitus in postmenopausal women. *American Journal of Public Health* 90(1):134–138.

Forhan, S. E., S. L. Gottlieb, M. R. Sternberg, F. Xu, S. D. Datta, S. Berman, and L. E. Markowitz. 2008. *Prevalence of Sexually Transmitted Infections and Bacterial Vaginosis Among Female Adolescents in the United States: Data from the National Health And Nutrition Examination Survey (NHANES) 2003–2004*. Paper presented at 2008 National STD Prevention Conference, Chicago, IL.

Foshee, V. A., K. E. Bauman, X. B. Arriaga, R. W. Helms, G. G. Koch, and G. F. Linder. 1998. An evaluation of safe dates, an adolescent dating violence prevention program. *American Journal of Public Health* 88(1):45–50.

Foshee, V., K. Bauman, S. Ennett, C. Suchindran, T. Benefield, and G. Linder. 2005. Assessing the effects of the dating violence prevention program "safe dates" using random coefficient regression modeling. *Prevention Science* 6(3):245–258.

Freedman, B. I. 2002. End-stage renal failure in African Americans: Insights in kidney disease susceptibility. *Nephrology, Dialysis, Transplantation* 17(2):198–200.

Friedmann, E., S. A. Thomas, F. Liu, P. G. Morton, D. Chapa, and S. S. Gottlieb. 2006. Relationship of depression, anxiety, and social isolation to chronic heart failure outpatient mortality. *American Heart Journal* 152(5):940.

Frost, J. J., L. B. Finer, and A. Tapales. 2008. The impact of publicly funded family planning clinic services on unintended pregnancies and government cost savings. *Journal of Health Care for the Poor and Underserved* 19(3):778–796.

Gammon, M. D., J. B. Schoenberg, S. L. Teitelbaum, L. A. Brinton, N. Potischman, C. A. Swanson, D. J. Brogan, R. J. Coates, K. E. Malone, and J. L. Stanford. 1998. Cigarette smoking and breast cancer risk among young women (United States). *Cancer Causes & Control* 9(6):583–590.

Glaser, R., J. Sheridan, W. B. Malarkey, R. C. MacCallum, and J. K. Kiecolt-Glaser. 2000. Chronic stress modulates the immune response to a pneumococcal pneumonia vaccine. *Psychosomatic Medicine* 62(6):804–807.

Glied, S., K. Jack, and J. Rachlin. 2008. Women's health insurance coverage 1980–2005. *Women's Health Issues* 18(1):7–16.

Gold, E. B., J. Bromberger, S. Crawford, S. Samuels, G. A. Greendale, S. Harlow, and J. Skurnick. 2001. Factors associated with age at natural menopause in a multiethnic sample of midlife women. *American Journal of Epidemiology* 153(9):865–874.

Gomez, C. A., and B. V. Van Oss Marin. 1996. Gender, culture, and power: Barriers to HIV-prevention strategies for women. *Journal of Sex Research* 33(4):355–362.

Goodpaster, B. H., S. Krishnaswami, T. B. Harris, A. Katsiaras, S. B. Kritchevsky, E. M. Simonsick, M. Nevitt, P. Holvoet, and A. B. Newman. 2005. Obesity, regional body fat distribution, and the metabolic syndrome in older men and women. *Archives of Internal Medicine* 165(7):777–783.

Gorman-Smith, D., and P. Tolan. 1998. The role of exposure to community violence and developmental problems among inner-city youth. *Development and Psychopathology* 10(01):101–116.

Greenfield, S. F. 2002. Women and alcohol use disorders. *Harvard Review of Psychiatry* 10(2): 76–85.

Gritz, E. R., I. R. Nielsen, and L. A. Brooks. 1996. Smoking cessation and gender: The influence of physiological, psychological, and behavioral factors. *Journal of the American Medical Women's Association* 51(1-2):35–42.

Guendelman, S., and B. Abrams. 1995. Dietary intake among Mexican-American women: Generational differences and a comparison with white non-Hispanic women. *American Journal of Public Health* 85(1):20–25.

Guide to Community Preventive Services. 2004. *Promoting Good Nutrition: School-Based Programs Promoting Nutrition and Physical Activity.* www.thecommunityguide.org/nutrition/school|programs.html (accessed August 28, 2009).

Guttmacher Institute. 2006. *Poorer U. S. Women Increasingly Likely to Face Unintended Pregnancies.* http://www.guttmacher.org/media/nr/2006/05/04/index.html (accessed August 28, 2009).

Hallman, T., G. Burell, S. Setterlind, A. Oden, and J. Lisspers. 2001. Psychosocial risk factors for coronary heart disease, their importance compared with other risk factors and gender differences in sensitivity. *Journal of Cardiovascular Risk* 8(1):39–49.

Hamajima, N., K. Hirose, K. Tajima, T. Rohan, E. E. Calle, C. W. Heath, Jr., R. J. Coates, J. M. Liff, R. Talamini, N. Chantarakul, S. Koetsawang, D. Rachawat, A. Morabia, L. Schuman, W. Stewart, M. Szklo, C. Bain, F. Schofield, V. Siskind, P. Band, A. J. Coldman, R. P. Gallagher, T. G. Hislop, P. Yang, L. M. Kolonel, A. M. Nomura, J. Hu, K. C. Johnson, Y. Mao, S. De Sanjose, N. Lee, P. Marchbanks, H. W. Ory, H. B. Peterson, H. G. Wilson, P. A. Wingo, K. Ebeling, D. Kunde, P. Nishan, J. L. Hopper, G. Colditz, V. Gajalanski, N. Martin, T. Pardthaisong, S. Silpisornkosol, C. Theetranont, B. Boosiri, S. Chutivongse, P. Jimakorn, P. Virutamasen, C. Wongsrichanalai, M. Ewertz, H. O. Adami, L. Bergkvist, C. Magnusson, I. Persson, J. Chang-Claude, C. Paul, D. C. Skegg, G. F. Spears, P. Boyle, T. Evstifeeva, J. R. Daling, W. B. Hutchinson, K. Malone, E. A. Noonan, J. L. Stanford, D. B. Thomas, N. S. Weiss, E. White, N. Andrieu, A. Bremond, F. Clavel, B. Gairard, J. Lansac, L. Piana, R. Renaud, A. Izquierdo, P. Viladiu, H. R. Cuevas, P. Ontiveros, A. Palet, S. B. Salazar, N. Aristizabel, A. Cuadros, L. Tryggvadottir, H. Tulinius, A. Bachelot, M. G. Le, J. Peto, S. Franceschi, F. Lubin, B. Modan, E. Ron, Y. Wax, G. D. Friedman, R. A. Hiatt, F. Levi, T. Bishop, K. Kosmelj, M. Primic-Zakelj, B. Ravnihar, J. Stare, W. L. Beeson, G. Fraser, R. D. Bullbrook, J. Cuzick, S. W. Duffy, I. S. Fentiman, J. L. Hayward, D. Y. Wang, A. J. McMichael, K. McPherson, R. L. Hanson, M. C. Leske, M. C. Mahoney, P. C. Nasca, A. O. Varma, A. L. Weinstein, T. R. Moller, H. Olsson, J. Ranstam, R. A. Goldbohm, P. A. van den Brandt, R. A. Apelo, J. Baens, J. R. de la Cruz, B. Javier, L. B. Lacaya, C. A. Ngelangel, C. La Vecchia, E. Negri, E. Marubini, M. Ferraroni, M. Gerber, S. Richardson, C. Segala, D. Gatei, P. Kenya, A. Kungu, J. G. Mati, L. A. Brinton, R. Hoover, C. Schairer, R. Spirtas, H. P. Lee, M. A. Rookus, F. E. van Leeuwen, J. A. Schoenberg, M. McCredie, M. D. Gammon, E. A. Clarke, L. Jones, A. Neil, M. Vessey, D. Yeates, P. Appleby, E. Banks, V. Beral, D. Bull, B. Crossley, A. Goodill, J. Green, C. Hermon, T. Key, N. Langston, C. Lewis, G. Reeves, R. Collins, R. Doll, R. Peto, K. Mabuchi, D. Preston, P. Hannaford, C. Kay, L. Rosero-Bixby, Y. T. Gao, F. Jin, J. M. Yuan, H. Y. Wei, T. Yun, C. Zhiheng, G. Berry, J. Cooper Booth, T. Jelihovsky, R. MacLennan, R. Shearman, Q. S. Wang, C. J. Baines, A. B. Miller, C. Wall, E. Lund, H. Stalsberg, X. O. Shu, W. Zheng, K. Katsouyanni, A. Trichopoulou, D. Trichopoulos, A. Dabancens, L. Martinez, R. Molina, O. Salas, F. E. Alexander, K. Anderson, A. R. Folsom, B. S. Hulka, L. Bernstein, S. Enger, R. W. Haile, A. Paganini-Hill, M. C. Pike, R. K. Ross, G. Ursin, M. C. Yu, M. P. Longnecker, P. Newcomb, A. Kalache, T. M. Farley, S. Holck, and O. Meirik. 2002. Alcohol, tobacco and breast cancer—collaborative reanalysis of individual data from 53 epidemiological studies, including 58,515 women with breast cancer and 95,067 women without the disease. *British Journal of Cancer* 87(11):1234–1245.

Harrison, H. R., E. R. Alexander, L. Weinstein, M. Lewis, M. Nash, and D. A. Sim. 1983. Cervical chlamydia trachomatis and mycoplasmal infections in pregnancy: Epidemiology and outcomes. *Journal of the American Medical Association* 250(13):1721–1727.

Hathaway, J. E., G. Willis, B. Zimmer, and J. G. Silverman. 2005. Impact of partner abuse on women's reproductive lives. *Journal of the American Medical Women's Association* 29(4):42–45.

Hawkley, L. C., and J. T. Cacioppo. 2004. Stress and the aging immune system. *Brain, Behavior, and Immunity* 18(2):114–119.

Hayes-Bautista, D. E., L. Baexconde-Garbanati, and B. H. Hayes-Bautista. 1994. Latino health in Los Angeles: Family medicine in a changing minority context. *Family Practice* 11(3):318–324.

Hegmann, K. T., M. F. Alison, R. P. Keaney, S. E. Moser, D. S. Nilasena, M. Sedlars, L. Higham-Gren, and J. L. Lyon. 1993. The effect of age at smoking initiation on lung cancer risk. *Epidemiology* 4(5):444–448.

Herman, D. R., G. G. Harrison, A. A. Afifi, and E. Jenks. 2008. Effect of a targeted subsidy on intake of fruits and vegetables among low-income women in the special supplemental nutrition program for women, infants, and children. *American Journal of Public Health* 98(1):98–105.

HHS (US Department of Health and Human Services). 1980. *The Health Consequences of Smoking for Women: A Report of the Surgeon General.* http://profiles.nlm.nih.gov/NN/B/B/R/T/_/nnbbrt. pdf (accessed September 10, 2009).

———. 2001. *Women and Smoking: A Report of the Surgeon General.* http://www.surgeongeneral. gov/library/womenandtobacco/index.html (accessed January 13, 2010).

———. 2004. *The Health Consequences of Smoking. A Report of the Surgeon General.* http:// surgeongeneral.gov/library/smokingconsequences (accessed August 15, 2009).

———. 2008a. *Treating Tobacco Use and Dependence 2008 Update.* Rockville, MD: Public Health Service.

———. 2008b. Adverse health conditions and health risk behaviors associated with intimate partner violence—United States, 2005. [see erratum]. *Morbidity and Mortality Weekly Report* 57(5): 113–117.

HHS and USDA (US Department of Agriculture). 2005. *Dietary Guidelines for Americans.* http://www. health.gov/dietaryguidelines/dga2005/document/default.htm (accessed January 13, 2010)

Hillis, S. D., and J. N. Wasserheit. 1996. Screening for chlamydia—A key to the prevention of pelvic inflammatory disease. *New England Journal of Medicine* 334(21):1399–1401.

Himle, J. A., R. E. Baser, R. J. Taylor, R. D. Campbell, and J. S. Jackson. 2009. Anxiety disorders among African Americans, blacks of Caribbean descent, and non-Hispanic whites in the United States. *Journal of Anxiety Disorders* 23(5):578–590.

Holmes, M. D., W. Y. Chen, D. Feskanich, C. H. Kroenke, and G. A. Colditz. 2005. Physical activity and survival after breast cancer diagnosis. *Journal of the American Medical Association* 293(20):2479–2486.

HRSA (Health Resources and Services Administration). 2008. *Women's Health USA 2008.* US Department of Health and Human Services.

Hsia, J., L. Wu, C. Allen, A. Oberman, W. E. Lawson, J. Torréns, M. Safford, M. C. Limacher, and B. V. Howard. 2005. Physical activity and diabetes risk in postmenopausal women. *American Journal of Preventive Medicine* 28(1):19–25.

Hu, F. B., R. J. Sigal, J. W. Rich-Edwards, G. A. Colditz, C. G. Solomon, W. C. Willett, F. E. Speizer, and J. E. Manson. 1999. Walking compared with vigorous physical activity and risk of type 2 diabetes in women: A prospective study. *Journal of the American Medical Association* 282(15):1433–1439.

Hu, F. B., M. J. Stampfer, G. A. Colditz, A. Ascherio, K. M. Rexrode, W. C. Willett, and J. E. Manson. 2000. Physical activity and risk of stroke in women. *Journal of the American Medical Association* 283(22):2961–2967.

Hu, F. B., J. E. Manson, M. J. Stampfer, G. Colditz, S. Liu, C. G. Solomon, and W. C. Willett. 2001. Diet, lifestyle, and the risk of type 2 diabetes mellitus in women. *New England Journal of Medicine* 345(11):790–797.

Hu, F. B., T. Y. Li, G. A. Colditz, W. C. Willett, and J. E. Manson. 2003. Television watching and other sedentary behaviors in relation to risk of obesity and type 2 diabetes mellitus in women. *Journal of the American Medical Association* 289(14):1785–1791.

Hu, G., J. Tuomilehto, K. Silventoinen, N. Barengo, and P. Jousilahti. 2004. Joint effects of physical activity, body mass index, waist circumference and waist-to-hip ratio with the risk of cardiovascular disease among middle-aged Finnish men and women. *European Heart Journal* 25(24):2212–2219.

Hudman, J., and M. O'Malley. 2003. *Policy Brief. Health Insurance Premiums and Cost-Sharing: Findings from the Research on Low-Income Populations.* Menlo Park, CA: Kaiser Family Foundation.

Huhman, M., L. D. Potter, F. L. Wong, S. W. Banspach, J. C. Duke, and C. D. Heitzler. 2005. Effects of a mass media campaign to increase physical activity among children: Year-1 results of the VERB campaign. *Pediatrics* 116(2):e277–e284.

Humpel, N., N. Owen, D. Iverson, E. Leslie, and A. Bauman. 2004. Perceived environment attributes, residential location, and walking for particular purposes. *American Journal of Preventive Medicine* 26(2):119–125.

Hvidtfeldt, U. A., J. S. Tolstrup, M. U. Jakobsen, B. L. Heitmann, M. Gronbaek, E. O'Reilly, K. Balter, U. Goldbourt, G. Hallmans, P. Knekt, S. Liu, M. Pereira, P. Pietinen, D. Spiegelman, J. Stevens, J. Virtamo, W. C. Willett, E. B. Rimm, and A. Ascherio. 2010. Alcohol intake and risk of coronary heart disease in younger, middle-aged, and older adults. *Circulation* 121(14):1589–1597.

IOM. 1997. *The Hidden Epidemic: Confronting Sexually Transmitted Diseases.* Washington, DC: National Academy Press.

———. 2000a. *Promoting Health: Intervention Strategies from Social and Behavioral Research.* Washington, DC: National Academy Press.

———. 2000b. *The Role of Nutrition in Maintaining Health in the Nation's Elderly.* Washington, DC: National Academy Press.

———. 2001a. *Health and Behavior: The Interplay of Biological, Behavioral, and Societal Influences.* Washington, DC: National Academy Press.

———. 2001b. *Crossing the Quality Chasm: A New Health System for the 21st Century.* Washington, DC: National Academy Press.

———. 2002a. *The Future of the Public's Health in the 21st Century.* Washington, DC: The National Academies Press.

———. 2002b. *Care Without Coverage: Too Little, Too Late, Insuring Health.* Washington, DC: The National Academies Press.

———. 2002c. *Health Insurance Is a Family Matter.* Washington, DC: The National Academies Press.

———. 2003. *Hidden Costs, Value Lost: Uninsurance in America, Insuring Health.* Washington, DC: The National Academies Press.

———. 2004a. *Health Literacy: A Prescription to End Confusion.* Edited by L. Nielsen-Bohlman, A. M. Panzer, and D. A. Kindig. Washington, DC: The National Academies Press.

———. 2004b. *Insuring America's Health: Principles and Recommendations, Insuring Health.* Washington, DC: The National Academies Press.

———. 2005a. *Estimating the Contributions of Lifestyle-Related Factors to Preventable Death.* Washington, DC: The National Academies Press.

———. 2005b. *Preventing Childhood Obesity: Health in the Balance.* Washington, DC: The National Academies Press.

————. 2005c. *Dietary Reference Intakes for Energy, Carbohydrate, Fiber, Fat, Fatty Acids, Cholesterol, Protein, and Amino Acids (Macronutrients).* Washington, DC: National Academies Press.

————. 2009a. *Combating Tobacco Use in Military and Veteran Populations.* Washington, DC: The National Academies Press.

————. 2009b. *America's Uninsured Crisis: Consequences for Health and Health Care.* Washington, DC: The National Academies Press.

————. 2010. *Strategies to Reduce Sodium Intake in the United States.* Washington, DC: The National Academies Press.

Jackson, J. S., I. Forsythe-Brown, and I. O. Govia. 2007. Age cohort, ancestry, and immigrant generation influences in family relations and psychological well-being among black Caribbean family members. *Journal of Social Issues* 63(4):729–743.

Jackson, R. D., A. Z. LaCroix, M. Gass, R. B. Wallace, J. Robbins, C. E. Lewis, T. Bassford, S. A. Beresford, H. R. Black, P. Blanchette, D. E. Bonds, R. L. Brunner, R. G. Brzyski, B. Caan, J. A. Cauley, R. T. Chlebowski, S. R. Cummings, I. Granek, J. Hays, G. Heiss, S. L. Hendrix, B. V. Howard, J. Hsia, F. A. Hubbell, K. C. Johnson, H. Judd, J. M. Kotchen, L. H. Kuller, R. D. Langer, N. L. Lasser, M. C. Limacher, S. Ludlam, J. E. Manson, K. L. Margolis, J. McGowan, J. K. Ockene, M. J. O'Sullivan, L. Phillips, R. L. Prentice, G. E. Sarto, M. L. Stefanick, L. Van Horn, J. Wactawski-Wende, E. Whitlock, G. L. Anderson, A. R. Assaf, D. Barad, and the Women's Health Initiative Investigators. 2006. Calcium plus vitamin D supplementation and the risk of fractures. *New England Journal of Medicine* 354(7):669–683.

Jemal, A., M. J. Thun, L. A. Ries, H. L. Howe, H. K. Weir, M. M. Center, E. Ward, X. C. Wu, C. Eheman, R. Anderson, U. A. Ajani, B. Kohler, and B. K. Edwards. 2008. Annual report to the nation on the status of cancer, 1975–2005, featuring trends in lung cancer, tobacco use, and tobacco control. *Journal of the National Cancer Institute* 100(23):1672–1694.

Jeon, C. Y., R. P. Lokken, F. B. Hu, and R. M. van Dam. 2007. Physical activity of moderate intensity and risk of type 2 diabetes: A systematic review. *Diabetes Care* 30(3):744–752.

Jirtle, R. L., and M. K. Skinner. 2007. Environmental epigenomics and disease susceptibility. *Nature Reviews. Genetics* 8(4):253–262.

Jolly, A. M., P. H. Orr, G. Hammond, and T. K. Young. 1995. Risk factors for infection in women undergoing testing for Chlamydia trachomatis and Neisseria gonorrhoeae in Manitoba, Canada. *Sexually Transmitted Diseases* 22(5):289–295.

Kaiser Family Foundation. 2007. *Women's Issue Brief. An Update on Women's Health Policy: Medicaid's Role for Women.* Menlo Park, CA.

————. 2009. *Women's Fact Sheet. Women's Health Insurance Coverage.* Menlo Park, CA.

Kalkhoff, R. K., A. H. Hartz, D. Rupley, A. H. Kissebah, and S. Kelber. 1983. Relationship of body fat distribution to blood pressure, carbohydrate tolerance, and plasma lipids in healthy obese women. *Journal of Laboratory and Clinical Medicine* 102(4):621–627.

Kallan, J. E. 1993. Race, intervening variables, and two components of low birth weight. *Demography* 30(3):489–506.

Kamphuis, C., K. Giskes, G. J. Bruinjn, W. Wendel-Vos, J. Brug, and J. V. Lenthe. 2006. Environmental determinants of fruit and vegetable consumption among adults: A systematic review. *British Journal of Nutrition* 96(4):620–635.

Kaplan, G., and J. Keil. 1993. Socioeconomic factors and cardiovascular disease: A review of the literature. *Circulation* 88(4):1973–1998.

Katz, L. F., J. R. Kling, and J. B. Liebman. 2001. Moving to opportunity in Boston: Early results of a randomized mobility experiment. *Quarterly Journal of Economics* 116(2):607–654.

Kawachi, I., G. A. Colditz, M. J. Stampfer, W. C. Willett, J. E. Manson, B. Rosner, D. J. Hunter, C. H. Hennekens, and F. E. Speizer. 1993. Smoking cessation in relation to total mortality rates in women. A prospective cohort study. *Annals of Internal Medicine* 119(10):992–1000.

Kelleher, C. J., L. D. Cardozo, V. Khullar, and S. Salvatore. 1997. A new questionnaire to assess the quality of life of urinary incontinent women. *British Journal of Obstetrics and Gynaecology* 104(12):1374–1379.

Kimm, S. Y., N. W. Glynn, C. E. Aston, E. T. Poehlman, and S. R. Daniels. 2001. Effects of race, cigarette smoking, and use of contraceptive medications on resting energy expenditure in young women. *American Journal of Epidemiology* 154(8):718–724.

Kimm, S. Y. S., N. W. Glynn, A. M. Kriska, B. A. Barton, S. S. Kronsberg, S. R. Daniels, P. B. Crawford, Z. I. Sabry, and K. Liu. 2002. Decline in physical activity in black girls and white girls during adolescence. *New England Journal of Medicine* 347(10):709–715.

King, A. C., D. Stokols, E. Talen, G. S. Brassington, and R. Killingsworth. 2002. Theoretical approaches to the promotion of physical activity: Forging a transdisciplinary paradigm. *American Journal of Preventive Medicine* 23(Suppl. 1):15–25.

Kirby, D. 2007. *Emerging Answers 2007: Research Findings on Programs to Reduce Teen Pregnancy and Sexually Transmitted Diseases.* Washington, DC: The National Campaign to Prevent Teen and Unplanned Pregnancy.

Kirby, D. B., B. A. Laris, and L. A. Rolleri. 2007. Sex and HIV education programs: Their impact on sexual behaviors of young people throughout the world. *Journal of Adolescent Health* 40(3):206–217.

Kissebah, A. H., N. Vydelinfum, R. Murray, D. J. Evans, A. J. Hartz, R. K. Kalkhoff, and P. W. Adams. 1983. Relation of body fat distribution to metabolic complications of obesity. *Obstetrical & Gynecological Survey* 38(1):41–43.

Kjerulff, K. H., K. D. Frick, J. A. Rhoades, and C. S. Hollenbeak. 2007. The cost of being a woman: A national study of health care utilization and expenditures for female-specific conditions. *Women's Health Issues* 17(1):13–21.

Kohler, P. K., L. E. Manhart, and W. E. Lafferty. 2008. Abstinence-only and comprehensive sex education and the initiation of sexual activity and teen pregnancy. *Journal of Adolescent Health* 42(4):344–351.

Kosiak, B., J. Sangl, and R. Correa-de-Araujo. 2006. Quality of health care for older women: What do we know? *Women's Health Issues* 16(2):89–99.

Kreuter, M. W., S. N. Lukwago, D. C. Bucholtz, E. M. Clark, and V. Sanders-Thompson. 2003. Achieving cultural appropriateness in health promotion programs: Targeted and tailored approaches. *Health Education & Behavior* 30(2):133–146.

Krishnan, S., Y. C. Cozier, L. Ronsenberg, and J. R. Palmer. 2010. Socioeconomic status and incidence of type 2 diabetes: Results from the Black Women's Health Study. *American Journal of Epidemiology* 171(5):564–570.

Kuhlmann, A. K., P. M. Dietz, C. Galavotti, and L. J. England. 2008. Weight-management interventions for pregnant or postpartum women. *American Journal of Preventive Medicine* 34(6):523–528.

Kushi, L. H., T. Byers, C. Doyle, E. V. Bandera, M. McCullough, A. McTiernan, T. Gansler, K. S. Andrews, and M. J. Thun. 2006. American Cancer Society guidelines on nutrition and physical activity for cancer prevention: Reducing the risk of cancer with healthy food choices and physical activity. *CA: A Cancer Journal for Clinicians* 56(5):254–281.

LaBrie, J. W., A. D. Thompson, K. Huchting, A. Lac, and K. Buckley. 2007. A group motivational interviewing intervention reduces drinking and alcohol-related negative consequences in adjudicated college women. *Addictive Behaviors* 32(11):2549–2562.

Laden, F., and D. J. Hunter. 1998. Environmental risk factors and female breast cancer. *Annual Review of Public Health* 19(1):101–123.

Lanphear, B. P., R. S. Byrd, P. Auinger, and S. J. Schaffer. 1998. Community characteristics associated with elevated blood lead levels in children. *Pediatrics* 101(2):264–271.

Lantz, P. M., J. S. House, J. M. Lepkowski, D. R. Williams, R. P. Mero, and J. Chen. 1998. Socioeconomic factors, health behaviors, and mortality: Results from a nationally representative prospective study of US adults. *Journal of the American Medical Association* 279(21):1703–1708.

Lara, M., C. Gamboa, M. I. Kahramanian, L. S. Morales, and D. E. Hayes Bautista. 2005. Acculturation and the Latino health in the United States: A review of the literature and its sociopolitical context. *Annual Review of Public Health* 26(1):367–397.

Laurent, S. L., S. J. Thompson, C. Addy, C. Z. Garrison, and E. E. Moore. 1992. An epidemiologic study of smoking and primary infertility in women. *Fertility and Sterility* 57(3):565–572.

Law, M. R., and A. K. Hackshaw. 1997. A meta-analysis of cigarette smoking, bone mineral density and risk of hip fracture: Recognition of a major effect. *British Medical Journal* 315(7112): 841–846.

Lee, V., J. M. Tobin, and E. Foley. 2006. Relationship of cervical ectopy to chlamydia infection in young women. *Journal of Family Planning and Reproductive Health Care* 32(2):104–106.

Leventhal, T., and J. Brooks-Gunn. 2003. Moving to opportunity: An experimental study of neighborhood effects on mental health. *American Journal of Public Health* 93(9):1576–1582.

Levi, J., S. Vinter, L. Richardson, R. St. Laurent, and L. M. Segal. 2009. *F as in Fat: How Obesity Policies Are Failing in America.* Washington, DC: Robert Wood Johnson Foundation and the Trust for America's Health.

Ley, C., B. Lees, and J. Stevenson. 1992. Sex- and menopause-associated changes in body-fat distribution. *American Journal of Clinical Nutrition* 55(5):950–954.

Li, C., E. S. Ford, L. C. McGuire, and A. H. Mokdad. 2007. Increasing trends in waist circumference and abdominal obesity among US adults. *Obesity* 15(1):216–224.

Li, T. Y., J. S. Rana, J. E. Manson, W. C. Willett, M. J. Stampfer, G. A. Colditz, K. M. Rexrode, and F. B. Hu. 2006. Obesity as compared with physical activity in predicting risk of coronary heart disease in women. *Circulation* 113(4):499–506.

Lieberman, M., L. Gauvin, W. M. Bukowski, and D. R. White. 2001. Interpersonal influence and disordered eating behaviors in adolescent girls: The role of peer modeling, social reinforcement, and body-related teasing. *Eating Behaviors* 2(3):215–236.

Lin, C. C., E. Rogot, N. J. Johnson, P. D. Sorlie, and E. Arias. 2003. A further study of life expectancy by socioeconomic factors in the National Longitudinal Mortality Study. *Ethnicity & Disease* 13(2):240–247.

Link, B. G., and J. Phelan. 1995. Social conditions as fundamental causes of disease. *Journal of Health and Social Behavior* Spec. No.:80–94.

Liu, S., J. E. Manson, M. J. Stampfer, K. M. Rexrode, F. B. Hu, E. B. Rimm, and W. C. Willett. 2000. Whole grain consumption and risk of ischemic stroke in women: A prospective study. *Journal of the American Medical Association* 284(12):1534–1540.

Logan, C., S. Holcombe, J. Ryan, J. Manlove, and K. Moore. 2007. *Childhood Sexual Abuse and Teen Pregnancy. A White Paper.* Washington, DC: Child Trends, Inc.

Luborsky, J. L., P. Meyer, M. F. Sowers, E. B. Gold, and N. Santoro. 2003. Premature menopause in a multi-ethnic population study of the menopause transition. *Human Reproduction* 18(1): 199–206.

Macintyre, S. 2000. The social patterning of exercise behaviours: The role of personal and local resources. *British Journal of Sports Medicine* 34(1):6.

Malik, S., S. B. Sorenson, and C. S. Aneshensel. 1997. Community and dating violence among adolescents: Perpetration and victimization. *Journal of Adolescent Health* 21(5):291–302.

Manlove, J., E. Terry-Humen, and E. Ikramullah. 2006. Young teenagers and older sexual partners: Correlates and consequences for males and females. *Perspectives on Sexual and Reproductive Health* 38(4):197–207.

Mann, T., A. J. Tomiyama, E. Westling, A. M. Lew, B. Samuels, and J. Chatman. 2007. Medicare's search for effective obesity treatments: Diets are not the answer. *American Psychologist* 62(3): 220–233.

Manson, J. E., F. B. Hu, J. W. Rich-Edwards, G. A. Colditz, M. J. Stampfer, W. C. Willett, F. E. Speizer, and C. H. Hennekens. 1999. A prospective study of walking as compared with vigorous exercise in the prevention of coronary heart disease in women. *New England Journal of Medicine* 341(9):650–658.

Marcus, B. H., D. M. Williams, P. M. Dubbert, J. F. Sallis, A. C. King, A. K. Yancey, B. A. Franklin, D. Buchner, S. R. Daniels, and R. P. Claytor. 2006. Physical activity intervention studies: What we know and what we need to know: A scientific statement from the American Heart Association Council on Nutrition, Physical Activity, and Metabolism (Subcommittee on Physical Activity); Council on Cardiovascular Disease in the Young; and the Interdisciplinary Working Group on Quality of Care and Outcomes Research. *Circulation* 114(24):2739–2752.

Martinez, M., E. Giovannucci, D. Spiegelman, D. Hunter, W. Willett, and G. Colditz. 1997. Leisure-time physical activity, body size, and colon cancer in women. Nurses' Health Study Research Group. *Journal of the National Cancer Institute* 89(13):948–955.

Maruti, S. S., W. C. Willett, D. Feskanich, B. Rosner, and G. A. Colditz. 2008. A prospective study of age-specific physical activity and premenopausal breast cancer. *Journal of the National Cancer Institute* 100(10):728–737.

McCauley, J., D. E. Kern, K. Kolodner, L. Dill, A. F. Schroeder, H. K. DeChant, J. Ryden, E. B. Bass, and L. R. Derogatis. 1995. The "battering syndrome": Prevalence and clinical characteristics of domestic violence in primary care internal medicine practices. *Annals of Internal Medicine* 123(10):737–746.

McComb, R. J. J., A. Tacon, P. Randolph, and Y. Caldera. 2004. A pilot study to examine the effects of a mindfulness-based stress-reduction and relaxation program on levels of stress hormones, physical functioning, and submaximal exercise responses. *Journal of Alternative and Complementary Medicine* 10(5):819–827.

McEwen, B. S. 2004. Protection and damage from acute and chronic stress: Allostasis and allostatic overload and relevance to the pathophysiology of psychiatric disorders. *Annals of the New York Academy of Sciences* 1032:1–7.

McEwen, B. S., and P. J. Gianaros. 2010. Central role of the brain in stress and adaptation: Links to socioeconomic status, health, and disease. *Annals of the New York Academy of Sciences* 1186:190–222.

McEwen, B. S., and E. Stellar. 1993. Stress and the individual: Mechanisms leading to disease. *Archives of Internal Medicine* 153(18):2093–2101.

McGinnis, J. M., and W. H. Foege. 1993. Actual causes of death in the United States. *Journal of the American Medical Association* 270(18):2207–2212.

McGinnis, J. M., P. Williams-Russo, and J. R. Knickman. 2002. The case for more active policy attention to health promotion. *Health Affairs* 21(2):78–93.

McGlynn, E. A., E. A. Kerr, and S. M. Asch. 1999. New approach to assessing clinical quality of care for women: The QA Tool system. *Women's Health Issues* 9(4):184–192.

McKinley, E. D., J. W. Thompson, J. Briefer-French, L. S. Wilcox, C. S. Weisman, and W. C. Andrews. 2002. Performance indicators in women's health: Incorporating women's health in the health plan employer data and information set (HEDIS). *Women's Health Issues* 12(1):46–58.

McNeely, M. L., K. L. Campbell, B. H. Rowe, T. P. Klassen, J. R. Mackey, and K. S. Courneya. 2006. Effects of exercise on breast cancer patients and survivors: A systematic review and meta-analysis. *Canadian Medical Association Journal* 175(1):34–41.

Mente, A., L. de Koning, H. S. Shannon, and S. S. Anand. 2009. A systematic review of the evidence supporting a causal link between dietary factors and coronary heart disease. *Archives of Internal Medicine* 169(7):659–669.

Miller, E., M. R. Decker, R. Elizabeth, A. Raj, J. E. Hathaway, and J. G. Silverman. 2007a. Male partner pregnancy-promoting behaviors and adolescent partner violence: Findings from a qualitative study with adolescent females. *Ambulatory Pediatrics* 7(5):360–366.

Miller, E., M. R. Decker, J. G. Silverman, and A. Raj. 2007b. Migration, sexual exploitation, and women's health. *Violence Against Women* 13(5):486–497.

Mokdad, A. H., M. K. Serdula, W. H. Dietz, B. A. Bowman, J. S. Marks, and J. P. Koplan. 1999. The spread of the obesity epidemic in the United States, 1991–1998. *Journal of the American Medical Association* 282(16):1519–1522.

Molyneux, M. 2006. Mothers at the service of the new poverty agenda: Progresa/Oportunidades, Mexico's conditional transfer programme. *Social Policy & Administration* 40(4):425–449.

Moore, L. V., and A. V. Diez Roux. 2006. Associations of neighborhood characteristics with the location and type of food stores. *American Journal of Public Health* 96(2):325–331.

Morales, L. S., M. Lara, R. S. Kington, R. O. Valdez, and J. J. Escarce. 2002. Socioeconomic, cultural, and behavioral factors affecting Hispanic health outcomes. *Journal of Health Care for the Poor and Underserved* 13(4):477–503.

Moreau, K. L., R. Degarmo, J. Langley, C. McMahon, E. T. Howley, D. R. J. Bassett, and D. L. Thompson. 2001. Increasing daily walking lowers blood pressure in postmenopausal women. *Medicine & Science in Sports & Exercise* 33(11):1825–1831.

Morland, K., S. Wing, and A. Diez Roux. 2002. The contextual effect of the local food environment on residents' diets: The atherosclerosis risk in communities study. *American Journal of Public Health* 92(11):1761–1767.

Mottola, M. F., and M. K. Campbell. 2003. Activity patterns during pregnancy. *Applied Physiology, Nutrition, and Metabolism* 28(4):642–653.

Mudd, L. M., S. Nechuta, J. M. Pivarnik, and N. Paneth. 2009. Factors associated with women's perceptions of physical activity safety during pregnancy. *Preventive Medicine* 49(2-3):194–199.

Murdey, I. D., N. Cameron, S. J. H. Biddle, S. J. Marshall, and T. Gorely. 2004. Pubertal development and sedentary behaviour during adolescence. *Annals of Human Biology* 31(1):75–86.

Mytton, J. A., C. DiGuiseppi, D. A. Gough, R. S. Taylor, and S. Logan. 2002. School-based violence prevention programs: Systematic review of secondary prevention trials. *Archives of Pediatrics & Adolescent Medicine* 156(8):752–762.

Nasim, A., R. Corona, F. Belgrave, S. O. Utsey, and N. Fallah. 2007. Cultural orientation as a protective factor against tobacco and marijuana smoking for African American young women. *Journal of Youth and Adolescence* 36(4):503–516.

The National Campaign to Prevent Teen Pregnancy. 2010. *Resources—Race/Ethnicity.* http://www.thenationalcampaign.org/resources/race_ethnicity.aspx (accessed May 2, 2010).

NCI (National Cancer Institute). 2008. *The Role of the Media in Promoting and Reducing Tobacco Use.* http://cancercontrol.cancer.gov/tcrb/monographs/19/docs/M19MajorConclusionsFactSheet.pdf (accessed September 10, 2009).

NCQA (National Committee for Quality Assurance). 2010. *HEDIS 2010 Measures.* http://www.ncqa.org/tabid/59/Default.aspx (accessed March 23, 2010).

Neumark-Sztainer, D. 2005. Preventing the broad spectrum of weight-related problems: Working with parents to help teens achieve a healthy weight and a positive body image. *Journal of Nutrition Education and Behavior* 37 (Suppl. 2):S133–S140.

Neumark-Sztainer, D., M. Story, M. D. Resnick, and R. W. Blum. 1998. Lessons learned about adolescent nutrition from the Minnesota Adolescent Health Survey. *Journal of the American Dietetic Association* 98(12):1449–1456.

NIAAA (National Institute on Alcohol Abuse and Alcoholism). 2008. *Alcohol: A Women's Health Issue.* http://pubs.niaaa.nih.gov/publications/brochurewomen/women.htm (accessed September 10, 2009).

NIAMS (National Institute of Arthritis, Musculoskeletal and Skin Diseases). 2009. *Osteoporosis: Peak Bone Mass in Women.* http://www.niams.nih.gov/Health_Info/Bone/Osteoporosis/bone_mass.asp (accessed August 5, 2009).

Nicholson, H. J., and L. T. Postrado. 1991. *Girls Incorporated Preventing Adolescent Pregnancy: A Program Development and Research Project.* New York: Girls Incorporated.

Ning, Y., M. A. Williams, J. C. Dempsey, T. K. Sorensen, I. O. Frederick, and D. A. Luthy. 2003. Correlates of recreational physical activity in early pregnancy. *Journal of Maternal-Fetal and Neonatal Medicine* 13(6):385–393.

NRC (National Research Council). 2005. *Does the Built Environment Influence Physical Activity? Examining the Evidence.* Transportation Research Board, Institute of Medicine of the National Academies. Washington, DC: The National Academies Press.

O'Donnell, D. A., M. E. Schwab-Stone, and A. Z. Muyeed. 2002. Multidimensional resilience in urban children exposed to community violence. *Child Development* 73(4):1265–1282.

O'Donnell, L., G. Agronick, R. Duran, U. A. Myint, and A. Stueve. 2009. Intimate partner violence among economically disadvantaged young adult women: Associations with adolescent risk-taking and pregnancy experiences. *Perspectives on Sexual and Reproductive Health* 41(2):84–91.

Ogden, C. L., M. D. Carroll, L. R. Curtin, M. A. McDowell, C. J. Tabak, and K. M. Flegal. 2006. Prevalence of overweight and obesity in the United States, 1999–2004. *Journal of the American Medical Association* 295(13):1549–1555.

Oguma, Y., and T. Shinoda-Tagawa. 2004. Physical activity decreases cardiovascular disease risk in women: Review and meta-analysis. *American Journal of Preventive Medicine* 26(5):407–418.

Oken, E., Y. Ning, S. L. Rifas-Shiman, J. S. Radesky, J. W. Rich-Edwards, and M. W. Gillman. 2006. Associations of physical activity and inactivity before and during pregnancy with glucose tolerance. *Obstetrics and Gynecology* 108(5):1200–1207.

Orr, D. P., C. D. Langefeld, B. P. Katz, and V. A. Caine. 1996. Behavioral intervention to increase condom use among high-risk female adolescents. *Journal of Pediatrics* 128(2):288–295.

Owen, N., N. Humpel, E. Leslie, A. Bauman, and J. F. Sallis. 2004. Understanding environmental influences on walking: Review and research agenda. *American Journal of Preventive Medicine* 27(1):67–76.

Ozer, E. J., and R. S. Weinstein. 2004. Urban adolescents' exposure to community violence: The role of support, school safety, and social constraints in a school-based sample of boys and girls. *Journal of Clinical Child & Adolescent Psychology* 33(3):463–476.

Page, J. B. 2005. The concept of culture: A core issue in health disparities. *Journal of Urban Health* 82(2 Suppl. 3):35–43.

Pallitto, C. C., J. C. Campbell, and P. O'Campo. 2005. Is intimate partner violence associated with unintended pregnancy? A review of the literature. *Trauma, Violence & Abuse* 6(3):217–235.

Pan, L., D. Galuska, B. Sherry, A. Hunter, G. Rutledge, W. Dietz, and L. Balluz. 2009. Differences in prevalence of obesity among black, white, and Hispanic adults—United States, 2006–2008. *Morbidity and Mortality Weekly Report* 58(27):740–744.

Pate, R. R., D. S. Ward, R. P. Saunders, G. Felton, R. K. Dishman, and M. Dowda. 2005. Promotion of physical activity among high-school girls: A randomized controlled trial. *American Journal of Public Health* 95(9):1582–1587.

Patrick, H., and T. A. Nicklas. 2005. A review of family and social determinants of children's eating patterns and diet quality. *Journal of the American College of Nutrition* 24(2):83–92.

Patrick, K., G. J. Norman, K. J. Calfas, J. F. Sallis, M. F. Zabinski, J. Rupp, and J. Cella. 2004. Diet, physical activity, and sedentary behaviors as risk factors for overweight in adolescence. *Archives of Pediatrics & Adolescent Medicine* 158(4):385–390.

Perez-Escamilla, R., and P. Putnik. 2007. The role of acculturation in nutrition, lifestyle, and incidence of type 2 diabetes among Latinos. *Journal of Nutrition* 137(4):860–870.

Perez-Stable, E. J., A. Nápoles-Springer, and J. M. Miramontes. 1997. The effects of ethnicity and language on medical outcomes of patients with hypertension or diabetes. *Medical Care* 35(12): 1212–1219.

Phelan, S. T. 2009. Obesity in minority women: Calories, commerce, and culture. *Obstetrics and Gynecology Clinics of North America* 36(2):379–392.

Phipps, S. A., and P. S. Burton. 1998. What's mine is yours? The influence of male and female incomes on patterns of household expenditure. *Economica* 65(260):599–613.

Pierce, J. P., M. L. Stefanick, S. W. Flatt, L. Natarajan, B. Sternfeld, L. Madlensky, W. K. Al-Delaimy, C. A. Thomson, S. Kealey, R. Hajek, B. A. Parker, V. A. Newman, B. Caan, and C. L. Rock. 2007. Greater survival after breast cancer in physically active women with high vegetable-fruit intake regardless of obesity. *Journal of Clinical Oncology* 25(17):2345–2351.

Pirkle, J. L., R. B. Kaufmann, D. J. Brody, T. Hickman, E. W. Gunter, and D. C. Paschal. 1998. Exposure of the US population to lead, 1991–1994. *Environmental Health Perspectives* 106(11): 745–750.

Pollitz, K., M. Kofman, A. Salganicoff, and U. Ranji. 2007. *Maternity Care and Consumer-Driven Health Plans.* Menlo Park, CA: Kaiser Family Foundation.

Poudevigne, M. S., and P. J. O'Connor. 2006. A review of physical activity patterns in pregnant women and their relationship to psychological health. *Sports Medicine* 36(1):19–38.

Prentice, R. L., and G. L. Anderson. 2008. The Women's Health Initiative: Lessons learned. *Annual Review of Public Health* 29:131–150.

Pulerwitz, J., S. Gortmaker, and W. DeJong. 2000. Measuring sexual relationship power in HIV/STD research. *Sex Roles* 42(7):637–660.

Pulerwitz, J., H. Amaro, W. De Jong, S. L. Gortmaker, and R. Rudd. 2002. Relationship power, condom use and HIV risk among women in the USA. *AIDS Care* 14(6):789–800.

Ranji, U. R., R. Wyn, A. Salganicoff, and H. Yu. 2007. Role of health insurance coverage in women's access to prescription medicines. *Women's Health Issues* 17(6):360–366.

Rasmussen, M., R. Krølner, K. I. Klepp, L. Lytle, J. Brug, E. Bere, and P. Due. 2006. Determinants of fruit and vegetable consumption among chidlren and adolescents: A review of the literature. Part 1: Quantitative studies. *International Journal of Behavioral Nutrition and Physical Activity* 3(22).

Rehle, T., S. Lazzari, G. Dallabetta, and E. Asamoah-Odei. 2004. Second-generation HIV surveillance: Better data for decision-making. *Bulletin of the World Health Organization* 82:121–127.

Reichert, V. C., V. Seltzer, L. S. Efferen, and N. Kohn. 2004. Women and tobacco dependence. *Medical Clinics of North America* 88(6):1467–1481.

Rejeski, W. J., A. Thompson, P. H. Brubaker, and H. S. Miller. 1992. Acute exercise: Buffering psychosocial stress responses in women. *Health Psychology* 11(6):355–362.

Reynoso, J., A. Susabda, and A. Cepida-Benito. 2005. Gender differences in smoking cessation. *Journal of Psychopathology and Behavioral Assessment* 27(3):227–234.

Rice, T., and K. Y. Matsuoka. 2004. Book review: The impact of cost-sharing on appropriate utilization and health status: A review of the literature on seniors. *Medical Care Research and Review* 61(4):415–452.

Robert, S. A., and L. W. Li. 2001. Age variation in the relationship between community socioeconomic status and adult health. *Research on Aging* 23(2):234–259.

Rolls, B. J., J. A. Ello-Martin, and B. C. Tohill. 2004. What can intervention studies tell us about the relationship between fruit and vegetable consumption and weight management? *Nutrition Reviews* 62(1):1–17.

Roye, C., P. P. Silverman, and B. Krauss. 2007. A brief, low-cost, theory-based intervention to promote dual method use by black and Latina female adolescents: A randomized clinical trial. *Health Education & Behavior* 34(4):608–621.

Ruderman, M. N., P. J. Ohlott, K. Panzer, and S. N. King. 2002. Benefits of multiple roles for managerial women. *Academy of Management Journal* 45(2):369–386.

Russo, I. H. 2002. Cigarette smoking and risk of breast cancer in women. *Lancet* 360(9339): 1033–1034.

Rustgi, S. D., M. M. Doty, and S. R. Collins. 2009. *Women at Risk: Why Many Women Are Forgoing Needed Health Care.* New York: Commonwealth Fund.

RWJF (Robert Wood Johnson Foundation). 2002. From coverage to care: Exploring links between health insurance, a usual source of care and access. In *Synthesis Project Report.* Washington, DC: Robert Wood Johnson Foundation. http://www.rwjf.org/publications/synthesis/reports%5Fand%5Fbriefs/pdf/no1%5Fresearchreport.pdf (accessed August 15, 2009).

———. 2009. *Deadly in Pink: Big Tobacco Steps Up Its Targeting of Women and Girls.* http://www.tobaccofreekids.org/deadlyinpink/downloads/deadlyinpink_02172009_media.pdf (accessed August 15, 2009).

Saftlas, A. F., N. Logsden-Sackett, W. Wang, R. Woolson, and M. B. Bracken. 2004. Work, leisure-time physical activity, and risk of preeclampsia and gestational hypertension. *American Journal of Epidemiology* 120(8):758–765.

Sakala, C., and M. P. Corry. 2007. Listening to mothers II reveals maternity care quality chasm. *Journal of Midwifery & Women's Health* 52(3):183–185.

Saksvig, B. I., J. Gittelsohn, S. B. Harris, A. J. G. Hanley, T. W. Valente, and B. Zinman. 2005. A pilot school-based healthy eating and physical activity intervention improves diet, food knowledge, and self-efficacy for native Canadian children. *Journal of Nutrition* 135(10):2392–2398.

Salganicoff, A., U. R. Ranji, and R. Wyn. 2005. *Women and Health Care: A National Profile. Key Findings from the Kaiser Women's Health Survey.* Menlo Park, CA: Kaiser Family Foundation.

Salganicoff, A., J. Cubanski, U. Ranji, and T. Neuman. 2009. Health coverage and expenses: Impact on older women's economic well-being. *Journal of Women, Politics & Policy* 30(2):222–247.

Sallis, J. F., and K. Glanz. 2009. Physical activity and food environments: Solutions to the obesity epidemic. *Milbank Quarterly* 87(1):123–154.

Sallis, J. F., J. J. Prochaska, and W. C. Taylor. 2000. A review of correlates of physical activity of children and adolescents. *Medicine & Science in Sports & Exercise* 32(5):963–975.

Salmeron, J., J. E. Manson, M. J. Stampfer, G. A. Colditz, A. L. Wing, and W. C. Willett. 1997. Dietary fiber, glycemic load, and risk of non–insulin-dependent diabetes mellitus in women. *Journal of the American Medical Association* 277(6):472–477.

Sandlund, E. A., and T. Norlander. 2000. The effects of Tai Chi Chuan relaxation and exercise on stress responses and well-being: An overview of research. *International Journal of Stress Management* 7(2):139–149.

Santelli, J. S., N. D. Brener, R. Lowry, A. Bhatt, and L. S. Zabin. 1998. Multiple sexual partners among US adolescents and young adults. *Family Planning Perspectives* 30(6):271–275.

Santiago, C. D., M. E. Wadsworth, and J. Stump. 2009. Socioeconomic status, neighborhood disadvantage, and poverty-related stress: Prospective effects on psychological syndromes among diverse low-income families. *Journal of Economic Psychology*, In Press, Corrected Proof.

Schmidt, M. D., P. Pekow, P. S. Freedson, G. Markenson, and L. Chasan-Taber. 2006. Physical activity patterns during pregnancy in a diverse population of women. *Journal of Women's Health* 15(8):909–919.

Schnoll, R. A., F. Patterson, and C. Lerman. 2007. Treating tobacco dependence in women. *Journal of Women's Health* 16(8):1211–1218.

Scholes, D., C. M. McBride, L. Grothaus, D. Civic, L. E. Ichikawa, L. J. Fish, and K. S. H. Yarnall. 2003. A tailored minimal self-help intervention to promote condom use in young women: Results from a randomized trial. *AIDS* 17(10):1547–1556.

Schwab-Stone, M. E., and T. S. Ayers. 1995. No safe haven: A study of violence exposure in an urban community. *Journal of the American Academy of Child & Adolescent Psychiatry* 34(10):1343.

Seeman, T., E. Epel, T. Gruenewald, A. S. Karlamangla, and B. S. McEwen. 2009. Socio-economic differentials in peripheral biology: Cumulative allostatic load. *Annals of the New York Academy of Sciences* 1186:223–239.

Shearer, C. L., S. J. Hosterman, M. M. Gillen, and E. S. Lefkowitz. 2005. Are traditional gender role attitudes associated with risky sexual behavior and condom-related beliefs? *Sex Roles* 52(5-6):311–324.

Shrier, L. A., R. Ancheta, E. Goodman, V. M. Chiou, M. R. Lyden, and S. J. Emans. 2001. Randomized controlled trial of a safer sex intervention for high-risk adolescent girls. *Archives of Pediatrics & Adolescent Medicine* 155(1):73–79.

Silagy, C., T. Lancaster, L. Stead, D. Mant, and G. Fowler. 2004. Nicotine replacement therapy for smoking cessation. *Cochrane Database of Systematic Reviews* 3:CD000146.

Silverman, J. G., A. Raj, and K. Clements. 2004. Dating violence and associated sexual risk and pregnancy among adolescent girls in the United States. *Pediatrics* 114(2):e220–e225.

Silverman, J. G., J. Gupta, M. R. Decker, N. Kapur, and A. Raj. 2007. Intimate partner violence and unwanted pregnancy, miscarriage, induced abortion, and stillbirth among a national sample of Bangladeshi women. *BJOG: An International Journal of Obstetrics & Gynaecology* 114(10):1246–1252.

Smith, J. P. 2004. Unraveling the SES: Health connection. *Population and Development Review* 30(Suppl. Aging, Health, and Public Policy):108–132.

Sorensen, T. K., M. A. Williams, I. M. Lee, E. E. Dashow, and M. L. Thompson. 2003. Recreational physical activity during pregnancy and risk of preeclampsia. *Hypertension Journal of the American Heart Association* 41:1273–1280.

Speca, M., L. E. Carlson, E. Goodey, and M. Angen. 2000. A randomized, wait-list controlled clinical trial: The effect of a mindfulness meditation-based stress reduction program on mood and symptoms of stress in cancer outpatients. *Psychosomatic Medicine* 62(5):613–622.

Spence, J. C., and R. E. Lee. 2003. Toward a comprehensive model of physical activity. *Psychology of Sport and Exercise* 4:7–24.

Stampfer, M. J., F. B. Hu, J. E. Manson, E. B. Rimm, and W. C. Willett. 2000. Primary prevention of coronary heart disease in women through diet and lifestyle. *New England Journal of Medicine* 343(1):16–22.

Stefanick, M. L., S. Mackey, M. Sheehan, N. Ellsworth, W. L. Haskell, and P. D. Wood. 1998. Effects of diet and exercise in men and postmenopausal women with low levels of HDL cholesterol and high levels of LDL cholesterol. *New England Journal of Medicine* 339(1):12–20.

Steptoe, A., L. Perkins-Porras, C. McKay, E. Rink, S. Hilton, and F. P. Cappuccio. 2003. Psychological factors associated with fruit and vegetable intake and with biomarkers in adults from a low-income neighborhood. *Health Psychology* 22(2):148–155.

Stern, M., and S. Haffner. 1986. Body fat distribution and hyperinsulinemia as risk factors for diabetes and cardiovascular disease. *Arteriosclerosis, Thrombosis, and Vascular Biology* 6(2):123–130.

Sternfeld, B., B. E. Ainsworth, and C. P. Quesenberry. 1999. Physical activity patterns in a diverse population of women. *Preventive Medicine* 28(3):313–323.

Sternfeld, B., J. Cauley, S. Harlow, G. Liu, and M. Lee. 2000. Assessment of physical activity with a single global question in a large, multiethnic sample of midlife women. *American Journal of Epidemiology* 152(7):678–687.

Stevens, J., J. Cai, K. R. Evenson, and R. Thomas. 2002. Fitness and fatness as predictors of mortality from all causes and from cardiovascular disease in men and women in the lipid research clinics study. *American Journal of Epidemiology* 156(9):832–841.

Sturm, R. 2003. Increases in clinically severe obesity in the United States, 1986–2000. *Archives of Internal Medicine* 163(18):2146–2148.

Suarez, L. M., A. J. Polo, C. N. Chen, and M. Alegria. 2009. Prevalence and correlates of childhood-onset anxiety disorders among Latinos and non-Latino whites in the United States. *Psicología Conductual* 17(1):89–109.

Taber-Chasan, L., P. S. Freedson, D. E. Roberts, M. D. Schmidt, and M. S. Fragala. 2007. Energy expenditure of selected household activities during pregnancy. *Research Quarterly for Exercise and Sport* 78(2):133–137.

Takeuchi, D. T., M. Alegría, J. S. Jackson, and D. R. Williams. 2007a. Immigration and mental health: Diverse findings in Asian, black, and Latino populations. *American Journal of Public Health* 97(1):11–12.

Takeuchi, D. T., N. Zane, H. Seunghye, D. H. Chae, G. Fang, G. C. Gee, E. Walton, S. Sue, and M. Alegría. 2007b. Immigration-related factors and mental disorders among Asian Americans. *American Journal of Public Health* 97(1):84–90.

Taylor, A. K., S. Larson, and R. Correa-de-Araujo. 2006. Women's health care utilization and expenditures. *Women's Health Issues* 16(2):66–79.

Taylor, S. E. 1990. Health psychology: The science and the field. *American Psychologist* 45(1):40–50.

Taylor, S. E., L. C. Klein, B. P. Lewis, T. L. Gruenewald, R. A. R. Gurung, and J. A. Updegraff. 2000. Biobehavioral responses to stress in females: Tend-and-befriend, not fight-or-flight. *Psychological Review* 107(3):411–429.

Terry, P. D., and T. E. Rohan. 2002. Cigarette smoking and the risk of breast cancer in women. *Cancer Epidemiology Biomarkers & Prevention* 11(10):953–971.

Theorell, T. 2000. The impact of job loss and retirement on health. In *Social Epidemiology*, edited by L. F. Berkman and I. Kawachi. New York: Oxford University Press.

Thorner, E. D., M. Jaszyna-Gasior, D. H. Epstein, and E. T. Moolchan. 2007. Progression to daily smoking: Is there a gender difference among cessation treatment seekers? *Substance Use & Misuse* 42(5):829–835.

Tjaden, P. G., and N. Thoennes. 1998. *Prevalence, Incidence, and Consequences of Violence Against Women: Findings from the National Violence Against Women Survey, Research in Brief.* Washington, DC: US Department of Justice, Office of Justice Programs, National Institute of Justice.

Tjaden, P., and N. Thoennes. 2000. *Full Report of the Prevalence, Incidence and Consequences of Violence Against Women: Research Report.* Washington, DC: US Department of Justice, Office of Justice Programs, National Institute of Justice.

Trenholm, C., B. Devaney, K. Fortson, L. Quay, J. Wheeler, and M. Clark. 2007. *Impacts of Four Title V, Section 510 Abstinence Education Programs.* Princeton, NJ: Mathematica Policy Research, Inc.

Trivedi, A., W. Rakowski, and J. Ayanian. 2008. Effect of cost sharing on screening mammography in Medicare health plans. *New England Journal of Medicine* 358(4):375.

Trost, S. G., N. Owen, A. E. Bauman, J. F. Sallis, and W. Brown. 2002. Correlates of adults' participation in physical activity: Review and update. *Medicine & Science in Sports & Exercise* 34(12):1996–2001.

United Nations. 1993. *Declaration on the Elimination of Violence Against Women.* New York: United Nations Department of Public Information.

US Department of State. 2009. *Trafficking in Persons Report.* Ft. Belvoir, VA: Defense Technical Information Center.

Valdez, A., J. Mikow, and A. Cepeda. 2006. The role of stress, family coping, ethnic identity, and mother-daughter relationships on substance use among gang-affiliated Hispanic females. *Journal of Social Work Practice in the Addictions* 6(4):31–54.

Vega, W. A., B. Kolody, S. Aguilar-Gaxiola, E. Alderete, R. Catalano, and J. Caraveo-Anduaga. 1998. Lifetime prevalence of DSM-III-R psychiatric disorders among urban and rural Mexican Americans in California. *Archives of General Psychiatry* 55(9):771–778.

Vitaliano, P. P., J. M. Scanlan, J. Zhang, M. V. Savage, and I. B. Hirsch. 2002. A path model of chronic stress, the metabolic syndrome, and coronary heart disease. *Psychosomatic Medicine* 64(3):418–435.

Walker, S. P., E. B. Rimm, A. Ascherio, I. Kawachi, M. J. Stampfer, and W. C. Willett. 1996. Body size and fat distribution as predictors of stroke among US men. *American Journal of Epidemiology* 144(12):1143–1150.

Wang, M. C., S. Kim, A. A. Gonzalez, K. E. MacLeod, and M. A. Winkleby. 2007. Socioeconomic and food-related physical characteristics of the neighbourhood environment are associated with body mass index. *Journal of Epidemiology and Community Health* 61(6):491–498.

Wang, Y., E. B. Rimm, M. J. Stampfer, W. C. Willett, and F. B. Hu. 2005. Comparison of abdominal adiposity and overall obesity in predicting risk of type 2 diabetes among men. *American Journal of Clinical Nutrition* 81(3):555–563.

Wardle, J., A. M. Haase, A. Steptoe, M. Nillapun, K. Jonwutiwes, and F. Bellise. 2004. Gender differences in food choice: The contribution of health belief and dieting. *Annals of Behavioral Medicine* 27(2):107–116.

Wasserman, M. R., D. E. Bender, S. Y. Lee, J. P. Morrisey, T. Mouw, and E. C. Norton. 2006. Social support among Latina immigrant women: Bridge persons as mediators of cervical cancer screening. *Journal of Immigrant and Minority Health* 8(1):67–84.

Watson, M., M. Saraiya, F. Ahmed, C. J. Cardinez, M. E. Reichman, H. K. Weir, and T. B. Richards. 2008. Using population-based cancer registry data to assess the burden of human papillomavirus-associated cancers in the United States: Overview of methods. *Cancer* 113(10 Suppl.):2841–2854.

Weinsier, R. L., G. R. Hunter, A. F. Heini, M. I. Goran, and S. M. Sell. 1998. The etiology of obesity: Relative contribution of metabolic factors, diet, and physical activity. *American Journal of Medicine* 105(2):145–150.

Weinstein, A. R., H. D. Sesso, I. M. Lee, N. R. Cook, J. E. Manson, J. E. Buring, and J. M. Gaziano. 2004. Relationship of physical activity vs body mass index with type 2 diabetes in women. *Journal of the American Medical Association* 292(10):1188–1194.

Weinstein, A. R., H. D. Sesso, I. M. Lee, K. M. Rexrode, N. R. Cook, J. E. Manson, J. E. Buring, and J. M. Gaziano. 2008. The joint effects of physical activity and body mass index on coronary heart disease risk in women. *Archives of Internal Medicine* 168(8):884–890.

Weisman, C. S. 2000. Advocating for gender-specific health care: A historical perspective. *Journal of Gender-Specific Medicine* 3(3):22–24.

Weiss, E., D. Whelan, and G. R. Gupta. 2000. Gender, sexuality and HIV: Making a difference in the lives of young women in developing countries. *Sexual and Relationship Therapy* 15(3): 233–245.

Wessel, T. R., C. B. Arant, M. B. Olson, B. D. Johnson, S. E. Reis, B. L. Sharaf, L. J. Shaw, E. Handberg, G. Sopko, S. F. Kelsey, C. J. Pepine, and C. N. Bairey Merz. 2004. Relationship of physical fitness vs body mass index with coronary artery disease and cardiovascular events in women. *Journal of the American Medical Association* 292(10):1179–1187.

Weuve, J., J. H. Kang, J. E. Manson, M. M. Breteler, J. H. Ware, and F. Grodstein. 2004. Physical activity, including walking, and cognitive function in older women. *Journal of the American Medical Association* 292(12):1454–1461.

Whitaker, R. C., J. A. Wright, M. S. Pepe, K. D. Seidel, and W. H. Dietz. 1997. Predicting obesity in young adulthood from childhood and parental obesity. *New England Journal of Medicine* 337(13):869–873.

WHO (World Health Organization). 2005. *WHO Multi-Country Study on Women's Health and Domestic Violence Against Women: Summary Report: Initial Results on Prevalence, Health Outcomes and Women's Responses.* Geneva, Switzerland: World Health Organization.

Wilcox, A. J. 1999. The quest for better questionnaires. *American Journal of Epidemiology* 150(12): 1261–1262.

Wilcox, S., D. Parra-Medina, M. Thompson-Robinson, and J. Will. 2001. Nutrition and physical activity interventions to reduce cardiovascular disease risk in health care settings: A quantitative review with a focus on women. *Nutrition Reviews* 59(7):197–214.

Williams, D. R. 1999. Race, socioeconomic status, and health. The added effects of racism and discrimination. *Annals of the New York Academy of Sciences* 896:173–188.

Williams, D. R., and C. Collins. 2001. Racial residential segregation: A fundamental cause of racial disparities in health. *Public Health Reports* 116(5):404–416.

Williams, D. R., H. M. Gonzalez, H. Neighbors, R. Nesse, J. M. Abelson, J. Sweetman, and J. S. Jackson. 2007. Prevalence and distribution of major depressive disorder in African Americans, Caribbean blacks, and non-Hispanic whites: Results from the National Survey of American Life. *Archives of General Psychiatry* 64(3):305–315.

Wing, R. R., K. A. Matthews, L. H. Kuller, E. N. Meilahn, and P. Plantinga. 1991. Waist to hip ratio in middle-aged women. Associations with behavioral and psychosocial factors and with changes in cardiovascular risk factors. *Arteriosclerosis, Thrombosis, and Vascular Biology* 11:1250–1257.

Wingood, G. M., and R. J. DiClemente. 1997. The effects of an abusive primary partner on the condom use and sexual negotiation practices of African–American women. *American Journal of Public Health* 87(6):1016–1018.

Wingood, G. M., R. J. DiClemente, K. F. Harrington, M. K. Oh, D. L. Lang, S. L. Davies, E. W. Hook, III, and J. W. Hardin. 2006. Efficacy of an HIV prevention program among female adolescents experiencing gender-based violence. *American Journal of Public Health* 96(6):1085–1090.

Winkleby, M., K. Sundquist, and C. Cubbin. 2007. Inequities in CHD incidence and case fatality by neighborhood deprivation. *American Journal of Preventive Medicine* 32(2):97–106.

Wolff, M. S., G. W. Collman, J. C. Barrett, and J. Huff. 1996. Breast cancer and environmental risk factors: Epidemiological and experimental findings. *Annual Review of Pharmacology and Toxicology* 36:573–596.

Wolin, K. Y., I. M. Lee, G. A. Colditz, R. J. Glynn, C. Fuchs, and E. Giovannucci. 2007. Leisure-time physical activity patterns and risk of colon cancer in women. *International Journal of Cancer* 121(12):2776–2781.

Wu, E., N. El-Bassel, S. S. Witte, L. Gilbert, and M. Chang. 2003. Intimate partner violence and HIV risk among urban minority women in primary health care settings. *AIDS and Behavior* 7(3):291–301.

Xie, B., F. D. Gilliland, Y. F. Li, and H. R. H. Rockett. 2003. Effects of ethnicity, family income, and education on dietary intake among adolescents. *Preventive Medicine* 36(2):30.

Yaffe, K., D. Barnes, M. Nevitt, L. Y. Lui, and K. Covinsky. 2001. A prospective study of physical activity and cognitive decline in elderly women: Women who walk. *Archives of Internal Medicine* 161(14):1703–1708.

Young, H. M., and B. B. Cochrane. 2004. Healthy aging for older women. *Nursing Clinics of North America* 39(1):131–143.

Yusuf, S., S. Hawken, S. Ounpuu, L. Bautista, M. G. Franzosi, P. Commerford, C. C. Lang, Z. Rumboldt, C. L. Onen, L. Lisheng, S. Tanomsup, P. Wangai, Jr., F. Razak, A. M. Sharma, and S. S. Anand. 2005. Obesity and the risk of myocardial infarction in 27,000 participants from 52 countries: A case–control study. *Lancet* 366(9497):1640–1649.

Zaher, C. 2002. When a woman's marital status determined her legal status: A research guide on common law doctrine of coverture. *Law Library Journal* 90(3):459–486.

Zhang, C., C. G. Solomon, J. E. Manson, and F. B. Hu. 2006. A prospective study of pregravid physical activity and sedentary behaviors in relation to the risk for gestational diabetes mellitus. *Archives of Internal Medicine* 166(5):543–548.

3

Research on Conditions with
Particular Relevance to Women

This chapter discusses women's health research of the last 2 decades according to conditions.[1] The committee limits its discussion according to its characterization of women's health in Chapter 1—conditions that are specific to women; that are more common or serious in women; that have distinct causes, manifestations, outcomes, or treatments in women; or that have high morbidity or mortality in women. Appendix B summarizes the incidence, prevalence, and mortality data and trends that, in part, guided committee selections.

Given the impossibility of presenting all research on women's health, the committee first discusses examples of successful research that contributed to progress in women's health. The committee assessed progress on the basis of decreases in incidence or mortality or on the basis of scientific innovations that led to major transformations in approaching a condition. The committee then discusses conditions on which some progress has been made and those on which little progress has been made and about which heightened awareness and further research are needed. Although aware of comorbidities and cross-cutting issues, the committee organized the data for this chapter by condition to reflect of predominant models of research funding and publications.

The committee is aware that the conditions do not include all health conditions that are important to women; a number of conditions that affect many women's quality of life—including arthritis, chronic fatigue syndrome, chronic pain, colorectal cancer, eating disorders, fibromyalgia, incontinence, irritable bowel syndrome, many pregnancy-related issues, melanoma, memory and cognitive changes associated with perimenopause, mental illness other than depression,

---

[1]For brevity, diseases, disorders, and conditions are sometimes referred to here as conditions.

95

migraines, sexual dysfunction, stress-related disorders, thyroid disease, and type 2 diabetes—are not discussed here. Because of the volume of literature available, the committee could not discuss the research on all health conditions important to women and on some conditions there was little research to discuss. Absence of discussion does not indicate that the committee thought it unimportant. The committee highlighted conditions to provide examples of successes and examples of less progress on which overarching conclusions and recommendations can be based.

The diseases on which there has been substantial progress are breast cancer, cardiovascular disease, and cervical cancer. Conditions on which there has been some progress are depression, human immunodeficiency virus/acquired immune deficiency syndrome (HIV/AIDS), and osteoporosis. The committee discusses research on other conditions—unintended pregnancy,[2] maternal mortality and morbidity, autoimmune diseases, alcohol and drug addiction, lung cancer, gynecologic cancers other than cervical cancer, non-malignant gynecological disorders, and dementia of the Alzheimer type (Alzheimer's disease)—on which little progress has been made.

Each condition is discussed with regard to a brief evaluation of advances in research; its relevance to women's health in terms of current incidence, prevalence, and mortality rates and trends therein; disparities in current incidence, prevalence, and mortality rates and trends therein among groups of women (see Box 3-1 for explanation of data on disparities); advances in research, particularly in relation to women's health encompassing research on the understanding of the biology, prevention,[3] and diagnosis of, screening, and treatment for it; research gaps; and lessons learned from the research and extent of progress. When discussing treatments, the committee focuses on conventional treatments and does not discuss complementary and alternative medicine (CAM) in detail. As discussed in a previous Institute of Medicine (IOM) report (2005), women are more likely than men to seek CAM therapies and, therefore, those therapies are important to consider when looking at women's health, from the perspective of potential therapies as well as their potential toxicities and interactions with other medications. The reader is referred to the previous IOM report for further details on CAM research (IOM, 2005).

It is important to note that trends in incidence need to be interpreted in the context of changes in diagnostic criteria and technologies, which can result in the appearance of an increased incidence of a condition (see Box 3-2). This chapter addresses questions 2, 3, and 4 from Box 1-4, whether women's health research is

---

[2]The committee considered whether to discuss unintended pregnancy as a health outcome or a determinant of health. It decided to discuss it as an outcome, along with maternal mortality and morbidity, and discuss the determinants that increase the rate of unintended pregnancies in Chapter 2.

[3]Non-biological determinants of health are mentioned only briefly in this chapter. Details of research on them are discussed in Chapter 2.

BOX 3-1
Data on Disparities

Incidence, prevalence, and trend data across races and ethnicities are presented as available. For some conditions for which there is active surveillance, such as cancer, data are routinely collected and presented by race or ethnicity. For other conditions, data are available from the published literature.

BOX 3-2
Interpretation of Changes in Incidence

In looking at changes in incidence, it is important to consider whether an increase or a decrease in a rate is due to a real trend in occurrence or to a change in diagnostic criteria, sensitivity of diagnostic tests, screening programs, or another external factor that changes the likelihood of finding a case and might make it *appear* that incidence is changing (Devesa et al., 1984). For example, some increases seen in breast-cancer incidence have been attributed to more intensive screening programs increasing the ascertainment of cases and not an increase in the secular trend (Seigneurin et al., 2008).

---

focused on the most appropriate and relevant conditions and end points, whether it is studying the most relevant groups of women, and whether the most appropriate research methods are being used.

CONDITIONS ON WHICH RESEARCH HAS CONTRIBUTED TO MAJOR PROGRESS

Breast Cancer

The committee considered a large and diverse body of scientific research on breast cancer to have contributed to major progress in understanding the basic biology of breast cancer and the identification of specific risk factors, which led to prevention efforts; in improvements in the detection and treatment of breast cancer; and ultimately in a decrease in mortality rates.

Incidence, Prevalence, and Mortality in Women

During the last 2 decades, there has been heavy investment in breast-cancer research owing in part to the lobbying efforts of breast-cancer survivors and advocates (IOM, 2004a). One example is the authorization by Congress of a new funding mechanism for breast-cancer research through the Department of Defense, initially focused on pursuing interservice research on breast-cancer screening and diagnosis for military women and dependents of military men (IOM, 2004a). Increased funding was also made available from the National Cancer Institute, other government agencies (such as the Centers for Disease Control and Prevention [CDC] and the Agency for Healthcare Research and Quality [AHRQ]), and individual statewide programs (such as the California Breast Cancer Research Program, funded with tobacco-tax funds). In parallel, the private philanthropic community—such as the Susan G. Komen Foundation, the Breast Cancer Research Foundation, and Avon—raised awareness and money for research to improve treatment and quality of life of the growing number of breast-cancer survivors.

After remaining relatively steady from 1975 to 1990, the overall invasive–breast-cancer mortality in women in the United States began a steady fall in 1990 and continued to drop each year between 1998 and 2007 (NCI, 2010a). The age-adjusted mortality[4] from invasive breast cancer dropped from 33.1 per 100,000 women in 1990 to 22.8 per 100,000 women in 2007 (NCI, 2010a). A consortium of investigators using 7 statistical models indicated that the portion of the reduction in mortality attributable to improved or increased screening varied from 28 to 65% (median, 46%), and the remainder was attributed to improved adjuvant therapies (Berry et al., 2005). Breast cancer, however, is still the second-leading cause of cancer deaths in women in the United States (ACS, 2009a; CDC, 2010).[5]

Despite many gains from research and regardless of the recent drop in mortality, the incidence of breast cancer in women is higher now than in 1975, and breast cancer is the most common non-skin cancer in women in the United States, estimated to account for about 28% of new cancer cases in 2010 (Jemal et al., 2010). The age-adjusted incidence of breast cancer was as high as 141.2 per 100,000 women in 1998 and 1999, and decreased to 124.7 per 100,000 women in 2007, up from about 100–105 per 100,000 women in 1975–1980 (NCI, 2010b). Much of the increase between 1980 and 1998 occurred during the 1980s and reflected increased detection of localized tumors through increased mammographic screening (Garfinkel et al., 1994; Miller et al., 1991; White et al., 1990). During those years, the incidence increased in every 4-year age group above 45 years. From 1999 to 2003, the age-specific incidence of breast cancer decreased in every age group over 45 years (Jemal et al., 2007). Jemal and colleagues (2007) con-

---

[4]Data are from US Mortality Files, National Center for Health Statistics, Centers for Disease Control and Prevention. Rates are age-adjusted to the 2000 US Standardized Population (19 age groups—Census P25-1130).

[5]Lung cancer is the leading cause of cancer death in women; cardiovascular disease is the leading cause of death overall in women (see Appendix B for data).

cluded that part of the decrease is "consistent with saturation in screening mammography." The large decreases in invasive estrogen-positive breast cancers seen after July 2002 have been attributed to the identification, through the Women's Health Initiative (WHI), of an increased risk of breast cancer associated with the use of menopausal hormone therapy and a precipitous decline in the number of hormone prescriptions filled after the rapid dissemination of that finding to women who were on hormone therapy (Chlebowski et al., 2009; Hausauer et al., 2009; Ravdin et al., 2007). Sharp decreases in breast cancer from 2002 to 2003 were seen in estrogen-positive tumors in women 50–69 years old (Jemal et al., 2007) and, in a study of white women, were largest in urban counties and counties that had low poverty rates (Hausauer et al., 2007).

Disparities Among Groups

Large disparities in breast-cancer incidence and mortality exist among different demographic groups (see Figure 3-1). Breast cancer is one of the few diseases whose incidence is higher in white women than in other ethnic groups; however, black women have higher mortality. Breast-cancer mortality increased in black women from 1975 to 1995—a period when breast cancer mortality in white women decreased (NCI, 2010b). Mortality in black women leveled off and began to decrease in 1995 (see Figure 3-1), but in 2005 mortality in black women (32.8 per 100,000) was still higher than in white women (23.3 per 100,000). The disparity is particularly high in black women under 50 years old (Baquet et al., 2008; DeSantis et al., 2008; Ghafoor et al., 2003; Grann et al., 2006). Both incidence and mortality are lower in Hispanic, Asian and Pacific Islander, and American Indian and Alaskan Native women than in white or black women (Ghafoor et al., 2003). Recently, Kinsey and colleagues (2008) examined breast-cancer mortality in black and white women in 1993–2001 as related to 4 levels of education. Mortality decreased by 1.4% in white women who had less than 12 years of education and by 4.3% in white women who had more than 16 years of education. In black women, a decrease (3.8%) was seen only in women who had more than 16 years of education; this shows an association of both race and education with breast-cancer mortality. American Indian and Alaskan Native women are also more likely to receive a diagnosis of late-stage disease than non-Hispanic white women (Wingo et al., 2008). Research has documented that Ashkenazi Jewish women have a genetic susceptibility to breast cancer (Rubinstein, 2004).

The high case-fatality rate from breast cancer in black women had been hypothesized as being due to differences in biologic factors and in access to timely screening and care (Ademuyiwa and Olopade, 2003; Shavers and Brown, 2002). The Carolina Breast Cancer Study showed that basal-like breast tumors were more prevalent among premenopausal African American women than among postmenopausal African American and non–African American women. That suggests a biologic cause of the excess mortality in young black women and leads

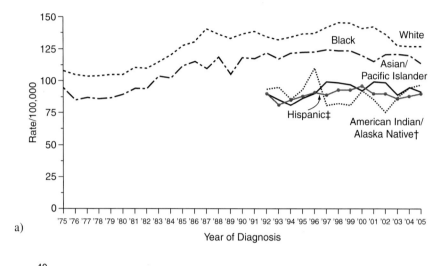

a)

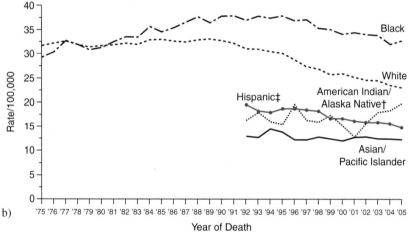

b)

FIGURE 3-1 Annual breast cancer (a) incidence and (b) mortality in the United States by race or ethnicity. Incidence source: Surveillance, Epidemiology, and End Results (SEER) Program, National Cancer Institute (NCI)—1975–1991, SEER 9; 1992–2005, SEER 13. Mortality source: US Mortality Files, National Center for Health Statistics, Centers for Disease Control and Prevention. Rates age-adjusted to the 2000 US standard population (19 age groups—Census P25-1130).

†Rates for American Indians and Alaska Natives based on Contract Health Service Delivery Area counties.

‡Hispanics are not mutually exclusive from whites, blacks, Asians and Pacific Islanders, and American Indians and Alaskan Natives. Incidence data on Hispanics are based on the North American Association of Central Cancer Registries Hispanic Identification Algorithm and exclude cases from the Alaska Native Registry. Mortality data on Hispanics do not include cases from Connecticut, Maine, Maryland, Minnesota, New Hampshire, New York, North Dakota, Oklahoma, and Vermont.

SOURCE: http://www.cdc.gov/cancer/breast/statistics/race.htm (accessed May 3, 2010).

to the option of more aggressive therapies for this patient cohort (see below for discussion of treatment options) (Carey et al., 2006). Issues related to access to screening and care are discussed in Chapter 2; more details on the biology of breast cancer are discussed below.

Research Advances in Knowledge of Biology

Epidemiologic research has identified a variety of factors that are associated with changes in reproductive hormones that are also associated with breast cancer, such as age at first full-term pregnancy, number of full-term pregnancies, breastfeeding, and age at menarche and menopause. Through many types of studies, research has uncovered the role of estrogen in breast-cancer pathogenesis. It is known that estrogen binds to nuclear estrogen receptor α and, with the addition of cofactors, stimulates cell proliferation (Hall and McDonnell, 2005), and it is thus a risk factor for breast cancer. During the last decade, a second estrogen receptor, estrogen receptor β was identified (Kuiper et al., 1996; Mosselman et al., 1996). It is thought that estrogen mediates estrogen–receptor–signaling cross-talk with insulin-like growth-factor receptors to mediate breast-cancer pathogenesis (Clemons and Goss, 2001; Lee et al., 1999).

A family history of breast cancer is also a risk factor for breast cancer, and genetic research has provided an understanding of many of the mechanisms that underlie breast cancer (Hua et al., 2008; Olopade et al., 2008). Mutations in two tumor-suppressor genes—*BRCA1* and *BRCA2*—are associated with breast cancer (Antoniou et al., 2008; Claus et al., 1998; Collins et al., 1995; Easton et al., 1993; Hall et al., 1990; Schubert et al., 1997) and responsible for 5–10% of breast cancers (ACS, 2010a). The germ-line *BRCA1* and *BRCA2* mutations are highly penetrant and greatly increase a person's risk of breast cancer (Easton et al., 1993; Rowell et al., 1994). *BRCA1* breast cancers are typically poorly differentiated, high-grade, infiltrating ductal carcinomas and are usually estrogen-receptor (ER)–negative, progesterone-receptor–negative, and Human Epidermal Receptor type 2 (HER2)/neu–negative (Bordeleau et al., 2010). *BRCA2* breast cancer is characterized by early age of onset, bilaterality, and association with a risk of ovarian cancer (Frank et al., 1998; Krainer et al., 1997). Later research has identified other gene mutations that are associated with an increased risk of breast cancer, including *TP53* (the human gene that encodes P53), *PTEN*, *CASP8*, *FGFR2*, *MAP3K1*, and *LSP1* (see Garcia-Closas and Chanock, 2008, for review). Most of those mutations are low-penetrance variants, and much of the genetic component of breast cancer is not accounted for by known gene mutations.

The understanding of the cellular biology of breast cancer has improved over the past 2 decades, contributing to the development of a number of therapies directed toward interrupting pathways in breast-cancer cells for the prevention and treatment of breast cancer. In particular, the roles of a number of receptors in breast-cancer cells have been identified. Approximately two-thirds of breast cancers express ER. There are two types of estrogen receptors (α and β), but at present only ERα has any known clinical significance. Withdrawal of estrogen (by oophorectomy) was shown to be an effective treatment for breast cancer in the 1890s (Beatson, 1896). Subsequently developed therapies directed toward interrupting the estrogen/ER pathway have been prime tools in treatment and prevention of breast cancer (see below).

HER2, also know as erbB2 and c-neu, is a member of the epidermal growth factor receptor family. Approximately 20–30% of breast cancers have amplified HER2 gene and/or over-express the protein (Cooke et al., 2001; Press et al., 1993; Slamon et al., 1987, 1989; Wolff et al., 2007; Zell et al., 2009). HER2 has been shown to be associated with poorer prognosis in women with newly diagnosed breast cancer, but it is also the target of specifically designed therapeutics directed toward it.

In addition to the ER and HER2 systems, several other important biologic pathways have been identified that have been shown or might serve as therapeutic targets in breast cancer. These include neo-angiogenesis, as mediated by the vascular endothelial growth factor (VEGF). This molecule is the target for bevacizumab, which has activity in the metastatic setting (Miller et al., 2007). Other investigational pathways include, but are not limited to, the insulin-like growth factors (IGFRs), mammalian target of rapamycin (M-TOR), AKT, PI3K, and MEK.

Research Advances in Prevention

Many factors and exposures that are associated with both increasing and decreasing risk of breast cancer can be addressed to help to decrease the incidence of breast cancer, including those presented in Box 3-3.

A major research finding from the WHI was the confirmation of an increased risk of breast cancer associated with the use of conjugated equine estrogen plus progestin (Prempro™) but not with estrogen alone (Premarin™) (Chlebowski et al., 2003; Writing Group for the Women's Health Initiative Investigators, 2002). The dissemination of that finding resulted in a rapid decrease in the use of menopausal hormone therapy (Haas et al., 2004; Hersh et al., 2004) and a later decrease in breast cancer incidence (Krieger et al., 2010; Ravdin et al., 2007). That decline, however, was not seen equally across all socioeconomic, racial, and ethnic groups (Krieger et al., 2010).

Alcohol, even in moderate amounts, can increase the risk of breast cancer[6] (see Suzuki et al., 2008, for meta-analysis), as can poor diet (see Norman et al., 2007, for review), and more specifically, obesity (Brown and Simpson, 2010; Schapira et al., 1994; Vainio and Bianchini, 2002a). Evidence suggests that the common mechanism whereby alcohol and obesity increase the risk of breast can-

---

[6]Both the adverse and beneficial effects of alcohol consumption are discussed further in Chapter 2.

BOX 3-3
Factors Associated with Breast Cancer

Factors Associated with Increased Risk of Breast Cancer
- Hormone therapy
- Ionizing radiation
- Obesity
- Alcohol
- Genetic factors

Factors Associated with Decreased Risk of Breast Cancer
- Exercise
- Early pregnancy
- Breastfeeding

Treatments Associated with Risk of Breast Cancer
- Selective estrogen-receptor modulators
- Aromatase inhibitors or inactivators
- Prophylactic mastectomy

SOURCE: National Cancer Institute. http://www.cancer.gov/cancertopics/pdq/prevention/breast/HealthProfessional (accessed August 3, 2010).

---

cer is an increase in estrogen, which stimulates the proliferation of breast tissue (Brown and Simpson, 2010; Cleary et al., 2010; Ginsburg et al., 1996). The relationship between smoking and breast cancer is not clear. As reviewed by Coyle (2009), although data on deoxyribonucleic acid (DNA) adducts provide biological plausibility for an association between smoking and breast cancer, epidemiology studies have either shown no association or an inverse association. There is some evidence, however, that smoking during a first pregnancy (Innes and Byers, 2001) and secondhand-smoke exposure are associated with an increased risk of breast cancer (Cal EPA, 2005). The research on relevant behavioral factors is discussed in more detail in Chapter 2.

Exposure to ionizing radiation can increase the risk of breast cancer, especially if it occurs before the age of 20 years (Ronckers et al., 2005). Most studies that showed an increased risk of breast cancer in association with exposure to ionizing radiation looked at radiation levels higher than occur in mammography (Nelson et al., 2009a).

However, exercise, early pregnancy, and number of pregnancies predict a decrease in breast cancer, again with some evidence of a role of estrogen in the altered risk (Bernstein, 2008; Britt et al., 2007; Monninkhof et al., 2007; Pines, 2009).

Preventive measures apart from modifying risk factors have been developed for people at high risk for breast cancer. Recommendations for preventive options for breast cancer depend on a person's risk (Guarneri and Conte, 2009; Sparano et al., 2009). In very high-risk people—those who have a germ-line mutation in *BRCA1* or *BRCA2* with lobular carcinoma in situ and a strong family history of breast cancer—prophylactic mastectomy is an option to consider to reduce the risk of breast cancer (Bermejo-Pérez et al., 2007; Kaas et al., 2010; Nusbaum and Isaacs, 2007; Zakaria and Degnim, 2007), as is prophylactic oophorectomy (Metcalfe, 2009; Rebbeck et al., 2009). For people who have a high risk because of family history, chemoprevention is available. During the last 2 decades, 2 large sequential breast-cancer-prevention trials of healthy women at high risk for breast cancer demonstrated that treatment with tamoxifen (a selective estrogen receptor modulator) for 5 years could reduce the risk of invasive breast cancer by at least 50% (Fisher et al., 1998; Veronesi et al., 2007). Tamoxifen also reduced the risk of recurrent breast cancer after treatment in both younger and older women (Cuzick et al., 2003; Lewis, 2007; Schrag et al., 2000). In a study of postmenopausal women with a mean age of 58.5 years, tamoxifen and raloxifene (a selective estrogen receptor modulator approved for prevention of osteoporosis) had similar efficacy in reducing the risk of invasive breast cancer (Vogel et al., 2006). As a result of that research, older women at high risk for breast cancer now have two US Food and Drug Administration (FDA)–approved medications that reduce the risk of breast cancer and of osteoporosis. Side effects, however, contribute to low acceptance and use of tamoxifen (Fallowfield, 2005). In addition, identifying at-risk people can pose a problem.

Research Advances in Diagnosis

A number of diagnostic and screening methods—screen-film mammography, digital mammography, ultrasonography, magnetic resonance imaging (MRI), and biopsy—can identify breast cancer at earlier stages and facilitate early treatment.

The most widely used imaging technology for breast-cancer screening is mammography. Eight randomized trials evaluated the effectiveness of screening mammography in the United States (Shapiro, 1988; Shapiro et al., 1988), Sweden (Andersson and Janzon, 1997; Bjurstam et al., 2003; Frisell and Lidbrink, 1997; Nystrom et al., 2002; Tabar et al., 1995), Canada (Miller et al., 2000, 2002), and the United Kingdom (Alexander et al., 1999). Although criticisms of those trials have been published (Gotzsche and Olsen, 2000; Olsen and Gotzsche, 2001), independent review concluded that there was strong evidence of the effectiveness of mammography for women over 50 years old (Fletcher and Elmore, 2003; Health Council of the Netherlands, 2002; US Preventive Services Task Force, 2002; Vainio and Bianchini, 2002b). According to a meta-analysis that included all the trials, 15-year mortality from breast cancer in women 50–69 years old was decreased by 20–35%, and the reduction was statistically significant; it was reduced in women between 40–49 years old by about 20% (Fletcher and Elmore, 2003). Results of individual trials and another meta-analysis suggest statistically significant reductions of 29–44% in the population 40–49 years old (Andersson and Janzon, 1997; Bjurstam et al., 2003; Hendrick et al., 1997). Some researchers have noted that screening mammography is associated with a high rate of false positives and overdiagnosis (that is, diagnosis of and treatment for some cancers that might not progress and cause morbidity or death) (Esserman et al., 2009). Such overdiagnosis results in patients being subjected to adverse effects of breast-cancer treatments and being labeled as having a "preexisting condition," which can affect insurance coverage[7] and raise emotional issues (Esserman et al., 2009). This points to the need to be able to differentiate between tumors that will progress and metastasize from those that will not. Recently, the US Preventive Services Task Force (2009) recommended "against routine screening mammography in women aged 40 to 49 years." Instead, the task force said the decision to have mammography before the age of 50 years should be an individual choice and take into account individual risks and "the patient's values regarding specific benefits and harms." Those guidelines, however, are very controversial, "have had a polarizing effect in the breast-cancer community," and have led to "confusion, fear, and anger on the part of patients with breast cancer, their families, and women's health advocates" (Partridge and Winer, 2009). The communication of those guidelines is discussed further in Chapter 5.

The technology associated with mammography has improved substantially since the first studies of its efficacy. Major developments included more-sensitive high-resolution image intensifiers and film, low-absorption cassettes, and dedicated film processors, all of which contributed to radiation-dose reductions for women (Price and Butler, 1970). Changes in mammography tubes (for example, the use of molybdenum targets and filters with beryllium windows and smaller focal spots and the use of moving grids) improved image quality (Haus, 1990; Muntz and Logan, 1979).

Digital mammography was developed to overcome the limitations of screen-film mammography, such as difficulty visualizing low-contrast objects against dense backgrounds (Pisano and Yaffe, 2005; Shtern, 1992). Clinical trials (without death as an end point) have demonstrated that its diagnostic accuracy is equivalent to that of film mammography for the general population (Lewin et al., 2002; Pisano et al., 2005; Skaane et al., 2007; Vinnicombe et al., 2009), but that digital mammography has better accuracy than film in premenopausal and perimenopausal women, women who have dense breasts, and women less than 50 years old (Pisano et al., 2005). As of August 2010, 68.5% of accredited US mammography units were digital (FDA, 2010)—up from 36% in January 2008

---

[7]Under the Patient Protection and Affordable Care Act (Public Law 111-148) insurers will be prohibited from denying or charging more because of preexisting illnesses.

(Karellas and Vedantham, 2008)—despite the high relative cost[8] (Tosteson et al., 2008). Individualized screening strategies with such technologies as MRI and ultrasonography are being developed for women who are at high risk for breast cancer (Berg, 2009).

MRI provides three-dimensional images of the breast and outstanding soft-tissue contrast. Nine studies (Hagen et al., 2007; Hartman et al., 2004; Kriege et al., 2006; Kuhl et al., 2005; Leach et al., 2005; Lehman et al., 2005, 2007; Sardanelli et al., 2007; Warner et al., 2004) of women who were at very high risk for breast cancer collectively showed an increase in the detection of tumors by combining mammography and MRI for an overall sensitivity of 92.7% and greater detection of smaller, node-negative tumors (see Berg, 2009, for review; Kriege et al., 2004). Those results and others led the American Cancer Society to issue new guidelines for breast-cancer screening with MRI for women who have a 20% or greater lifetime risk of breast cancer[9] (Saslow et al., 2007). Many women, however, cannot undergo MRI because of claustrophobia, obesity, renal insufficiency, or the presence of metallic implants (Berg, 2009). In addition, the false-positive MRI results that lead to unnecessary biopsy may limit its acceptability (Tillman et al., 2002).

Sonography is more available, better tolerated, and less expensive than is MRI as a supplemental tool to mammography (Berg, 2009). In high-risk women, mammography combined with sonography has a sensitivity of only 52% compared with 92.7% for mammography with MRI (Berg, 2009; Buchberger et al., 2000; Crystal et al., 2003; Gordon and Goldenberg, 1995; Hartman et al., 2004; Kaplan, 2001; Kelly et al., 2009; Kolb et al., 2002; Kuhl et al., 2005; Leconte et al., 2003; Lehman et al., 2005; Sardanelli et al., 2007; Warner et al., 2004). The supplemental breast-cancer detection rate of sonography in several studies has been consistently reported as 2.7–4.6 per 1,000 women screened (see Berg, 2009; Berg et al., 2008). Cancers found with screening sonography were almost always invasive and node-negative and had a median size of 9–11 mm (Buchberger et al., 2000; Corsetti et al., 2008; Crystal et al., 2003; Gordon and Goldenberg, 1995; Kaplan, 2001; Kolb et al., 2002; Leconte et al., 2003).

Newer technologies—such as tomosynthesis (Gur et al., 2009; Niklason et al., 1997; Poplack et al., 2007), digital subtraction mammography (Diekmann

---

[8]The rationale may be that it is not practical for most breast-imaging practices to maintain support for two types of mammography-screening technologies (Berg, 2009), especially in the context of the conversion of the rest of radiology practice from analogue to digital radiography.

[9]The populations included in this recommendation are known *BRCA*-mutation carriers, first-degree relatives of carriers who are untested, and those with a lifetime risk of breast cancer as defined by *BRCA*PRO (Berry et al., 2002) or other models that depend primarily on family history, such as Tyrer-Cuzick and BOADICEA (Antoniou et al., 2008; Tyrer et al., 2004). Other groups identified as eligible for augmented screening in the guidance document are those who have genetic syndromes, such as Li-Fraumeni and Cowden, and their first-degree relatives, and women who have a history of radiation therapy to the chest at the ages of 10–30 years (Saslow et al., 2007).

et al., 2005; Dromain et al., 2006; Jong et al., 2003), dedicated breast computed tomography (Boone et al., 2001, 2006; Yang et al., 2007), positron-emission mammography (Berg et al., 2006), scintimammography (Khalkhali et al., 2000; Liberman et al., 2003), and magnetic resonance spectroscopy (Bartella et al., 2007; Huang et al., 2004; Meisamy et al., 2005)—have not yet been evaluated well enough in a screening setting to warrant their widespread adoption either adjunctively or as replacements for mammography.

It is important to note that all studies of screening with new technologies assess imaging end points, not mortality. The presupposition is that finding more cancers than are found with film mammography (at a less advanced stage) will lead to reduced mortality if implemented on a population-wide basis (Smith et al., 2004). As with other screening methods, there are adverse outcomes associated with false positives and overdiagnosis. In addition to stress and unnecessary biopsies conducted because of false positives, there is evidence that some breast tumors that would not progress to breast cancer are diagnosed as breast cancer through screening programs (Esserman et al., 2009).

Research Advances in Treatment

One of the earliest treatments for breast cancer, surgery with radical mastectomy and complete lymph-node removal, is disfiguring. A randomized clinical trial comparing 5-year survival after mastectomy, lumpectomy (tumor removal only), and lumpectomy with radiation showed that patients who underwent lumpectomy plus radiation had the same survival as those who underwent radical mastectomy (Komaki et al., 1990). Those results gave women options for breast cancer surgery.

Assessing breast-cancer metastases with sentinel lymph-node biopsy (SLNB) began in the middle 1990s, has replaced axillary lymph-node dissection (ALND) for determining the extent of spread of breast cancer, and has shown decreased posttreatment morbidity (Kell and Kerin, 2004; Lyman et al., 2005; Olson et al., 2008; Quan and McCready, 2009; Schrenk et al., 2000). A number of studies have demonstrated that SLNB is as accurate for staging breast cancer and is followed by similar short-term survival alone as in conjunction with ALND (Quan and McCready, 2009); large randomized controlled trials with longer followup are underway to evaluate SLNB further (Quan and McCready, 2009).

Surgery (lumpectomy or mastectomy) remains the primary treatment for breast cancer. Before and after surgery, adjuvant chemotherapy is an important component of breast-cancer treatment (NCI, 2009a). There has been development of many agents and combinations of agents and testing in clinical trials to assess survival and side effects in women who have breast cancer at different stages. The development of effective adjuvant therapies for early-stage breast cancer has greatly improved survival rates.

Several chemotherapeutic agents are available to treat patients with metastatic breast cancer, resulting in substantial palliation and some survival benefits (Chia et al., 2007). More importantly, several trials have demonstrated that using chemotherapy to prevent recurrences in women with early-stage disease has had an enormous impact on mortality (Early Breast Cancer Trialists' Collaborative Group, 2005). Early trials were principally focused on cyclophosphamide, methotrexate and 5-flourouracil (Buzdar et al., 1988). Later studies demonstrated that the addition of the anthracyclines (doxorubicin and epirubicin) and the taxanes (paclitaxel and docetaxel) improve outcomes even further (Early Breast Cancer Trialists' Collaborative Group, 2005; Henderson et al., 2003; Martin et al., 2005).

As mentioned previously, therapies that interrupt the estrogen/ER pathway have been prime tools in treatment and prevention of breast cancer. Of these, the selective ER modulator (SERMs), tamoxifen, has been most influential in much of the decline in breast cancer mortality observed in the Western world over the last 25 years (Osborne, 1998). More recently, complete inhibition of estradiol synthesis in postmenopausal women has been affected by specific aromatase inhibitors (AIs), which are now known to be slightly more effective than tamoxifen in both the metastatic and adjuvant settings (Winer et al., 2005). Tamoxifen, and a similar SERM compound, raloxifene, have both been proven to prevent new ER-positive breast cancers in women at modestly high risk for the disease, and studies are underway to test the worth of AIs in this setting (Fisher et al., 1998; Vogel et al., 2006).

Trastuzumab is a monoclonal antibody that interferes with HER2 and has been shown to reduce mortality in both metastatic and adjuvant settings (Mariani et al., 2009). More recently, studies have demonstrated that a small molecular weight tyrosine kinase inhibitor, lapatinib, has activity in patients with HER2-positive metastatic breast cancer who have progressed on trastuzumab (Di Leo et al., 2008; Geyer et al., 2006). These two agents are now being compared, alone or in combination, in ongoing randomized adjuvant clinical trials.

Increased understanding of the genotypes and phenotypes of different breast cancers has allowed clinicians to individualize treatment in many ways. Studies in the 1970s and 1980s demonstrated that women with ER-positive breast cancer benefit from endocrine treatments, like tamoxifen and, therefore, those treatments should be used in those women (Early Breast Cancer Trialists' Collaborative Group, 2005). In contrast, patients with HER2-negative breast cancers appear to gain little, if any, benefit from trastuzumab or lapatinib (Press et al., 2008; Slamon and Pegram, 2001). More recently, gene or protein expression assays combining ER, HER2, markers of proliferation, and other factors, have been shown to identify women who might forego chemotherapy or for whom chemotherapy might not work (Albain et al., 2010; Fong et al., 2009; van't Veer et al., 2005). More recently, studies of tumors that do not express either ER or HER2 have demonstrated that another pathway, the poly (adenosine diphosphate [ADP]–ribose) polymerase pathway, is involved in DNA repair and, therefore, in tumor survival and in resistance to chemotherapy. In early trials inhibitors of this pathway have been reported to have antitumor activity, and large prospective randomized trials to determine their clinical utility are now underway (Fong et al., 2009).

Genetic research has also helped to move toward personalized medicine for women who have breast cancer. Women with low cytochrome P450 2D6 activity do not effectively metabolize tamoxifen to its active metabolite, and identification of those poor metabolizers helps assess the benefits of tamoxifen in individual breast-cancer patients (Desta et al., 2004; Kiyotani et al., 2010; Rooney et al., 2004). In additional, gene-expression profiles can identify women who will or will not benefit from the use of anthracyclines and other therapies, thus avoiding exposure of women who would not benefit from that toxic class of drugs.

More recently, other agents—such as AIs, which interfere with postmenopausal women's ability to produce the estrogen—have been shown in large-scale clinical trials to be superior to tamoxifen in extending survival in women who have metastatic disease and in preventing recurrence when used as primary adjuvant therapy (Sparano et al., 2009). In addition, treatment with AIs after a full course of tamoxifen continues to improve recurrence-free survival compared with cessation of hormone therapy (Goss et al., 2003; Winer et al., 2005), and they are approved to treat postmenopausal women for breast cancer (Winer et al., 2005).

Another significant advance was discontinuing the use of an ineffective treatment. Before 2000, bone-marrow transplantation was commonly used in combination with high-dose chemotherapy despite the absence of a randomized controlled trial that demonstrated its efficacy. A randomized controlled trial showed that the combined treatment did not improve survival in women who had metastatic breast cancer (Stadtmauer et al., 2000; Weiss, 1999); the finding was confirmed in other studies (Farquhar et al., 2003). The use of bone-marrow transplantation was abandoned in the late 1990s (Welch and Mogielnicki, 2002).

Knowledge Gaps

Scientific research, spurred by demands by and involvement of breast-cancer survivors and advocates, has improved survival of women who receive a diagnosis of breast cancer (IOM, 2006). There are now about 2.5 million women with a history of breast cancer either living disease free or undergoing treatments (ACS, 2010a). Although research has demonstrated that generally these women recover and lead relatively normal lives, some of the survivors may suffer serious sequelae, such as persistent fatigue, cognitive changes, musculoskeletal aches and pains, sexual difficulties, and secondary malignancies. Sequelae arise from the toxicity of therapies, from the psychological and emotional aspects following treatment (for example, mastectomies), and from concerns over recurrence. Leading-edge research is now focused on understanding the biopsychosocial mechanisms that underlie these persistent problems, and new therapies are being developed to help in their management with a goal of improving the survivors' lives (Bower, 2008; IOM, 2006, 2008; Miller et al., 2008). Despite those gains, more than 40,000 US women died in 2009 from breast cancer (see Table B-2). In addition, the gains against breast cancer have not been seen among all demographics groups, and the reasons for the higher mortality in black women needs to be better understood and addressed. The ability to differentiate between tumors that will progress and metastasize from those that will not is needed.

Lessons Learned

Breast cancer is an example of a serious disease for which the risks, and consequences have been decreased through advances in scientific research. Research has led to improved overall prevention, detection, survival of, and treatments for breast cancer, but there is a need to focus research programs on quality-of-life issues as well as mortality. If one looks at the overall progress made in the health of women who have breast cancer and at the research findings, the successes can not be attributed to a single aspect of the research but rather to multi-pronged research, including molecular, cellular, and animal experiments; improving diagnostic techniques; implementation of widespread screening programs; observational studies; and clinical trials. The disparities that remain highlight the need to focus research on groups that have the highest risks and burdens of disease. In addition, the increased risk of breast cancer from the use of hormone therapy (conjugated equine estrogen plus progestin) and the lack of efficacy of bone-marrow transplantation point to the need to conduct clinical research to demonstrate the efficacy and safety of treatments before widespread public use.

Cardiovascular Disease

Cardiovascular disease—considered here as a group that includes heart disease and stroke—has seen major progress in women, as reflected in a decrease in mortality. Despite that progress and all that has been learned over the last 2 decades about cardiovascular disease in general, and about the potential differences in cardiovascular disease between women and men, in the United States cardiovascular disease is still the leading cause of death among women of almost all races and ethnicities,[10] and it is a major contributor to morbidity and a decrease in quality of life in women (AHA, 2009).

---

[10]Heart disease is the leading cause of death in white, black, and Hispanic women. It is the second-leading cause of death in Asian and Pacific Islander and in American Indian and Alaska Native women (see Appendix B).

Incidence, Prevalence, and Mortality in Women

Cardiovascular disease in general used to be thought of more in relation to men than women, and most of the earlier cardiovascular research focused solely on men (AHRQ, 2009), which could be why some women underestimate their risk of cardiovascular disease and overstate their risk of breast cancer (Erblich et al., 2000). Statistics, however, show that cardiovascular disease has been the leading cause of mortality in US women since 1989 (see Appendix B). In 2006, one-third of US women had cardiovascular disease (Lloyd-Jones et al., 2009) and over 3 million women were discharged from short-stay hospitals with their first listed diagnosis as cardiovascular disease (AHA, 2009).

Since 1984, the non–age-adjusted number of deaths in women due to cardiovascular disease has exceeded the number in men; in 2005, nearly 0.5 million women died from cardiovascular disease—52.6% of all people who died from cardiovascular disease (AHA, 2009). Taking age into account, however, shows a different picture. The incidence is lower in women than in men in all age groups, and the prevalence is lower in women than men or the same in women as men between 20–79 years old, but higher in women 80 years old or older (Lloyd-Jones et al., 2009). Although cardiovascular disease in women remains a substantial problem, success can be seen in the recent decreases in mortality from cardiovascular disease. The age-adjusted rate fell by 48.9% in women (from 263.3 to 134.4 per 100,000) and by 50.8% in men (from 542.9 to 266.8 per 100,000) (Ford et al., 2007).

Cardiovascular disease can be classified as coronary heart disease,[11] stroke, and non-ischemic heart disease (for example, mitral valve disease). Coronary heart disease and stroke are discussed here as examples of cardiovascular disease in women. The majority of cardiovascular disease in women is coronary heart disease, most of which is caused by atherosclerotic coronary disease or atherosclerosis. Coronary heart disease can manifest as angina (chest discomfort), ischemic heart disease (reduced blood supply to the heart) or acute myocardial infarction (heart attack). In 2006, about 8 million women in the United States were living with coronary heart disease (Lloyd-Jones et al., 2009). Data from the National Health and Nutrition Examination Survey (NHANES) indicate that the prevalence of acute myocardial infarction in women has increased over the last 2 decades but decreased in men (Towfighi et al., 2009). Of women 40 years old or older who have a recognized myocardial infarction, 23% die within a year compared with 18% of men (Lloyd-Jones et al., 2009). Younger, but not older, women have higher mortality during hospitalization after myocardial infarction than do men of the same age. The younger the patients, the higher is women's mortality relative to men's (Vaccarino et al., 1999).

---

[11]Coronary heart disease is a condition in which there is inadequate circulation of blood to the heart.

Chronic coronary heart disease is a major contributor to heart failure in women. Almost 600,000 women are discharged from short-stay hospitals each year, and 2.5 million women are living with heart failure (AHA, 2009). The number of women living with chronic heart conditions is rising and is expected to continue doing so because of improved acute treatments for coronary heart disease, the aging of the population, and other advances in medical therapies.

Stroke, when considered separately from other cardiovascular conditions, is the third-leading cause of death among women, and about 4 million women survivors are estimated to be alive today (Lloyd-Jones et al., 2009). Each year, about 55,000 more women than men have strokes (Lloyd-Jones et al., 2009). Although it is attributable primarily to women's longer life expectancy (Lloyd-Jones et al., 2009), more women have strokes even when compared with men in the same age group. One study analyzed NHANES data from 1999–2004 and found that self-reported stroke prevalence in women 45–54 years old was double that of men in the same age group (Towfighi et al., 2007).

Disparities Among Groups

With respect to cardiovascular disease as a group, 46.9% of black women 20 years old and older and 34.4% of white women had cardiovascular disease in 2006 (Lloyd-Jones et al., 2009).

Mortality from coronary heart disease was higher in black women than in white women (141 vs 110 per 100,000 age-adjusted population) in 2005. Black women in all age groups had a higher incidence of first heart attacks and overall heart attacks than white women. In 2006, the prevalence of coronary heart disease in women 20 years old or older was 6.9% in white women, 8.8% in black women, and 6.6% in Mexican American women (Lloyd-Jones et al., 2009).[12]

Data from 1998 indicate that the age-adjusted mortality rate from coronary heart disease and specifically from acute myocardial infarction is lower in Hispanic, Asian and Pacific Islander, and American Indian and Alaskan Native women than in either black or white women (CDC, 2001). Like mortality from most other cardiovascular diseases, mortality from stroke is substantially higher in black women than in white women (60.7 vs 44.0 per 100,000 age-adjusted population) (AHA, 2009). Low socioeconomic status is also related to higher mortality. Among women 60 years old or older with cardiovascular disease, those without a high school degree were twice as likely to die from their disease as were high school graduates (Lee et al., 2005). In one study that looked at age-adjusted death rates from cardiovascular disease in both black and white women, death rates are higher in those with less education and in those with less income (Pappas et al., 1993).

---

[12]The prevalence takes into account survivors.

Research Advances in Knowledge of Biology

Research over the last 20 years has demonstrated that women have cardiovascular disease, and determining whether there are sex differences in cardiovascular disease and underlying biologic differences between women and men that could underlie the differences in disease is an active area of research (Rosenfeld, 2006; Shaw et al., 2009). A recent pooled analysis of data from 11 studies of acute coronary syndrome concluded that women have higher 30-day mortality; this may be largely explained by clinical differences on presentation (for example, women are older and have more comorbidities and risk factors than men) and differences in the severity of angiographically documented disease (Berger et al., 2009).

The Women's Ischemia Syndrome Evaluation (WISE) study, sponsored by the National Heart, Lung, and Blood Institute, was conducted to evaluate diagnostic tests for heart disease in women and to determine whether evidence of myocardial ischemia occurs in the absence of obstructive coronary disease in women. Data from WISE highlight the role of microvascular dysfunction, subendocardial ischemia, inflammation, genetic predisposition, and neurohormonal imbalance in imparting risk in women (Bairey Merz et al., 2006; Quyyumi, 2006). Of the 7,603 women with symptoms screened, however, 936 (less than 5%) were enrolled in the study; women with a diagnosis of coronary artery disease on angiography and women with a previous coronary event (i.e., myocardial infarction, stroke, or revascularization) were excluded (Gulati et al., 2009). The WISE study only included females so sex-differences cannot be directly assessed. Differences in responses to ischemia are seen at the cellular level; different pathways trigger programmed cell death after ischemia in male and female rats and mice from birth (Bae and Zhang, 2005; Elsasser et al., 2000; Lang and McCullough, 2008; Vannucci et al., 2001). The clinical implications of those findings in humans and animals are unknown.

Research Advances in Prevention

Two-thirds of women who die suddenly from coronary heart disease had no previous symptoms (compared with half of men) (AHA, 2009). That suggests that primary prevention must be a key strategy to reduce the burden of coronary heart disease in women.

Smoking is the leading cause of cardiovascular disease, and the risk decreases quickly on smoking cessation. Hormone therapy (estrogen alone and estrogen plus progestin), as well as the selective estrogen-receptor modulators tamoxifen and raloxifene have been shown in a number of studies—the WHI, the Raloxifene Use for the Heart (RUTH) trial, and the Study of Tamoxifen and Raloxifene (STAR) trial—to increase the risk of stroke or fatal stroke in women (Nelson et al., 2009b; Stefanick, 2006; Writing Group for the Women's Health Initiative Investigators, 2002). On the basis of the findings of the WHI, which was designed to study the use of menopausal hormone therapy for primary prevention of cardiovascular disease, menopausal hormone therapy is not recommended to prevent cardiovascular disease (Wassertheil-Smoller et al., 2003; Writing Group for the Women's Health Initiative Investigators, 2002). Behavioral factors (for example, smoking, eating habits, physical activity) that affect the risk of cardiovascular disease are discussed in Chapter 2.

An important sex difference in the prevention of stroke is the use of aspirin. Aspirin has been shown to prevent ischemic strokes in women (primarily among those over age 65) but not in men (Bailey et al., 2010; Ridker et al., 2005). The risk of hemorraghic stroke and gastrointestinal bleeding, however, may be increased by aspirin use, and because women often have uncontrolled blood pressure and stroke as they age, stroke and bleeding are particularly important health issues for older women (Bailey et al., 2010; Ridker et al., 2005). National guidelines recommend that those risks be weighed against the benefits of aspirin, and that age be taken into account in decisions about aspirin chemoprevention (Mosca et al., 2007).

In an early clinical trial, statins (3-hydroxy-3-methyl-glutaryl coenzyme A reductase inhibitors) were shown to be effective in lowering cholesterol in a Scottish trial in men (Shepherd et al., 1995). The absence of women in that and other statin trials led to questions about extrapolating the data to women and thus a delay in their use in women, even those who had previously had a coronary event. A meta-analysis of data from those trials later demonstrated the efficacy of statins in women (LaRosa et al., 1999). A large-scale trial (JUPITER) showed that primary prevention benefits from statins are similar in women 60 years old or older and men 50 years old or older (Mora et al., 2010), however, the number needed to treat (that is, the number of patients who would have to be treated to prevent a single outcome event) and side effects might be higher in women than men (Ridker et al., 2009). A 2009 meta-analysis showed benefits of statin therapy in both women and men at risk for cardiovascular disease (Brugts et al., 2009), and a meta-analysis of trials (not specifically in women) comparing early statin therapy after acute coronary syndrome with placebo or usual care at 1 and 4 months following showed no reduction in deaths, myocardial infarction, or stroke with statin therapy (Briel et al., 2006). A prospective cohort study showed an increased risk of cataracts, kidney failure, and liver dysfunction in both men and women with statin treatment (Hippisley-Cox and Coupland, 2010). Further research is needed to define the risk–benefit ratio of statins for primary prevention in diverse populations of women with varying risks of cardiovascular disease.

Patient, physician, health-system, and societal factors can all contribute to gender and racial disparities in cardiovascular-disease outcomes, but their relative contribution is not known. In a survey of 500 physicians (300 primary care physicians, 100 obstetricians/gynecologists, and 100 cardiologists), primary care physicians were significantly more likely to place women, who according to their Framingham risk score were in an intermediate-risk category, in a lower risk category than they did for men (Mosca et al., 2005). That rating affected the recommendations the physicians provided for lifestyle and preventive pharmacotherapy. Earlier studies also indicated that physicians may manage women's chest pain less aggressively, particularly black women (Schulman et al., 1999). Gender-based disparities in cardiovascular care have been documented in commercial health plans and the greatest disparity is present among those who had recent acute cardiac events (Chou et al., 2007a,b).

The American Heart Association (AHA) reviewed what is known about the use and effectiveness of percutaneous coronary interventions and adjunctive pharmacotherapy in men and women and concluded that invasive percutaneous coronary interventions are "performed less frequently and with greater delays in women" (Lansky et al., 2005). Rates of reperfusion therapy are also lower in women than in men, and "there is no evidence that the gap has narrowed in recent years" (Vaccarino et al., 2005). Greater complications and early mortality have been detected in women as compared to men following revascularization (bypass surgery and percutaneous coronary interventions) and, therefore, the lower number of procedures might be beneficial to women (Kim et al., 2007).

Studies have shown a higher risk of death or acute myocardial infarction in women who have unstable angina and an increase in non–ST-segment myocardial infarctions in women after invasive treatment than in women after conservative treatment.[13] A meta-analysis of eight trials indicated that invasive strategies benefit high-risk women—that is, those who have increased concentrations of the biomarkers creatine kinase MB or troponin—but do not benefit and possibly increase risk in women who do not have increased concentrations of those biomarkers (O'Donoghue et al., 2008). Similarly, invasive treatment has been shown to benefit high-risk women who have acute coronary syndrome, but study results indicate no benefits of and even harm after invasive treatment in non–high-risk women who have acute coronary syndrome (Lansky et al., 2005).

AHA published sex-specific evidence-based guidelines for the prevention of cardiovascular disease in women in 2004 (Mosca et al., 2004), but the extent to which they have changed practice is not established. Most physicians are aware of the guidelines, but few state that they implement the guidelines (Mieres et al., 2005).

Research Advances in Diagnosis

Sex and gender differences in the presentation of cardiovascular disease have been studied over the last 2 decades, including studies looking for differences in clinical features (Canto et al., 2007; Correa-de-Araujo, 2006; Correa-de-Araujo and Clancy, 2006; DeCara, 2003; Dracup, 2007). The initial presentation of coronary heart disease is about 10 years later in women than in men (Mikhail, 2005). For myocardial infarction, the most common symptom for women is chest

---

[13]Percutaneous coronary interventions would be considered invasive treatments. Pharmacologic management and later coronary angiography if symptoms recur would be a conservative treatment.

pain, although myocardial infarction in women does occur in the absence of chest pain (AHA, 2010). Other symptoms of myocardial infarction include feeling out of breath; pain that runs along the neck, jaw, or upper back; nausea; vomiting or indigestion; unexplained sweating; sudden or overwhelming fatigue; and dizziness (AHA, 2010). Statistically, women who have myocardial infarctions are less likely than men to have coronary disease (Shaw et al., 2009). That chest pain is more common in men and is considered a "typical" symptom of heart disease may contribute to the finding that women are less likely to undergo diagnostic evaluation for symptoms and may have their conditions misdiagnosed (Brieger et al., 2004; Canto et al., 2007). Some evidence suggests that women and men experience cardiac pain differently, and that this affects the diagnosis of cardiovascular conditions and events (O'Keefe-McCarthy, 2008).

Women who have coronary heart disease are more likely to present with angina and fatigue, nausea and vomiting, and shortness of breath, whereas men are more likely to present with acute myocardial infarction or coronary heart disease death (DeCara, 2003). Women also have more atypical chest pain related to angina than men and more nausea, back pain, and jaw pain (Brieger et al., 2004; Canto et al., 2007; Kudenchuk et al., 1996; Milner et al., 1999).

Women and men vary in the predictive strength of risk factors, and this complicates the diagnosis of coronary arterial disease in women. Diabetes has been shown to be a stronger predictor of risk in women than in men (Scheidt-Nave et al., 1991). In a study of premenopausal women who underwent coronary angiography for suspected ischemia, diabetes was associated with hypothalamic hypoestrogenemia, increased prevalence and severity of angiographic coronary artery disease, and a slight increased risk of major adverse cardiovascular events (Ahmed et al., 2008). Isolated systolic hypertension is more common and more predictive in women than in men (Rich-Edwards et al., 1995), whereas a high concentration of low-density lipoproteins is more predictive of coronary arterial disease in men than in women (Rich-Edwards et al., 1995). An increase in triglycerides is a risk factor for cardiovascular disease in women (Evangelista and McLaughlin, 2009).

C-reactive protein has been suggested for use as a risk marker, particularly in women (Cook et al., 2006; Ridker et al., 2003). Research on the clinical relevance of C-reactive protein is ongoing. The US Preventative Task Force concluded that although data are convincing that C-reactive protein is associated with coronary heart disease, evidence that its use as a risk marker improves risk estimates is weak, and evidence that reducing C-reactive protein levels protects against coronary heart disease is lacking for either women or men (Buckley et al., 2009).

Sex differences have sometimes been reported in the sensitivity and specificity of diagnostic tests for cardiovascular disease. Kim and colleagues (2001) conducted a meta-analysis and found sex differences in the diagnostics. An AHA consensus statement in 2005 concluded that the present approach to diagnostic testing may require some variation when applied to women (Mieres et al., 2005). DeCara (2003) reviewed noninvasive cardiac testing in women and found a high rate of false positives for coronary arterial disease with exercise electrocardio-graphic (ECG) stress testing in women (Hung et al., 1984; Mieres et al., 2005) and female-specific outcomes have been developed for exercise ECGs (Gulati et al., 2005). A systematic review for AHRQ, however, did not find sex differences in the accuracy of exercise myocardial perfusion imaging for diagnosis of coronary heart disease and found little difference in the accuracy of exercise myocardial perfusion imaging and exercise echocardiography for diagnosis of coronary heart disease in women (Grady et al., 2003).

Differences in the diagnosis of cardiovascular disease in women, if present, could bias the results of clinical trials. If trials are based on symptoms of coronary heart disease and cardiovascular disease that are more commonly seen in men than in women, and female cases will be missed.

Research Advances in Treatment

Research laid the groundwork for a number of important pharmacologic breakthroughs in treating patients with cardiovascular disease. The use of beta-blockers and aspirin as soon as possible after a myocardial infarction quickly became the standard of care for men; however, women were not receiving that care and it took a few years for the use of beta-blockers and aspirin in women to approach that in men (Berger et al., 2009). The use of stents in women lagged behnd their use in men because the size of the stent was based on male blood vessels, which are typically larger than in women (Lansky et al., 2005).

As summarized by Lansky and colleagues (2005), the current use of stents does not appear to differ between the sexes. In addition, the mortality associated with their use is similar in women and men unless confounding risk factors are present in women (Chauhan et al., 2005; Mehilli et al., 2000).

Research has demonstrated that adjunctive pharmacotherapy is beneficial in women who are undergoing percutaneous coronary intervention as secondary prevention, including the use of aspirin, ADP–receptor antagonist antiplatelet agents (clopidogrel and ticlopidine), glycoprotein (GP) IIb/IIa inhibitors, the antithrombin agents unfractionated heparin and low-molecular-weight heparin, and direct thrombin inhibitors (Antithrombotic Trialists Collaboration, 2002; Braunwald et al., 2002; Fernandes et al., 2002; Kong et al., 2002; Steinhubl et al., 1999; Stone et al., 2002; Wong et al., 2003; Yusuf et al., 2003). Because of women's risk of bleeding complications at baseline (Lenderink et al., 2004), and because of risks of overdosing with GP IIb/IIIa inhibitors in women, care must be taken to avoid complications (Alexander et al., 2006).

Knowledge Gaps

Despite research advances in scientific knowledge related to diagnosis, risk factors, preventive interventions, and effective therapies for coronary heart disease in women, progress might have happened sooner if women had been better represented in earlier studies of cardiovascular disease. More recently women have been enrolled in cardiovascular trials; however, a lack of knowledge about sex differences remains, in part because of a lack of sex-specific analysis and reporting of sex-specific results, with only 25% of trials of cardiovascular disease reporting on sex-specific results (Blauwet and Redberg, 2007; Blauwet et al., 2007; Grady et al., 2003). Because women have been consistently under-enrolled in cardiovascular-disease clinical trials (Grady et al., 2003; Kim and Menon, 2009; Sharpe, 2002), studies were not powered sufficiently to provide statistical significance on data for women, so meta-analyses have been used to determine whether the results obtained in men can be extrapolated to women (Grady et al., 2003). Because of their limitations, however, meta-analytic methods can not overcome a lack of enrollment or data on women, and they are not optimal for addressing the leading cause of mortality in women. A major limitation of evaluating data from eligible studies was that findings were often not stratified by sex, and little evidence was available to answer key questions about the disease in women (and in racial and ethnic minorities). Women continue to be inadequately represented in cardiovascular-disease clinical trials; this could be due in part to entry criteria that are based on symptoms seen more commonly in men (Grady et al., 2003). Cardiovascular disease may be a category in which sex-specific studies can be used to fill in the gaps (Lansky et al., 2005; O'Donoghue et al., 2008; Shaw et al., 2009).

Much also remains both to be learned about the biologic sex differences that underlie cardiovascular disease in men and to be done to use the information to develop sex-specific diagnostic, preventive, therapeutic, and rehabilitative approaches. Sex-specific diagnostic tools, especially for identifying subclinical disease, are needed as is a strategy for avoiding the delay in screening for, diagnosis of, and treatment of cardiovascular disease in women. Furthermore, the reasons for the disparities in mortality in different groups of women and how to address those disparities are also needed.

Although awareness of cardiovascular disease as the leading cause of death has nearly doubled among women since national educational programs, such as the Heart Truth and Red Dress campaigns, have been targeted to women—in 1997, only 30% of women recognized cardiovascular disease as the leading killer of women, significantly less than the 57% and 54% of women who recognized cardiovascular disease as the leading killer of women in 2006 and 2009, respectively (Mosca et al., 2010)—but awareness continues to lag among racial and ethnic minorities. Work is needed to raise awareness of the problem of cardiovascular diseases among women and their health-care providers, especially because awareness of cardiovascular-disease risk has been linked to the taking of preventive action (Christian et al., 2007; Mosca et al., 2006). Translation and communication issues are discussed in Chapter 5.

Lessons Learned

A major lesson was the recognition, not only by researchers but also by clinicians and the public, that cardiovascular disease is a major cause of morbidity and mortality in women. Part of the delay in recognizing that was lack of awareness, but other factors in the delay might be related to potential sex differences in the presentation (for example, age at presentation) of cardiovascular disease in women and men. That highlights the importance of recognizing the signs and symptoms of a disease in women, and ensuring that health practitioners and women are aware of those signs and symptoms. Sex-specific research on cardiovascular disease has shown potential sex-specific differences that affect everything from risk factors to diagnosis to treatment. Evidence indicates that behavioral factors are important for the prevention of cardiovascular disease (see Chapter 2 for a more detailed discussion), so research needs to go beyond the pathophysiology of the disease to the level of identifying effective interventions to modify people's behaviors to prevent disease. Comorbidities with cardiovascular disease have also been seen and highlight the impact that comorbidities can have on diagnosis and treatment. Another major lesson is the importance of the translation of research findings into practice and policies to benefit all.

Cervical Cancer

The committee considered cervical cancer to be a disease where research findings have led to major advances in prevention and detection of the disease. There have been large decreases in incidence of and mortality from cervical cancer in the United States, mostly because of the use of the Papanicolaou (Pap) smear and the Bethesda rating system, both of which were developed before the period of our review. Cervical-cancer incidence and mortality continued to decrease during the last 20 years, and there are now improved treatment options for early-stage cervical cancer. Cervical-cancer research has also resulted in the development of a vaccine against human papilloma virus (HPV), an infectious agent that causes most cases of cervical cancer. The vaccine has the potential to protect women against cervical cancer, the leading cause of cancer death in women worldwide.

Incidence, Prevalence, and Mortality in Women

Cervical cancer was once one of the leading causes of cancer death in women in the United States, but its incidence and mortality in the United States decreased by about 74% from 1955 to 1992 and continues to decrease (ACS, 2009b). In the United States in 2010, it is estimated that 12,200 women will be diagnosed with cervical cancer, and 4,210 women will die from it (NCI, 2010c). The decreases in incidence and mortality are attributed mainly to regular cytology-based cervical-cancer prevention programs, which were introduced in the United States in the 1960s (Wright, 2007; Zeferino and Derchain, 2006). In 2002–2007, the median age at diagnosis in the United States was 48 years; the median age at death was 57 years (NCI, 2010c).

Disparities Among Groups

Cervical-cancer incidence and mortality decreased in the United States from 1996 to 2005 in all races and ethnicities on which there are surveillance data (see Figure 3-2) (NCI, 2008). Disparities among races and ethnicities persist despite those gains (Barnholtz-Sloan et al., 2009). The age-adjusted average incidence (cases per 100,000) in 2001–2005 was highest, at 13.7, in Hispanic women, followed by 10.8 in black women and about 8 in white and Asian and

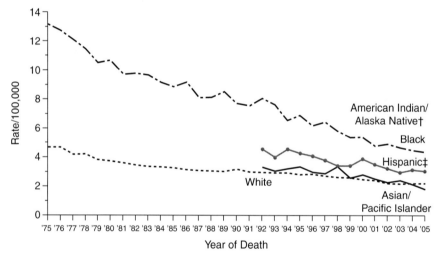

FIGURE 3-2 Cervical-cancer mortality in 1975–2005 by race.
Mortality source: US Mortality Files, National Center for Health Statistics, Centers for Disease Control and Prevention.
Rates per 100,000 and age-adjusted to 2000 US standard population (19 age groups—Census P25-1130).
†Rates for American Indians and Alaska Natives not displayed, because fewer than 16 cases were reported for at least 1 year within interval.
‡Hispanics not mutually exclusive from whites, blacks, Asians and Pacific Islanders, and American Indians and Alaska Natives. Mortality data on Hispanics do not include cases from Connecticut, Maine, Maryland, Minnesota, New Hampshire, New York, North Dakota, Oklahoma, and Vermont.
SOURCE: http://www.cdc.gov/cancer/cervical/statistics/race.htm (accessed May 5, 2010).

Pacific Islander women. In contrast, the average mortality (deaths per 100,000) in the same years was highest in black women at 4.7, followed by 3.2 in Hispanic women and 2.0 in white and Asian and Pacific Islander women. Possible reasons why advances are not translated to decreased mortality among all populations of women are discussed in Chapter 5. Incidence varies within racial and ethnic categories. For example, although overall Asian women are less likely to receive a diagnosis of cervical cancer than white women, within this subgroup Vietnamese American women are approximately 5 times more likely to be diagnosed with cervical cancer than white women (Taylor et al., 2004).

Research Advances in Knowledge of Biology

Epidemiologic, animal, and molecular studies have elucidated the role of HPV in cervical cancer and laid the groundwork for the novel diagnostic techniques and development of a vaccine discussed below and, ultimately, for the prevention of cervical cancer (Lehtinen and Paavonen, 2004; Olsson et al., 2009; zur Hausen, 2009).

The association between HPV type 16 and cervical cancer was found over 2 decades ago (Dürst et al., 1983, 1987). Research during the 1990s and early 2000s demonstrated that HPV is present in over 90% of premalignant cervical lesions and over 95% of cervical cancers and confirmed HPV as causal and necessary for cervical cancer (Bosch et al., 2002; Ferenczy and Franco, 2002; Franco et al., 2001; Muñoz, 2000; Muñoz et al., 2003; Walboomers et al., 1999). HPV 16 and 18 are responsible for cervical cancer (Schlecht et al., 2001; Woodman et al., 2007). Muñoz and colleagues (2003) demonstrated that HPV 16, 18, 31, 33, 35, 45, 52, and 58 account for 95% of squamous-cell carcinomas that are positive for HPV. Researchers also examined the structure of the virus particles; engineered proteins, called the L1 proteins, that reform to virus-like particles (or capsids); and demonstrated that the reformed L1 virus-like particles trigger an immune response in animals (Breitburd et al., 1995; Campo, 2002; Kirnbauer et al., 1992, 1993; Suzich et al., 1995; Zhou et al., 1991). The improved understanding of the relationship between HPV and cervical cancer laid the groundwork for the development of an HPV vaccine.

Research Advances in Prevention

It has been noted for centuries that cervical cancer is associated with sexual activity and sexual contacts (see Chapter 2 for discussion of sexual risk behavior) (zur Hausen, 2009), and limiting the number of sexual partners and using condoms have long been recommended for primary prevention of cervical cancer. Because sexual activity is a risk factor for cervical cancer, behaviors during teenage years and early adulthood can affect the risk of cervical cancer later in life. There is recent evidence that condom use greatly reduces the risk of genital HPV infections (Winer et al., 2006).

The identification of the HPV virus as the causative agent in cervical cancer and the characterization of the virus and its components provided the basis of the development of a vaccine for the primary prevention of HPV infection and cervical cancer (Kulski et al., 1998). After trials to test safety (Harro et al., 2001) and antibody response (Carter et al., 2000; Petter et al., 2000), Koutsky and colleagues (2002) conducted a randomized controlled trial of an HPV 16 L1 virus-like particle vaccine in 2,392 women. A median of 17.4 months later, the vaccine had 100% efficacy in protecting against HPV 16 infection.[14] Harper and colleagues (2004) conducted a randomized controlled trial of the efficacy of a bivalent HPV 16/18 virus-like particle vaccine against HPV 16 and HPV 18 infections in 1,113 women 15–25 years old. The vaccine was over 90% effective against incident and persistent infection with HPV 16/18. Relatively few minor and no serious adverse events were reported.

Gardasil®, a prophylactic vaccine containing the virus-like particle for HPV 6/11/16/18, has since been approved by FDA for girls and women 9–26 years old (FDA, 2008). Studies with the vaccine demonstrated safety; relatively few adverse events were reported. In one study the vaccine prevented 100% of cervical intraepithelial neoplasia (CIN), adenocarcinoma in situ or cancer, and vaginal, vulvar, perineal, and perianal intraepithelial lesions associated with vaccine-type HPV in women with no evidence of previous HPV infection (Garland et al., 2007). When the vaccine was administered to subjects who had no evidence of previous exposure to either HPV 16 or 18, the prophylactic HPV vaccine was 98% effective in preventing HPV 16– and 18–related CIN 2/3 and adenocarcinoma in situ (FUTURE II Study Group, 2007). In women with evidence of HPV infection, regardless of the type of HPV infection, the vaccine reduced the incidence of vulvar, vaginal, and perianal lesions by 34% and of cervical lesions by 20% (Garland et al., 2007). The efficacy of the vaccine in preventing HPV 16– or 18–related CIN2/3 and adenocarcinoma in situ was lower (44%) in women who had been previously exposed to HPV types 6/11/16/18. The estimated efficacy of the vaccine against all high-grade cervical lesions regardless of the causal HPV type was 17% (FUTURE II Study Group, 2007). In October 2009 FDA approved Cervarix™ an additional vaccine to prevent cervical cancer and precancerous lesions caused by HPV types 16 and 18 (FDA, 2009a).

In October 2009 FDA approved one form of the vaccine in boys and men aged 9–26 for prevention of genital warts (HHS, 2009). The approval did not address the prevention of transmission of HPV to girls and women, and there has been much debate on whether boys and men should be vaccinated to decrease the prevalence of HPV in girls and women (Campos-Outcalt, 2009; Cuschieri, 2009; Hibbitts, 2009; Hull and Caplan, 2009).

---

[14]Trials of the vaccines were funded by Merck and by GlaxoSmithKline.

Despite the evidence indicating safety and efficacy, a number of controversial issues have arisen around the implementation of HPV vaccination programs. Those issues are discussed in Chapter 5.

Although HPV infection is the major risk factor for cervical cancer, other risk factors have been studied. In general, diet does not appear to modify risks greatly. Diets rich in beta-carotene, or high in vegetables, however, have been linked to lower risk in a few studies (Hirose et al., 1998; La Vecchia et al., 1988), and antioxidants, such as carotenoids, have been shown to decrease HPV persistence in women (Giuliano et al., 1997, 2003). Smoking is associated with an increased risk of cervical cancer, although the extent to which the association is independent of HPV is not known (CDC, 2002a). Some research studies have shown an increased risk of cervical cancer associated with exposure to second-hand smoke (Tay and Tay, 2004; Trimble et al., 2005), but most reviews have concluded that there is inadequate or only suggestive evidence of an association (Office of Environmental Health Hazard Assessment, 2005; Office of the Surgeon General, 2006).

Research Advances in Diagnosis

The consistent use of conventional Pap tests (in which cervical cells are smeared on a slide) for decades in the United States to screen for cervical cancer and precancerous lesions has drastically reduced the incidence of and mortality from cervical cancer (Jansson et al., 1998; Mathew and George, 2009; Schiffman and Castle, 2005; Sherman et al., 2005). Revised screening techniques have the goal of improving the sensitivity (false negatives), and specificity (false positives) of screening, which are suboptimal because of sampling, preparation, detection, and interpretation (Siebers et al., 2009). Liquid preparations allow cytologic screening, computer-assisted reading, and testing for HPV DNA using a single sample preparation (Sherman et al., 1997). In 1996, FDA approved the first liquid-based medium for gynecologic cytology, ThinPrep® (Guidos and Selvaggi, 1999). Early studies showed that liquid-based cytology was at least as good as the conventional Pap test in detecting low-grade squamous intraepithelial lesions and other epithelial-cell abnormalities (Austin and Ramzy, 1998; Bishop et al., 1998; Linder, 1998; Sherman et al., 1998; Vassilakos et al., 1998). Other studies, however, did not yield convincing evidence of improved results of liquid-based cytology, and systematic reviews cited a lack of well-designed comparative studies (that is, studies that used randomized design, biopsy-confirmed cervical lesions, blinded verification, and adequate power) to determine which method was superior (Arbyn et al., 2008; Davey et al., 2006; Klinkhamer et al., 2003). A recent randomized controlled trial that evaluated over 84,000 Dutch women showed that liquid-based cytology does not detect cervical-cancer precursors better than the conventional Pap test (Siebers et al., 2009). The American Congress of Obstetricians and Gynecologists (ACOG) concluded that liquid-based and conventional methods of cervical cytology are both acceptable for use in testing (ACOG, 2003), and the American Cancer Society recommends the conventional Pap test or liquid-based cytology with different frequencies depending on age (ACS, 2009c). In recently released evidence-based guidelines, ACOG increased the recommended age at first screening and decreased the recommended frequency of cervical-cancer screening but not of pelvic examination (ACOG, 2009).

With the identification of the HPV types responsible for most cervical cancers, high-throughput DNA testing provides DNA diagnostic tests for HPV types associated with cervical cancer. Several FDA-approved HPV DNA diagnostic tests for high-risk types of HPV are effective in detecting HPV. Current guidelines for the management of women with abnormal cervical-cancer screening results have incorporated the use of HPV DNA testing as an adjunct to cytologic screening in their algorithms (Wright et al., 2007). Whether HPV DNA testing can replace cervical cytology remains to be seen.

Research Advances in Treatment

Precancerous lesions are often detected through routine Pap tests and affected cells are removed or destroyed before the development of cervical cancer (for example, with a loop electrosurgical excision procedure, cryosurgery, laser surgery, or cone biopsy).

Once a woman receives a diagnosis of cervical cancer, she can have surgery, radiation therapy, chemotherapy, or some combination of the three. The choice depends on the stage at diagnosis and on patient and physician preference. Clinical trials over the last 2 decades have provided information on the comparative efficacy and toxicity of different treatment regimens to allow evidence-based decisions on treatment protocols and improved quality of life after treatment for some stages of the disease.

Hysterectomy and radical hysterectomy, which were the standard treatments for early-stage (non-metastisized) cervical cancer, have good survival rates but were associated with major morbidity and eliminated the possibility of pregnancy (Chan and Naik, 2008). Over the last 2 decades, research has demonstrated the effectiveness of other surgical procedures or combination therapies that provide a better posttreatment quality of life than radical hysterectomy (Chan and Naik, 2008). For example, trachelectomy (removal of the cervix) is a fertility-sparing surgical option for younger women who have the disease, and laparoscopic radical hysterectomy has the potential of better postoperative recovery and cosmetics than traditional radical hysterectomy (Chan and Naik, 2008). Improvements in imaging also inform decision making for individual cases and allow more specific surgical treatments for localized advanced cancer (Sundar et al., 2005). Despite that progress, however, White (2008) noted that late effects of cervical-cancer treatments include bowel and bladder dysfunction and sexual difficulties.

Historically, radiation therapy (external radiation or brachytherapy where the radioactive material is sealed in a container or wire and is placed directly into or near the tumor) was not given in combination with chemotherapy, but clinical trials demonstrated the advantage of administering cisplatin-based chemotherapy during radiation in some patients who had stage I or more advanced cervical cancer (Gibbons and Keys, 2000; Lukka et al., 2002; Morris et al., 1999; Peters et al., 2000; Rose et al., 1999). Increased toxicity, however, is seen with the addition of chemotherapy (Eifel, 2006; Loizzi et al., 2008).

Chemotherapeutic options for recurrent and metastatic cervical cancer have been reviewed (Moore, 2006; Tao et al., 2008). Cisplatin chemotherapy has been used since the 1980s against advanced cervical cancer in people who cannot be treated with surgery or radiation and against recurrent cervical cancer (Alberts and Mason-Liddil, 1989). The prognosis with that treatment is poor; its goal is to slow the progression of the disease (that is, palliation), and it has high toxicity. During the 1990s, other platin analogues and combination therapies that contained cisplatin and non–platin-related compounds (for example, mitolactol and ifosfamide) were used in clinical trials with the hope of improving survival and decreasing the toxicity associated with chemotherapy, but they had little success (Moore, 2006). Trials of combinations of other chemotherapeutic agents (such as paclitaxel and topotecan) with cisplatin in the 1990s and early 2000s showed promising results, including a decrease in toxicity and, in the case of topotecan, an increase in progression-free survival compared with cisplatin alone (Moore et al., 2004; Rose et al., 1999), but overall survival was unchanged (McQuellon et al., 2006; Moore et al., 2004). More recent research is investigating agents that target the vasculature of tumors and is developing drugs that target molecular pathways that are abnormal in cancer cells, including cervical cancer (Herrera et al., 2008). In addition, some HPV vaccines are showing potential as therapeutic agents by inducing HPV-specific antitumor immune responses in animal models (Hung et al., 2008).

Despite the research, the prognosis of late-stage cervical cancer is poor, and stage IVB cervical cancer is usually considered incurable (ACS, 2009b). As Moore (2006) pointed out, it is of note that the study by McGuire and colleagues (1996) used validated instruments to assess patient-reported quality of life and was the first randomized controlled study of palliative treatments for advanced cervical cancer to consider quality of life as an end point. Given the palliative nature of the treatments, the toxicity associated with the agents, and the importance of quality of life to women, quality of life is an important consideration in the development of future treatment, as it is in relation to other conditions and treatments. Greater attention to the impact of treatments on quality of life may help women make more informed choices among options for treatment and increase the effectiveness of the treatment they choose.

Knowledge Gaps

Despite the wide use of cytology-based screening, cervical cancer continues to be an important issue among women in the United States, especially among particular racial and ethnic groups. The biggest limitation of cervical cytology is its poor sensitivity, and liquid-based cytology has not improved sensitivity (Ronco et al., 2006).

Advances in treatments have decreased posttreatment morbidity associated with early-stage cervical cancer, but a lack of effective treatments for advanced and recurrent cervical cancer leaves 5-year survival in these cases extremely rare. In addition, research is needed to understand the factors that contribute to acceptance and use of the HPV vaccine, especially in miniority groups at the greatest risk for cervical cancer, since prevention of this disease is now possible (see Chapter 5 for further discussion).

Lessons Learned

The decreases in the incidence of and mortality from cervical cancer highlight the importance of the availability of appropriate diagnostic tests and screening for the prevention of or early treatment for some diseases. The combination of epidemiologic, animal, and cellular research on the etiology of cervical cancer, the role of HPV in cervical cancer, and an understanding of the disease and associated virus itself allowed the development of a vaccine against this cancer. The identification of quality of life as an important outcome in evaluating a therapeutic agent is another important lesson from the research on cervical cancer. The higher incidence and mortality still seen in some populations highlights the need to target translation and communication efforts to reach people who are at greatest risk for the disease.

CONDITIONS ON WHICH RESEARCH HAS CONTRIBUTED TO SOME PROGRESS

Depression

There has been some progress on the development of improved therapies for the treatment for depression over the last 2 decades. Shortcomings in diagnosis and in the use of those therapies, however, have limited the implementation of those treatments and diminished progress against the disease.

Incidence, Prevalence, and Mortality in Women

The prevalence of major depression in the United States is estimated to be 16% over a lifetime (Kessler et al., 2003). The rate in women is estimated to be up to twice that in men (Kessler et al., 2003). The sex difference occurs in relation to the onset of depression (Marcus et al., 2005); chronicity and recurrence are similar between the sexes. Sex differences first emerge at the ages of 11–14 years and persist into adulthood (Angold et al., 1998). Pregnant women and nonpregnant controls have similar rates of depression (Gotlib et al., 1989), although the rates of major depression may increase during the postpartum period (Gotlib et al., 1989; Wisner et al., 1993). Women who have a strong family history of depression have a much higher risk of onset of first depression during the postpartum period (Sichel and Drischoll, 1999).

The etiology of gender differences in depression has been studied to help understand the greater vulnerability of women to depression. Stressful life events lead to an increased risk for depression (Mazure, 1998). Although it is not clear whether or not women experience more stressful life events than do men, women do experience more physical and sexual abuse than do men (Koss et al., 2003). Abuse is a risk factor for depression not only just after the abuse occurs, but throughout the lifetime following such abuse (Weiss et al., 1999). The lower social status of women compared with men is also implicated in rates of depression. Poverty is the chronic stressor most often associated with depression (Belle and Doucet, 2003). Women are more likely to live in poverty than are men. In addition, women appear more reactive to stressful life events than are men. Specifically, women are more likely to experience depression after a stressful life event than are men (Kessler and McLeod, 1984; Nazroo et al., 1997; Uhlenhuth and Paykel, 1973). Finally, two personality factors may predispose women to depression more than men. Women are more likely to score higher on measures on interpersonal dependency than do men, and such dependency is related to depression (Clark et al., 1992; Hammen, 1999; Mazure et al., 2000). Also, women tend to ruminate more in response to sadness than do men (Nolen-Hoeksema et al., 1999; Tamres et al., 2002). Those who ruminate are more likely to be diagnosed with major depression than are those who do not ruminate (Nolen-Hoeksema, 2004). In sum, women's socioeconomic and social status may influence women's increased likelihood of becoming depressed through abuse, chronic stress, and interpersonal dependency.

In both women and men, depression often coexists with other psychiatric disorders (such as anxiety disorders), with substance abuse, and with medical illnesses, such as cancer, HIV/AIDS, and diabetes. Depression can worsen the symptoms of those illnesses (NIMH, 2009).

Because of its high prevalence and its onset early in life, depression is estimated to be a leading cause of disease-related disability in women throughout the world (Murray and Lopez, 1997). The early onset contributes to problematic early-life decisions, poor parenting, lower work functioning, and intense personal pain in young women. Data on people who have early-onset major depression indicate that it adversely affects the educational attainment of women but not of men (Berndt et al., 2000). For example, "a randomly selected 21-year-old woman who had early-onset major depression in 1995 could have expected to earn 12–18% less per year than a randomly selected woman whose major depression occurred after the age of 21 years" (Berndt et al., 2000).

Disparities Among Groups

Rates of depression differ by ethnicity. Rates are lower among Latinos, blacks, Asians, and American Indians than among whites; differences might be due, at least in part, to underdetection (Alegría et al., 2008; Beals et al., 2005; Takeuchi et al., 2007; Williams et al., 2007). Among Mexican Americans, rates of depression in immigrants are lower than in those born in the United States; rates of depression begin rising among immigrants after 13 years of living in the United States (Vega et al., 1998). Similarly, rates of depression are lower among blacks who immigrated to the United States from Africa or the Caribbean than among blacks born in the United States (Miranda et al., 2005). Despite the lower rates, evidence suggests that minority-group members who are depressed are less likely to get depression treatment than are white Americans (Williams et al., 2007). Furthermore, they are less likely to get high-quality care if they do get care when depressed. The lack of care has led to longer, more severe bouts of depression in blacks than in white Americans, who are much more likely to obtain care when it is needed. African Americans report greater stigma associated with treatment for mental health, which could be related to the decreased likelihood of treatment (Menke and Flynn, 2009).

Research Advances in Knowledge of Biology

For many decades, the role of the central monoaminergic system dominated pharmaceutical and academic research on depression. That focus followed findings in the 1950s that the monoamine oxidase inhibitors were effective antidepressants, later development of the tricyclic antidepressant imipramine, and the identification of their mechanisms of action and development of reserpine and amphetamine in the 1960s (Slattery et al., 2004). The delay seen in the action of antidepressants (it can take weeks for them to become effective) suggests that the acute effects of the agents on serotonin, dopamine, and other neurotransmitters are not directly mediating the antidepressive actions, and over the last 15 years animal models and studies in humans have investigated a number of novel targets for antidepressants. As discussed in review articles, there is evidence that disruption of neurotrophic factors—such as brain-derived neurotrophic factor, IGFR, the neuropeptide VGF, and VEGF—their receptors or alterations in neuronal structure, glial number, and other changes could be involved in depression (Elhwuegi, 2004; Kugaya and Sanacora, 2005; Malberg and Monteggia, 2008; Pav et al., 2008; Tanis and Duman, 2007; Warner-Schmidt and Duman, 2008). The hypothalamic–pituitary–adrenal axis and stress hormones could also play a role (Cohen et al., 2007; Hindmarch, 2002; Pariante and Miller, 2001). The understanding of depression gained from those studies provides the potential for development of future pharmacologic treatments for depression.

Onset of depression in girls often occurs at the ages of 11–14 years, and this raises questions about the role of sex hormones in the increased risk of depression in women (Angold et al., 1998). Systematic reviews, however, consistently fail to find that rates of major depression are associated with other hormone-related events, including menopause, use of oral contraceptives, and hormone therapy (Kessler, 2003). Interestingly, perimenopause is associated with onset of depression (Schmidt, 2005) and there is some data to suggest the effectiveness of estradiol in perimenopausal depression.

Research Advances in Prevention

Cuijpers and colleagues (2008) reviewed available data on prevention of depression and conducted a meta-analysis of preventive programs. As discussed by the authors, although some studies have investigated treatment and intervention options, only a few have examined prevention of incident mental disorders, looking mostly at targeted populations or conditions (including postpartum depression, depression in school settings, and patients who have physical disorders).[15] The meta-analysis indicated that some prevention programs decrease the incidence of depressive disorders (Cuijpers et al., 2008). Because gender differences in depression appear early on, those school programs targeted at preventing depression in adolescent girls are particularly important and worthy of further study and dissemination.

No therapeutic interventions have been identified for primary prevention of incident depression, although a number of the therapeutic agents discussed below are used to prevent the recurrence of depression.

Research Advances in Diagnosis

Recent evidence suggests there a need to revise current diagnostic criteria for depression. In a review of randomized, placebo-controlled trials, the value of antidepressant medications was found to increase with increasing severity of depression. The benefit of antidepressant medications for those who had mild or moderate symptoms was minimal or nonexistent whereas medications were substantially beneficial for those who had severe symptoms (Fournier et al., 2010).

---

[15]Preventive programs evaluated were classified as universal programs (for example, school programs and mass-media campaigns), selective programs (aimed at people in high-risk groups), or individual preventive programs (aimed at people who had subclinical symptoms of depression). Interventions that were examined were classified as cognitive–behavioral therapy, interpersonal psychotherapy, and other (for example, debriefing, problem solving, mutual support).

That finding suggests that the Diagnostic and Statistical Manual of Mental Disorders (DSM) criteria for depression, which includes those with mild or moderate symptoms as well as severe symptoms, may not be appropriate for indicating who is likely to benefit from currently available medications.

Research Advances in Treatment

The development of animal models has guided the design of drugs to act on neurobiological targets recognized as involved in the pathophysiology of depression and has led to substantial advances in pharmacologic management of depression. The first of the targeted drugs are the selective serotonin reuptake inhibitors (SSRIs), followed more recently by norepinephrine uptake inhibitors and serotonin receptor antagonists (for example, trazodone and nefazodone). The newer dual-action antidepressants act by inhibiting the reuptake of both serotonin and norepinephrine. They appear to reduce depression and its associated symptoms with greater rapidity, although some trials have indicated similar efficacy and tolerability (Papakostas et al., 2007).

In the last 15 years, researchers have identified targeted nonpharmceutical therapies that are effective in treating for depression. Both interpersonal psychotherapy and cognitive–behavioral therapy can be as effective as medications in the acute treatment of depressed outpatients (Compton et al., 2004; DeRubeis et al., 1999; Frank et al., 2005; Hollon et al., 2005). Medication typically has a rapid and robust effect and can prevent symptom return for as long as it is continued or maintained, but it does little to reduce risk once its use is terminated (Hollon et al., 2005). Interpersonal psychotherapy may improve social functioning, and cognitive–behavioral therapy appears to have an enduring effect that reduces later risk (DeRubeis et al., 1999; Frank et al., 1990, 2005). Gender differences are seen in treatment-seeking behaviors (Dwight-Johnson et al., 2000).

Studies of programs to improve the effectiveness of treatment of depression in primary care suggest that collaborative care improves the quality of care and health outcomes of depressed patients (Katon et al., 1999; Vera et al., 2010); that more efficient methods, such as telephone case management, improve outcomes (Simon et al., 2000, 2004); that multimodal strategies that include case management tend to be more effective than improving clinician knowledge or skills alone (Cunningham and Zayas, 2002; Gensichen et al., 2006); that such programs can improve outcomes of adolescents (Asarnow et al., 2005) and elderly persons (Unutzer et al., 2002); and that active outreach strategies help to engage low-income and minority groups in such care (Revicki et al., 2005). The President's New Freedom Commission on Mental Health, established by President George W. Bush in April 2002, recommended implementing high-quality improvement programs for depression (Hogan, 2003). Current systems do not often reimburse for telephone case management and, in general, improvement of care has not occurred (Netting and Williams, 1996).

The Sequenced Treatment Alternatives to Relieve Depression (STAR*D) study is a 7-year study of over 4,000 patients (64% of patients were women) designed to assess the effectiveness of depression treatments in patients diagnosed with major depressive disorder in both primary and specialty care settings (Rush et al., 2004). A large number of reports have been published from STAR*D. One study reported sex differences in response to citalopram; women were more responsive to the SSRI citalopram than men (Young et al., 2009).

Unfortunately, there are a number of side effects associated with antidepressants that can require careful monitoring of patients and that decrease adherence to medications. Side effects of antidepressants range in severity and depend upon the class of antidepressant, but can include sexual side effects, weight gain, and an increased risk of suicidal thinking and behavior in young adults (18–24 years old) (Khawam et al., 2006).

Knowledge Gaps

Delivering evidence-based care for depression is challenging owing to organizational and financial factors (such as limited coverage of psychotherapy and diversity in third-party management of services) (Goldman et al., 1999; Sharftsein, 1999), clinical features of depression (such as social withdrawal) (Kornstein and Schneider, 2001), societal factors (such as social stigma, limited public knowledge and language barriers) (Goldman et al., 1999; Lewis-Fernandez et al., 2005; Sirey et al., 2001), and clinician factors (such as limited knowledge and experience) (Gallo et al., 1999; Goldman et al., 1999; Meredith et al., 2001). For example, while antidepressant medication use rose over the last decade, many in need of depression care did not receive counseling, medications, or referral. There are many barriers to provision of evidence-based psychotherapy, such as lack of criteria for licensing providers in such treatments (Patel et al., 2006b). Outside of organized group practices, coordination between primary and mental health care is often difficult, given widespread use of "carve-out" behavioral health management companies that operate largely independently of health plans or medical practices (Patel et al., 2006b). Public-sector mental-health agencies prioritize clients with severe and persistent illness, while public-sector primary-care agencies are not organized or financed to support ongoing mental-health care (HHS, 1999; Patel et al., 2006b).

A major gap in depression research is the development of models of treatment that can be disseminated and sustained within current systems of care. A focus on getting care to underserved populations is particularly needed.

Although treatment for depression in women is generally similar to that in men, Grigoriadis and Robinson (2007) note the need for sex and gender issues to be evaluated. Pharmacotherapy for depression during pregnancy and during the postpartum period requires an assessment of the risks and benefits to the fetus (Ward and Zamorski, 2002). Studies of tricyclic antidepressants and SSRIs have generally indicated that they are safe for pregnant women, but the evidence is far from conclusive (Källén, 2007; Way, 2007). FDA continues to rate most antidepressants at level C, noting that the risk to the fetus cannot be ruled out (Hackley, 2010). Postpartum women who have depression can be treated similarly to those who have nonpuerperal depression, unless they are breastfeeding. Few data on antidepressants in breast milk are available (Birnbaum et al., 1999; Weissman et al., 2004). The American Academy of Pediatrics Committee on Drugs concluded that antidepressants are drugs whose effects on nursing infants are unknown but may be of concern (Birnbaum et al., 1999); the risks to the newborn from potential exposure to antidepressants in breast milk need to be weighed against the benefits of nursing and against the risks of the mother foregoing treatment with antidepressants.

In addition, comorbidities are often seen with depression (Huang et al., 2010). For example, associations have been seen between depression and obesity (Luppino et al., 2010), diabetes (Anderson et al., 2001), cancer (Goldberg, 1981), and some chronic diseases in old age (Huang et al., 2010).

Lessons Learned

Although there are effective interventions for depression, many people, particularly minority-group members, fail to get effective treatment. Effective treatment often requires either well-defined psychotherapies, medications, or both managed with careful followup. The more complex interventions are often difficult to disseminate and pay for within current health-care systems and therefore often do not reach women who need care. The occurrence of comorbidities with depression highlights the need to look for comorbidities when treating women. The sex differences in depression further highlight the broad range of sex differences in health outcomes to include neurological disorders. Furthermore, early intervention, particularly preventive interventions for adolescent girls, may well be an important factor in eliminating the high rates of depression among girls and women.

HIV/AIDS

Over the last 20 years, there have been major advances in the treatment of HIV/AIDS, including new treatments that have led to substantial reductions in mortality and morbidity and a major decline in maternal–fetal transmission of HIV. Although much of the initial HIV/AIDS research (particularly clinical trials) has been focused on men, and the proportion of women infected with HIV/AIDS has increased, especially in some groups, the advances have improved the treatment of HIV/AIDS in women as well as men. The committee therefore considers that on balance HIV/AIDS is a condition where scientific advances have led to progress in women's health.

Incidence, Prevalence, and Mortality in Women

An estimated 1 million people live with HIV/AIDS in the United States (Hall et al., 2008; Kaiser Family Foundation, 2009). HIV/AIDS-related morbidity and mortality have decreased substantially in both men and women due to the development of effective combination antiretroviral therapies over the past 15 years (Bailey and Fisher, 2008; Palella et al., 1998). Although it is more prevalent in men, the rate of HIV/AIDS in women is increasing. In the US, women accounted for only 9% of AIDS cases in 1987 but account for over 27% today (Figure 3-3) (CDC, 2008a; Kaiser Family Foundation, 2009). As is discussed below, the increase is greatest in minority women.

Disparities Among Groups

In 2006, black women had an HIV incidence rate about 15 times that of white women, and Hispanic women had an HIV incidence rate about 4 times that of white women (CDC, 2008b). Among women living with HIV/AIDS, 64% are black and 15% are Hispanic (CDC, 2008c). In 2006, black and Hispanic women accounted for the majority of newly infected HIV women, 61% and 16%, respectively (CDC, 2008b). In 2006, the estimated HIV prevalence (per 100,000) among black women and Hispanic women was 1,122 and 263, respectively—almost 18 and 4 times that among white women (CDC, 2008d). According the CDC 2004 data (CDC, 2008c), HIV was the leading cause of death of black women 25–34 years old, the third-leading cause of death of black women 35–44 years old, and the fourth-leading cause of black women 45–54 years old. For Hispanic women, HIV was the fourth-leading cause of death of women 35–44 years old.

HIV/AIDS is increasingly a disease of lower socioeconomic groups and underserved minorities that have not uniformly accessed early or preventive care (CDC, 2003; IOM, 2001a). HIV prevalence and HIV-risk behaviors are disproportionately high in incarcerated women (De Groot, 2000; Dean-Gaitor and Fleming, 1999; Fogel and Belyea, 1999). The associations between mental-health disorders and HIV (Bing et al., 2001; Rosenberg et al., 2001; Stoskopf et al., 2001; Walkup et al., 1999), and between substance abuse and HIV, are also documented (Bing et al., 2001; CDC, 2002b; HHS, 2008).

Research Advances in Knowledge of Biology

In 1983, the first studies that suggested an association between the retrovirus HIV and AIDS were published (Barre-Sinoussi et al., 2004; Essex et al., 1983; Gallo et al., 1983; Gelmann et al., 1983). Work by Gallo and colleagues (1983) established HIV infection as causal for AIDS, and much research has characterized the life cycle of the virus (see De Clercq, 2007, for review). Over the last 20 years, basic research has further elucidated the etiology of and biology underlying

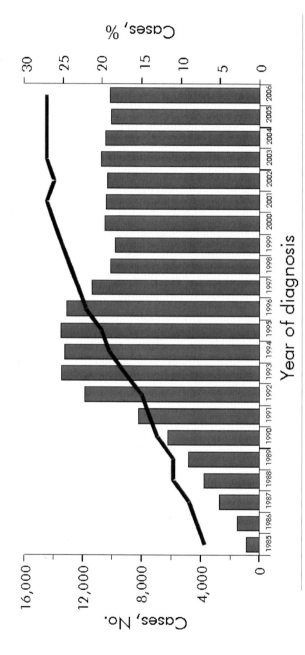

FIGURE 3-3 Estimated number and proportion* of all AIDS cases, in female adults and adolescents, 1985–2006.
NOTE: Data have been adjusted for reporting delay.
*Proportion of all cases that were diagnosed among women.
SOURCE: http://www.cdc.gov/hiv/topics/surveillance/resources/slides/women/slides/Women.ppt (accessed April 22, 2010).

AIDS. Women have benefited from that research, although much of it was conducted in men and there are some reports that progression from HIV to AIDS may differ by sex (Farzadegan et al., 1998; Nicastri et al., 2005). In addition, women are more likely than men to contract HIV during sexual intercourse (European Study Group on Heterosexual Transmission of HIV, 1992; Kaiser Family Foundation, 2009; Padian et al., 1991), and some sexually transmitted infections (STIs) in women have been associated with higher rates of HIV transmission and acquisition (Greenblatt et al., 1988; Plummer et al., 1991; Smith-McCune et al., 2010; Wasserheit, 1992). Two major studies—the HIV Epidemiology Research Study (HERS) and the Women's Interagency Health Study (WIHS)—have increased our understanding of the natural history of HIV infection in women (Barkan et al., 1998; Harlow et al., 2000; Smith et al., 1997).

The interaction between HIV/AIDS and pregnancy has been studied. Pregnancy does not accelerate the decline in CD4 counts, and studies have not shown that pregnancy affects progression or survival in HIV-infected women, especially in developed countries (Alliegro et al., 1997; French and Brocklehurst, 1998; Minkoff et al., 2003). As the first generation of HIV-infected women reaches menopause, issues related to HIV and menopause assume greater relevance, and there is a paucity of data on the relationship. Differences have been seen between premenopausal and postmenopausal women who have AIDS. In some studies, postmenopausal women have lower CD4 lymphocyte counts (van Benthem et al., 2002), and maximum CD4-cell response to antiretroviral therapy decreases with age (Manfredi et al., 2003; Viard et al., 2001). Other studies did not show age-related differences in viral-load decreases (the study population was 33% women; no sex-specific analysis) (Tumbarello et al., 2003) or menopause-related immunologic and virologic responses (Patterson et al., 2009).

Research Advances in Prevention

Despite the increased understanding of the underlying virus, no vaccine or preventive treatment for HIV/AIDS is available (Flexner, 2007). Prevention focuses primarily on decreasing high-risk sexual behaviors that are associated with HIV/AIDS (see Chapter 2 for discussion). It is important to remember that many women are infected with HIV not because of their own high-risk sexual behaviors but because of the risk behavior of their partners (CDC, 2008c; Hader et al., 2001; Varghese et al., 2002). In part because of the lack of awareness of risk, those women often present for HIV testing with acute symptoms late in the course of infection.

Research Advances in Diagnosis

There has been no substantial improvement in the early diagnosis of HIV/AIDS in newly infected people (men and women) since the 1990s. In September

2006, the CDC recommended routine HIV testing for adults, adolescents, and pregnant women (13–64 years old) in health-care settings to "foster earlier detection of HIV infection; identify and counsel persons with unrecognized HIV infection and link them to clinical and prevention services; and further reduce perinatal transmission of HIV in the United States" (CDC, 2006).

Research Advances in Treatment

Major progress has been made in the treatment of HIV/AIDS over the last 15 years, and, as stated by Bailey and Fisher (2008), "antiretroviral therapy for HIV infection has transformed it from a terminal illness to a chronic manageable condition." Detailed reviews of the development of HIV/AIDS drugs have been published (see Bailey and Fisher, 2008; De Clercq, 2007; Sturmer et al., 2009). In 1987, 4 years after the first studies suggested an association between the retrovirus HIV and AIDS (Barre-Sinoussi et al., 2004; Essex et al., 1983; Gallo et al., 1983; Gelmann et al., 1983), zidovudine (AZT), the first antiretroviral treatment, was approved for use in the United States (FDA, 2009b). Highly active antiretroviral therapy—a combination of nucleoside reverse transcriptase inhibitors (NRTIs), nonnucleoside reverse transcriptors (NNRTIs), and protease inhibitors—was in use by the middle 1990s (Bailey and Fisher, 2008). As of 2008, there are six classes of antiretroviral agents that work against HIV—viral reverse transcriptase enzyme inhibitors (NRTIs and NNRTIs), protease inhibitors, fusion inhibitors, entry inhibitors, and integrase inhibitors—and more than 20 drugs are available on the market (Bailey and Fisher, 2008). Although much of the research has been conducted in men, studies indicate that there are no major sex differences in immunologic and virologic response to effective combination antiretroviral therapy (Moore et al., 2003).

The underrepresentation of women in clinical trials has contributed to problems in addressing treatment toxicity. Most studies have not had adequate power to determine sex differences, but an overall review of the literature suggests that the severity and rate of toxicity of some antiretroviral drugs present unique challenges for women, including comorbidities and side effects associated with long-term HIV treatment, such as diabetes (Dube and Sattler, 2010; Nicastri et al., 2005), lipodystrophy (Sattler et al., 2001; Tien et al., 2007), metabolic syndrome (Sobieszczyk et al., 2008), and bone density (Dolan et al., 2004; Sobieszczyk et al., 2008). There is consistent evidence that the toxicity of NRTIs, such as potentially life-threatening lactic acidosis and acute pancreatitis, is more frequent in women (DeMeo et al., 2002; Moore et al., 2001) and that the risk of grade 4 anemia caused by AZT was significantly higher in women (Ssali et al., 2006). Other studies have found an increased prevalence of long-term metabolic abnormalities, such as lipodystrophy and dyslipidemia, in women (Bonfanti et al., 2003; Heath et al., 2002; Pernerstorfer-Schoen et al., 2001; Tien et al., 2003). The occurrence of skin rash (Antinori et al., 2001; Bersoff-Matcha et al., 2001; Mazhude et al., 2002; Wong et al., 2001) and hepatotoxicity (Sobieszczyk et al., 2008) caused by nevirapine is more common in women. The underlying mechanisms of sex differences in the rate of adverse events are unknown, but it has been suggested that pharmacokinetic sex differences may play a major role (Modjtahedi et al., 2006).

The effects of HIV/AIDS treatments on contraception and pregnancy and the effects of pregnancy on the results of HIV/AIDS treatments have been studied. Treatments can decrease the effectiveness of some hormonal contraceptives, but the contraceptive medroxyprogesterone was not affected by nevirapine, efavirenz, or nelfinavir (Cohn et al., 2007). Deaths from hepatic failure have been reported in pregnant women receiving nevirapine in combination antiretroviral therapy (Hitti et al., 2004; Lyons et al., 2006), and there have been reports of maternal deaths due to lactic acidosis during exposure to ddI and d4T with other antiretroviral agents (CDC, 2002c). Women who have CD4 counts greater than $250/mm^3$ have greater rates of nevirapine-associated rash (Antinori et al., 2001; Bersoff-Matcha et al., 2001; Mazhude et al., 2002; Moore et al., 1996) and hepatic toxicity (Sanne et al., 2005). Drug-resistance rates appear similar in pregnant and nonpregnant HIV-infected women (Juethner et al., 2003; Palumbo et al., 2001).

Maternal–fetal transmission of HIV greatly affects a woman's reproductive decisions, and advances in treatments reducing transmission are allowing women to bear children more safely. Where treatments and interventions are available, they have greatly decreased the likelihood that HIV infection will be transmitted to offspring. Research has identified risk factors[16] for HIV transmission (Fawzi et al., 1998; Garcia et al., 1999; Groginsky et al., 1998; Landesman et al., 1996; Minkoff, 1997; Minkoff and Mofenson, 1994; Reinhardt et al., 1995) and interventions, such as elective cesarean section (Read, 2000), that effectively decrease the risks and increase women's reproductive options. The transmission rate decreased from about 25% to 1–2% with advances in the care and treatment of pregnant HIV-infected women, including perinatal antiretroviral therapy (Cooper et al., 2002; The International Perinatal HIV Group, 1999; Mandelbrot et al., 1998; Read, 2000).

Knowledge Gaps

The recent failure in HIV-prevention strategies, including microbiocides and vaccines, in both women and men remains a serious problem in the control of HIV/AIDS (Buchbinder, 2009; Padian et al., 2007; Vandamme, 2008). Research

---

[16]Risk factors include maternal plasma viral load, advanced disease, low CD4 count, poor maternal nutrition, maternal drug use, concomitant sexually transmitted diseases, vaginal delivery, prolonged rupture of membranes, invasive fetal monitoring, chorioamnionitis, low birth weight, prematurity, and possibly genetic susceptibility and characteristics of the virus. About two-thirds to three-quarters of transmission occur during or close to the intrapartum period. In limited resource settings, breastfeeding accounts for a significant proportion of postnatal HIV transmission up to 42% (Kojic and Cu-Uvin, 2007).

is needed on prevention strategies, especially in black and Latina women on viral, host, and immune factors that may influence HIV transmission and acquisition in women throughout their lives, on disease progression, mortality, comorbidities; and on efficacy, safety, pharmacology, and side effects that are associated with medications in HIV-infected women that are different from those in men.

Lessons Learned

HIV/AIDS provides an example of how women can benefit but also be at a disadvantage when research is conducted mainly in men. HIV and AIDS highlight disparities among women of different races and ethnicities and the need to assess the disparities to target effective prevention, diagnosis, and treatment activities. Those differences occur even for the side effects of antiretroviral agents. In addition, the complications that occur in pregnancy (and the potential complications for treatment of women and of the offspring) are important, especially given the stage of life at which infection with HIV often occurs.

Osteoporosis and Fragility Fractures

Falls by elderly people are a major cause of morbidity and greatly affect women because of their longevity (Francis, 2008), and osteoporosis makes women more susceptible to fractures following a fall (Gallagher, 2007). Over the last 20 years there have been advances in the knowledge of the basic science underlying osteoporosis and in the diagnosis and treatment of osteoporosis. The committee considers it to be a condition on which there has been some progress.

Incidence, Prevalence, and Mortality in Women

It is estimated that 10 million Americans have osteoporosis and another 34 million have low bone mass; 80% of them are women (NOF, 2002).[17] Compared with women who have normal bone mineral density (BMD), women with osteoporosis and osteopenia had a rate ratio of sustaining a fragility fracture of 4.03 and 1.80 per 100 person-years, respectively (Siris et al., 2001). Only 18% of documented fragility fractures occurred among women who met BMD criteria for osteoporosis; 52% of women who had fractures had a BMD in the osteopenic range (T score, −1 to −2.5) in the preceding year (Siris et al., 2004).

Fragility fractures typically occur in the hips, wrists, and vertebrae and result in substantial morbidity and mortality (Cauley et al., 2000; Kado et al., 1999). Nearly one-fourth of those who fracture a hip die within 1 year (OTA, 1994), and elderly survivors of such fractures spend about 17% of their remaining life

---

[17]Men have an equivalent risk of osteoporosis and related fractures about a decade later than women (Melton et al., 1992).

in nursing facilities (Braithwaite et al., 2003). Hip fractures occur with higher frequency than spine fractures (Taylor et al., 2010).

The lifetime risk of osteoporosis and fragility fracture rises exponentially with age, with most fractures occurring in women 70 years old or older (Kiel et al., 1987; Melton et al., 1989). The risk increases linearly with the number of fractures that a person has had (Kado et al., 1999). The incidence of hip fractures increased during the 1990s, but incidence decreased more recently in some countries, including the United States and Canada (Brauer et al., 2009; Leslie et al., 2009).

Disparities Among Groups

Among whites and Asians over 50 years old, women have higher fracture risk than men. However, among Hispanics 50–59 years old, men have higher risk than women; after the age of 60 years, Hispanic women have a higher risk than men. Among blacks up to the age of 70 years, men have a higher fracture risk than women; after that women have a higher risk. The risk of fracture increases exponentially with age in all groups (Kanis, 2002).

Research Advances in Knowledge of Biology

Understanding of the pathophysiology of osteoporosis has improved over the last 2 decades (Close et al., 2006; Dennison et al., 2005; Sambrook and Cooper, 2006). That includes the identification of genes whose expression affects the risk of osteoporosis (Huang and Kung, 2006).

A number of factors that lead to an imbalance in bone-forming osteoblast and bone-resorbing osteoclast activity have been delineated (Ikeda, 2008). In mice, expression of the runx2 gene—which is necessary for osteoblast differentiation—decreases in bone tissue and osteoblasts with age; expression of peroxisome–proliferator–activated receptor $\gamma 2$—which inhibits osteoblasts—increases with age (Moerman et al., 2004). In contrast, changes in osteoclast generation with age have not been established (Pietschmann et al., 2009). Decreasing estrogen also plays a role in bone loss, possibly through effects on cytokines and inflammation (Pietschmann et al., 2009).

Research Advances in Diagnosis

Osteoporosis is often undetected and undertreated. One study estimated that only one-third of women who are at high risk of fracture are told that they have osteoporosis, and only one-fourth receive appropriate treatment (Gehlbach et al., 2007). Another study funded by Merck, the National Osteoporosis Risk Assessment, followed over 200,000 community-dwelling postmenopausal women who had no known history of osteoporosis and found that 7.2% of them met criteria for osteoporosis and 39.6% met criteria for osteopenia at study entry (Siris et al., 2001).

A number of new markers of bone remodeling are available, but identifying women at high risk of fracture to target effective treatments remains challenging (Blumsohn, 2003). Traditionally, fracture risk was based almost exclusively on BMD as measured with dual x-ray absorptionometry (DXA). There are not uniform standards for DXA machines, however, so results vary by machine and operator. In addition, DXA is insensitive because BMD is only one of several fracture risk factors—bone architecture is also important. Composite multivariable risk-prediction models (Cummings and Black, 1995; WHO, 2010) have enabled the identification of patients at higher risk for fracture on the basis of a combination of BMD, age, and other risk factors. For example, the FRAX model[18] predicts the 10-year probability of hip fracture and other major osteoporotic fractures on the basis of sex, age, body-mass index, tobacco use, previous fracture, parental fracture, and glucocorticoid use. Although there is variability among models, the most important fracture risk factors appear to be previous fracture, advancing age, female sex, low BMD, prolonged use of glucocorticoids, and family history of fracture.

It is now routine to screen for BMD in women 65 years old or older and in younger women who have risk factors (Buencamino et al., 2009). As screening for osteoporosis with DXA has become more readily available, more women and their physicians face the dilemma of how to respond to DXA results that fall in the osteopenic range.

Explorations of new imaging techniques (such as high-resolution computed tomography) have not added substantially to the ability to identify women who are most likely to have fractures (Genant et al., 2008).

Appropriate clinical followup of women who begin pharmacologic treatment for osteoporosis is controversial. Repeat DXA scans have been routinely performed 2–3 years after treatment initiation, but the value of such testing has been called into question. A recent study found that among healthy older postmenopausal women, repeating BMD assessments for up to 8 years added little value to the initial BMD measurement (Hillier et al., 2007).

Research Advances in Prevention

One difficulty in preventing osteoporosis is the timeframe of the potential risk factors. Determinants of older women's bone strength may date back to their adolescence. Bone mass typically increases until a woman is in her 40s, and the most rapid rise occurs during adolescence (Ensrud et al., 2000; Hannan et al., 2000). Dietary factors (such as high calcium consumption and adequate vitamin D) and doing weight-bearing exercise during adolescence and teenage years decrease the risk of osteoporosis, but teenage girls are not likely to be thinking

---

[18]See http://www.shef.ac.uk/FRAX (accessed September 1, 2010).

about their future bone health (Lloyd et al., 2000). In the first 1–2 years after menopause, bone loss accelerates (Garnero et al., 1996), and this is followed by an annual rate of loss of about 1% (Cooper and Melton, 1992). Low peak bone mass is thought to be associated with an increased risk of osteoporotic fracture, but the evidence is sparse (Cooper et al., 2006). Low body-mass index is a risk factor for fracture (De Laet et al., 2005).

There is controversy about the appropriate intake of vitamin D, including dosing levels and the possible role of calcium, for fracture prevention (Bischoff-Ferrari et al., 2007; Boonen et al., 2007; Cranney et al., 2007; Tang et al., 2007). There has never been a dose-ranging randomized controlled trial of vitamin D in susceptible populations. A meta-analysis of 12 double-blind trials (in which 89% of the participants were women) found that a high dose (over 400 IU/day) decreased the risk of nonverteral fractures (relative risk [RR], 0.80; 95% confidence interval [CI], 0.72–0.89) and the risk of hip fractures (RR, 0.82; 95% CI, 0.69–0.97). The effect was independent of calcium supplementation (Bischoff-Ferrari et al., 2009).

Several guidelines for prevention of and treatment for low BMD have emerged, most of which are consistent in their key treatment recommendations (Solomon et al., 2005). The guidelines have resulted in changes in clinical practice (Buencamino et al., 2009).

Research Advances in Treatment

Before the late 1990s, hormone therapy (estrogen or estrogen plus progestin) was the only treatment available to preserve bone density. There are now several types of treatment to choose from, including bisphosphonates, selective ER modulators (such as raloxifene), the parathyroid hormone analogue teriparatide, and calcitonin (Chesnut et al., 2000; Quattrocchi and Kourlas, 2004). Patients who have osteoporosis and demonstrate good long-term medication adherence have substantially lower risk of fracture (Emkey and Ettinger, 2006). Side effects, inconvenience, costs, and complexity of some dosing regimens have limited long-term adherence. Dosing intervals for bisphosphonates have been extended from a once-daily to a once-weekly, once-monthly, and even once-yearly schedule to improve adherence (Cramer and Silverman, 2006). Although that can improve adherence, the consequence of missing a dose or taking an incorrect dose is greater. Although they are considered rare, side effects of bisphosphonates, including severe musculoskeletal pain and osteonecrosis of the jaw, have been reported (Watts and Diab, 2010). In addition, there are some case reports of atypical subtrochanteric femur fractures while on bisphosphonates, but following a review of the data FDA concluded that bisphosphonates do not increase the risk of those fractures (HHS, 2010). Drug "holidays" are recommended depending on the fracture risk of patients (Watts and Diab, 2010).

The WHI found that postmenopausal women randomized to daily calcium and vitamin D experienced a small but significant improvement in hip bone density. However, calcium and vitamin D did not significantly reduce hip fracture (Jackson et al., 2006). The mean followup of 7 years might have limited the ability to detect significant differences.

Nonpharmacologic treatments, such as bone-loading physical activity, could be used to prevent osteoporosis and later fractures in elderly people (Borer, 2005; Gregg et al., 2000; Wilkins and Birge, 2005). Exercise has also been shown to increase bone mass in rats (Iwamoto et al., 2005).

Relatively few women who have osteoporosis or osteopenia receive medications that have been proved to prevent new fractures. In one study, only 30% of 6,311 patients at high risk for fracture received medication for osteoporosis (Solomon et al., 2004). In addition to (male) sex, factors associated with nontreatment included age over 74 year or under 55 years, black race, having more than one comorbid condition, and (for women) being seen by a male physician.

Knowledge Gaps

Progress has been made in the prevention of and treatment for osteoporosis. Some organizations have developed position statements for treatment (Ettinger et al., 2006), but no formal treatment guidelines have been developed despite having been called for since the middle 1990s (Abbott et al., 1996; Goldhahn et al., 2008). The best approach for targeting young girls to decrease their risk of osteoporosis in the future is not known.

The most beneficial time to take osteoporosis drugs and the most appropriate screening (that is, whether hip or spine bone density is the best indicator of osteoporosis) (Dennison et al., 2005) are still not clear, and quality standards for bone-density scans are needed (Leslie and Manitoba Bone Density Program, 2006).

The details of the relationship between bone density and fall outcome remain unknown (Geusens et al., 2002), and some models indicate that factors other than bone density, such as age and sex, should also be taken into account in estimating the risk of bone fracture (Kanis et al., 2005).

Lessons Learned

The challenges around osteoporosis highlight the quality-of-life issues that are a problem particularly for women as a result of their longevity. In addition, the effects of lifestyle choices (such as eating habits) at an early age on the risk of osteoporosis at a later age emphasize the need to consider a woman's full life span in evaluating risks of adverse health events.

CONDITIONS ON WHICH LITTLE PROGRESS HAS BEEN MADE

This section discusses a number of conditions on which little progress or improvement in health outcomes has been made. Numerous conditions could fit in this category. Instead of a comprehensive review of research on all conditions of concern to women, the committee discusses a few conditions as examples from which it draws broad conclusions.

First, the committee discusses two conditions related to pregnancy: unintended pregnancy and maternal morbidity and mortality. Other conditions considered to have little progress—alcohol and drug addiction, autoimmune diseases, dementia and Alzheimer's disease, gynecologic cancers (other than cervical), gynecologic disorders (nonmalignant), and lung cancer—are then discussed.

Unintended Pregnancy

The committee considers that there has been no major progress in prevention of unintended pregnancy in light of the lack of decrease in rates over time and in comparison with rates in other countries. Pregnancy constitutes a condition with implications for the health of the pregnant woman as well as of the newborn. Whereas the management of the newborn has seen great progress resulting in a marked reduction of neonatal mortality, many obstetrical syndromes remain poorly understood and are mostly the subject of palliation rather than etiologic cure. Rates of unintended pregnancy have not declined over time and rates of unintended pregnancy remain substantially higher in the United States than in other countries. Unintended pregnancy is associated with increased morbidity for the mother as well as risks to the fetus. Although the committee has included unintended pregnancy and its potential health consequences with health outcomes, unintended pregnancy could also be considered a determinant of health. The ability to space and time children effectively benefits women, men, children, families, and society as a whole (IOM, 2004b). Although not all unintended pregnancies are unwanted, often unintended pregnancy is associated with increased morbidity in the mother and risks to infants and children born from unintended pregnancies, such as risks posed by delay in prenatal care, by tobacco use, by alcohol consumption, and by drug abuse. Infants and children born from unintended pregnancies are also at risk for lower birth weight, death in the first year of life, child abuse, and insufficient resources for a healthy environment. The mother is at risk for depression and physical abuse herself and for dissolution of her relationship with her partner. Both parents may experience economic hardship and failure to achieve their educational and career goals, and these are also challenges to maintaining a strong family unit (IOM, 2009).

Unintended pregnancy occurs for a variety of reasons, including lack of availability of and access to acceptable methods of contraception, failure of chosen contraceptive methods, less than optimal patterns of contraceptive use or lack of use, and lack of adequate motivation to prevent pregnancy (IOM, 2009). Sexual risk behaviors and sexual assault are also associated with unintended pregnancy and are discussed in Chapter 2.

Incidence, Prevalence, and Mortality in Women

The rate of unintended pregnancies in the United States is among the highest in the developed world (Trussell and Wynn, 2008), despite the fact that decreasing the rate of unintended pregnancies is an objective of Healthy People 2010 (Klerman, 2000) and that family planning has been considered by CDC to be one of the 10 greatest public-health achievements of 20th century (CDC, 1999). About half (49%) of pregnancies are unintended, that is, unwanted or mistimed (Finer and Henshaw, 2006). Women are considered at risk for unintended pregnancy if they have sexual intercourse, are fertile (neither partner has been contraceptively sterilized or is infertile for any other reason), are not intentionally pregnant and have not been trying to conceive during any part of the year (IOM, 1995). Given those factors, of the 50 million sexually active women 18–44 years old, 28 million (56%) are at risk for unintended pregnancy (Frost et al., 2008). Some 74% of pregnancies among unmarried women in 2001 were unintended compared with 27% of those among married women (Finer and Henshaw, 2006).

Disparities Among Groups

The rate of unintended pregnancy is substantially higher among poor women (112 unintended pregnancies per 1,000 women with an income below the poverty level, or 62% of pregnancies) than among women who live at or above 200% of the poverty level (29 unintended pregnancies per 1,000 women or 38% of pregnancies) (Finer and Henshaw, 2006). Higher-income women were more likely to abort an unintended pregnancy than women below the poverty level, and the rate of unintended births in women below the poverty level (58 per 1,000 women) was higher than that of higher-income women (11 per 1,000 women at or above 200% of the poverty level). Women aged 18–19 years old (108 per 1,000 women) and 20–24 years old (104 per 1,000 women) are at highest risk (Finer and Henshaw, 2006). The percentage of pregnancies that are unintended was highest at earlier ages: 100% in those under 15 years old, 82% in those aged 15–19 years old, and 60% in those aged 20–24 years old (Finer and Henshaw, 2006). Unintended pregnancy is most likely to occur among women who are young, unmarried, of low income, or members of racial or ethnic minorities; black and Hispanic women have higher rates of unintended pregnancy than white women (Finer and Henshaw, 2006).

Research Advances in Prevention

Advances in social and behavioral interventions to prevent unintended pregnancy were discussed in Chapter 2 in relation to sexual risk behaviors. New contraceptive methods have become available over the last few decades, and the safety of oral contraceptives, which were first marketed in the United States in 1960, has improved over the same period as doses of the steroid hormones (estrogens and progestins) used in them have been continually reduced (Batur et al., 2003; Benagiano et al., 2007; Swica, 2007). Although there is evidence of an increased risk of venous thromboemoblism and pulmonary embolism in women taking oral contraceptives, especially in smokers (Chasan-Taber and Stampfer, 1998; Middeldorp, 2005), numerous studies have demonstrated the remarkable safety of current formulations of oral contraceptives, which for nearly all young, healthy women are safer than pregnancy (Beral et al., 1999; Chasan-Taber and Stampfer, 1998). New delivery systems for combined estrogen–progestin hormonal contraceptive preparations have been developed, including transdermal patches and vaginal rings. In addition, progestin-releasing implants and intrauterine devices that release progestin are now available (Tolaymat and Kaunitz, 2007). Another advance in contraceptive technology is the development of a female condom that, as do male condoms, has the potential to prevent not only pregnancy but also STIs, including HIV, when used consistently and correctly (Warren, 2000). Focus groups of girls and boys age 15–20 years, however, did not classify the female condom as "female controlled" (Latka et al., 2008).

Research Advances in Treatment

About half of unintended pregnancies end in abortion; therefore, contraception could reduce not only unintended pregnancy rates but also abortion rates and rates of STIs with some methods (IOM, 1995). The IOM report *The Best Intentions: Unintended Pregnancy and the Well-Being of Children and Families* discussed some of the potential medical and psychologic complications of surgical abortion. It stated that "whatever the risks associated with legal abortion in the United States, it remains a far less risky medical procedure for the woman than childbirth; over the 1979–1985 interval, for example, the mortality associated with childbirth was more than 10 times that of induced abortion" (IOM, 1995). It also stated that "abortion in the first trimester of pregnancy carries fewer risks to health than abortion in the second trimester of pregnancy and beyond." As reported by IOM (1995), "data show a total complication rate of induced abortion of less than 1 percent (Hakim-Elahi et al., 1990)."

A previous IOM committee, the Committee on Antiprogestins: Assessing the Science, reviewed the literature on the use of mifepristone (RU486) and other antiprogestins as medical abortifacients and for other potential uses (IOM, 1993). At the time, RU-486 in combination with prostaglandin was approved for early-pregnancy abortions in France, Sweden, and the United Kingdom, and the committee noted the "vast world literature with more than 60,000 patients treated in France" and stated that "repetition of large Phase 3 trials in the United States (to demonstrate efficacy and document side effects) does not appear necessary." For second-trimester pregnancies, that committee recommended "conducting clinical trials in the United States to compare the established surgical procedure of dilation and evacuation (D&E) both to antiprogestins in combination with prostaglandins and to prostaglandins used alone" (IOM, 1993). FDA approved mifepristone as an abortifacient in 2000. Since that time four medical abortion regimens—mifepristone and misoprostol pills, mifepristone pills and vaginal misoprostol, methotrexate and vaginal misoprostol, and vaginal misoprostol alone—have received FDA approval for use in the United States. A number of studies have been conducted to compare the safety and efficacy of different forms of medical abortions (Creinin et al., 1997).

Knowledge Gaps

Substantial advances have been made in contraceptive technology, but rates of unintended pregnancy remain high in the United States. In 2001, the 49% of all pregnancies that were unintended resulted in 1.4 million births, 1.3 million induced abortions, and an estimated 400,000 miscarriages (Frost et al., 2008). The United States has higher rates of unintended pregnancy than other developed countries, such as France (33%) and Scotland (28%) (Trussell and Wynn, 2008). The rates are highest in black and Hispanic women. The reason for the discrepancy in rates between the United States and other developed countries is not well understood (IOM, 2009).

Despite the development of modern contraceptive methods over the last several decades, high rates of unintended pregnancy are unabated, and it is clear that there is a need not only to develop new and improved contraceptive methods, including non-hormonal contraceptives, but also to ensure that existing methods are more available and accessible and used more effectively. The IOM (2004b) has created a blueprint for action on contraceptive development that this committee endorses. The blueprint includes recommendations for setting priorities for research and other activities in three main categories: (1) identifying and validating novel contraceptive targets; (2) enhancing contraceptive drug discovery, development, and clinical testing; and (3) facilitating and coordinating implementation of contraceptive research and development. Development of new contraceptives remains slow even after the publication of that report, and decreased research and development activities at pharmaceutical companies provide little optimism that new contraceptives are on the horizon (Aitken et al., 2008). The IOM (2009) has also evaluated the Title X program, which is the only federal program in the United States that is devoted exclusively to providing family-planning services. In addition to the recommendations in the 2009 report, which the present committee endorses, the committee urges more research on how to strengthen services for the provision of contraceptive methods especially in women at greatest risk. Such health-services research should set priorities for the strengthening of service delivery systems not only through Title X, Medicaid, and the rest of the public sector, but also through the private sector. Important research gaps also remain in understanding the behavioral issues surrounding successful contraceptive use, and further behavioral-science research to address these gaps is warranted in both men and women.[19] The work should include studies of the use of contraceptive methods for dual protection, that is, protection against both pregnancy and STIs, including HIV. Finally, although numerous epidemiologic investigations have demonstrated the safety of available contraceptives for healthy women, few studies of the safety of contraceptive use by women with medical disorders are available, and this gap should be addressed.

Lessons Learned

Unintended pregnancy is an example of a condition for which safe and effective prevention and treatment are available, but these are enmeshed in social and political controversies that are barriers to their use. A high proportion of pregnancies in the United States are unintended (unwanted or mistimed). Reducing that proportion will improve the health of women and children and will have important benefits to families and society in general. Progress in reducing unintended pregnancies will require not only making contraceptive methods more available, accessible, and acceptable through improved services, but also the development of new methods that meet additional needs.

Maternal Mortality and Morbidity

Although the US maternal mortality and morbidity rates have declined dramatically during the 20th century, they have decreased little over the past 2 decades. The committee, therefore, considers maternal mortality and morbidity to be a condition for which research over the past 2 decades has made little progress.

Incidence, Prevalence, and Mortality in Women

Although the United States experienced marked reductions in maternal mortality in the last century—from 607.9 deaths per 100,000 live births in 1915 to 12.1 in 2003 (Hoyert, 2007)—1 to 2 women die each day of pregnancy complications in the United States (CDC, 2008e). Recently maternal mortality in the

---

[19]Some determinants of unintended pregnancy, including violence against women and sexual risk behavior, are discussed as determinants in Chapter 2.

United States has been increasing—12.1 per 100,000 live births in 2003, 13.1 in 2004, and 15.1 in 2005—although it is unclear whether the increase is real or a result of improved reporting.[20] As many as half of all pregnancy-related deaths in the United States are preventable (CDC, 2008e). The leading causes of pregnancy-related death in the United States are embolism, hemorrhage, and other medical conditions (Berg et al., 2003).

Of the nearly 4 million women in the United States who give birth each year, nearly 30% experience complications (Berg et al., 2009). Little progress is noted in achieving the Healthy People 2010 objective of no more than 24 deliveries with intrapartum complications per 100 deliveries. A study of maternal morbidity based on data from the National Hospital Discharge Survey for 1993–1997 and 2001–2005 concluded that the rate of obstetrical complications remained unchanged at 28.6% (Berg et al., 2009). In addition, surveys show increases in the rate of pregnancies complicated by preexisting medical conditions and in the rate of cesarean deliveries (from 21% of births during the mid-1990s to 32% in 2007) (Menacker and Hamilton, 2010).

Disparities Among Groups

Marked disparities in the risk of maternal death remain in the United States. In 2007, in non-Hispanic blacks there were 28.4 deaths per 100,000 live births compared to 10.5 among non-Hispanic whites and 8.9 among Hispanic women (Xu et al., 2010).

Knowledge Gaps

Every effort should be made to ensure that the outcome of each and every labor and delivery in the United States is a healthy newborn–mother tandem, and Healthy People 2010 strives for no more than 3.3 maternal deaths (defined as deaths or complications leading to death that occur within 42 days of birth or the termination of pregnancy) per 100,000 live births (HHS, 2000). That goal, and goals for maternal morbidity, remains unattained. Determining the best ways to reduce maternal mortality and morbidity should have high priority in research.

Alcohol- and Drug-Addiction Disorders

There has been some progress in understanding sex and gender differences in alcohol- and drug-addiction disorders over the last 20 years, but the prevalence of addiction in women has not decreased and in some groups has increased. There

---

[20]It is likely that the introduction of the *International Classification of Diseases, Tenth Revision* in 1999, and the addition of a question regarding pregnancy to the Standard Certificate of Death, have improved the reporting of maternal deaths in the United States.

is a dearth of well-designed studies on gender-specific approaches to addiction treatment, and knowledge gained from research has not been applied.

Incidence, Prevalence, and Mortality in Women

According to the Office of National Drug Control Policy (2006), there has been a dramatic increase in substance use and misuse, delinquency, and health problems in girls and women since 1992. Although illicit-drug abuse and alcohol- and drug-addiction disorders have traditionally been more prevalent in men than in women, the gap has narrowed over the last decades (Holdcraft and Iacono, 2004; Keyes et al., 2008). Women now make up 40% of cocaine users, and this reflects a sharp increase in the last decade (SAMHSA, 2005). Although generally women begin using substances later than men, women have consistently been found to have heightened vulnerability to the adverse effects of substance abuse (Brady et al., 2009), and they move more quickly to dependence (telescoping) and manifestation of the adverse health effects of alcohol (Diehl et al., 2007; Greenfield, 2002).

The prevalence of alcohol dependence or addiction is higher in men than in women; 5.42–10.4% and 2.32–4.9%, respectively (Grant et al., 2004; Tetrault et al., 2008). Grant and colleagues (2004) found an increase in dependence rates in black women 18–29 years old. With respect to drug abuse or addiction, 2007 data indicate that drug dependence or abuse is higher in men than in women (3.8% and 1.8%, respectively) (SAMHSA, 2008).

Disparities Among Groups

The prevalence of alcohol dependence and addiction in women varies with race and ethnicity. American Indian women have the highest rate, 4.49%, followed by 2.39, 2.37, 1.94, and 1.34% in black, white, Hispanic, and Asian women, respectively (Grant et al., 2004). Trends indicate a convergence in the male:female ratio for alcohol abuse and dependence in the younger cohorts that is seen in all races and ethnicities except blacks (Grant et al., 2004; Keyes et al., 2008). While there is no consistent evidence of racial/ethnic disparities in rates of drug abuse or dependence, the consequences (e.g., HIV/AIDS, incarceration) of drug abuse and dependence appear to be more severe among racial/ethnic minorities (HHS, 2003). Similarly, although the rates of alcohol abuse are lower among older populations, the risks for morbidity and mortality from alcohol abuse are greater in this group (Cummings et al., 2008).

Research Advances in Knowledge of Biology

A number of physiologic sex differences have been explored to explain those differences. Animal studies have shown the role of sex hormones in the brain affecting, for example, the hippocampus, the amygdala, the anterior cingulate cortex, and the orbital frontal cortex (Goldstein et al., 2002). Human studies using functional imaging find differences in neural responses of men and women to rewards that are mediated, in part, by sex steroids and by different responses to drug cues between men and women with cocaine addictions (Kilts et al., 2004).

Neuroactive gonadal steroid hormones (such as estradiol, estriol, estrone, and dehydroepiandrosterone) also mediate effects in the brain. For example, evidence suggests that the extent of cocaine dependence (that is, the extent of cravings) in cocaine-dependent women correlates with the concentrations of progesterone and estradiol during the different phases of the menstrual cycle (Fox et al., 2008). Stress-induced relapses occur more frequently in women than in men, and the physiologic response to stress is different between cocaine-addicted men and women and between cocaine-addicted people and controls (Fox et al., 2005).

Sex differences have been found in pharmacokinetics and pharmacodynamics of alcohol. The difference is mainly due to sex differences in the activity of a key biotransformation enzyme (alcohol dehydrogenase) that is responsible for alcohol metabolism (Baraona et al., 2001). Women also have a slower transit time in the gastrointestinal tract (Baraona et al., 2001).

Research Advances in Prevention

Risk factors for drug abuse among women and girls include depression, posttraumatic stress disorder, self-destructive tendencies, delinquent predisposition, physical and mental health problems, family and social environment, having a partner who uses drugs, and childhood trauma and abuse (Becker and Grilo, 2006; Bukstein et al., 1992; Chatham et al., 1999; Hser et al., 1987; Langan and Pelissier, 2001).

Because alcohol use often co-occurs with use of other substances, many interventions are designed to prevent substance use and abuse in general. The Center for Substance Abuse Prevention funded 25 projects on substance-abuse prevention for adolescent girls. Qualitative data suggested that girls responded favorably to the programs, but significant changes in substance use were not found, possibly because of insufficient power and lack of specificity (Guthrie and Flinchbaugh, 2001). Currently the Substance Abuse and Mental Health Services Administration (SAMHSA) National Registry of Evidence-Based Programs and Practices lists only one program, the Athletes Targeting Healthy Exercise and Nutrition Alternatives (ATHENA) program, which is specifically designed for and targeted to girls. The school-based program targets middle- and high-school female athletes with interventions for substance abuse and other unhealthy behaviors, such as eating disorders. Reports to SAMHSA show that marijuana and alcohol use at 1-year followup were statistically lower in the schools with ATHENA than in those without it (HHS, 2007).

There is a paucity of research on gender differences in intervention effectiveness (Blake et al., 2001). Existing substance-use prevention does not systematically address risk factors for girls and young women, or the etiological factors related to substance use and misuse, delinquency and related health problems by gender (Kumpfer et al., 2008). Adolescent girls have not been recruited for interventions at the same rate as boys and have had lower retention in prevention interventions (Guthrie and Flinchbaugh, 2001). The efficacy of prevention approaches may vary by gender. The ALERT Plus program for at risk adolescents was efficacious only for girls (Longshore et al., 2007), while a universal prevention educational curriculum showed lower benefits for girls than for boys (Vigna-Taglianti et al., 2009).

Research Advances in Diagnosis and Treatment

There have not been any major advances in the diagnosis or treatment of substance-use disorders in women. The same DSM criteria are used for both men and women. Gender differences in treatment need, use, and outcomes have been found but have not been translated into new treatments in women.

Although 10% of women of reproductive age need treatment for substance-use problems, 85% of those who need treatment do not receive or perceive the need for treatment. Not being ready to stop use, not being able to pay for treatment, and the stigma associated with addiction are the major reasons why women do not receive treatment (SAMHSA, 2008). A higher proportion of men than of women are referred into treatment through the criminal-justice system (Grella, 2008) and receive family support for entering treatment (Grella and Joshi, 1999). In contrast, more women access treatment by referrals from community agencies and by referrals associated with receiving a diagnosis of antisocial personality disorder, having engaged in sex work, or having initiated treatment oneself (Grella, 2008). Women rely more on public insurance for payment, and this makes them more vulnerable to public-policy changes that reduce eligibility and funding (Grella, 2008).

Although women enter treatment after fewer years of substance use than men, they tend to have more severe clinical profiles, particularly mood and anxiety disorders; more family conflict and parenting challenges; a much greater proportion of past and current physical and sexual abuse; and more problems related to lack of employment, education, and vocational skills (Brady et al., 1993; Stewart et al., 2003).

Minority-group women and men receive a lower level of care than non-Hispanic whites and are more likely to get such services via the criminal-justice system and informal sectors of substance-abuse treatment (Perron et al., 2009).

Women's treatment adherence and retention has been associated with patient demographics (for example, marital status), psychosocial characteristics (for example, psychiatric comorbidity and history of trauma), and treatment-program characteristics (Greenfield and Pirard, 2009). Clinical studies that investigated the possibility of sex differences in treatment retention and completion have shown mixed results, and population-based studies have reported few or no differences in treatment retention (Greenfield and Pirard, 2009).

There is little evidence that gender is an important predictor of treatment outcomes, but there is evidence of gender differences in the factors that predict treatment outcomes (Greenfield, 2002; Grella, 2008). Co-occurring mental-health disorders and history of abuse are two factors that might have more adverse effects on the prognosis of substance-abuse disorders in women (Greenfield and Pirard, 2009).

Women might benefit more from some services, for example receipt of mental-health services has a positive effect in posttreatment, reducing drug use by women but not by men (Marsh et al., 2004). A number of other gender differences have been reported in factors related to risk of relapse. Relapse in women is associated with not living with their children, depression, stressful marital relationships, and partners' pressure to use substances (Grella, 2008).

Gender-specific addiction treatment has been developed and some studies suggest that women in programs that provide gender-specific treatment of addiction may stay in treatment longer and have better outcomes than those in non–gender-specific programs (Grella, 2008). Treatment completion and outcomes are better in women who receive residential services where they can be housed with their children, and in outpatient treatment that includes family therapy, family services, individual counseling, comprehensive support services, health and social services, and transportation (Grella, 2008).

Few studies have adequately assessed the effectiveness of gender-specific compared with mixed-gender treatments in women. Controlled randomized studies of treatment outcomes have not been conducted, only a small number of treatment outcomes have been studied, there is a lack of standardized measures and definitions of treatment factors and outcomes, and few studies have assessed long-term outcomes (Greenfield and Pirard, 2009; Grella, 2008).

Knowledge Gaps

There has been a dearth of research on the efficacy of gender-specific approaches for prevention of and treatment for addiction disorders, and there is a substantial gap in research on the efficacy of existing prevention and treatment approaches for racial and ethnic minorities populations. Social and cultural differences among subgroups of women are highly relevant for the course of addiction, its treatment, and the recovery process, and how to best address those differences is not known. Finally, there is a clear need to develop and test approaches that facilitate access to and increase use of treatment services by girls and women who need such services.

Lessons Learned

Research on drug addiction highlights the importance of co-occurring disorders and history of trauma in women, and of women's social roles as mothers and their lower socioeconomic status in relation to vulnerability to addiction and to its treatment.

In addition, although the specific roles of sex differences in brain anatomy, neurobiology, pharmacokinetics and pharmacodynamics, menstrual cycle, gonadal steroid hormones, and stress response in addiction are not yet elucidated, these research avenues highlight how much can be learned about a disease and its pathophysiology by exploring sex differences at many diffent levels. The value of diverse studies—of cells, animals, and humans—is evident from the breadth and depth of information generated not only on addiction, but on sex differences and brain function in general.

Autoimmune Diseases

As a group, autoimmune diseases are the third-most common diseases in the United States, following heart disease and cancer. They affect 5–8% of the population,[21] and over 78% of those affected are women (Fairweather et al., 2008). By the age of 50 years, 5–10% of women in the United States have autoimmunity. There have been advances in knowledge over the last 15–20 years about the etiology and pathophysiology of autoimmune diseases in women, but they have not yet led to effective treatments beyond treating for the symptoms. The diseases remain a major cause of morbidity in women. The committee discusses autoimmune diseases in general in this section, using examples when appropriate. The committee considers autoimmune diseases to be a category on which there has been little progress.

Incidence, Prevalence, and Mortality in Women

Many forms of autoimmunity affect women almost exclusively (see Table 3-1). Ulcerative colitis, diabetes mellitus, and myocarditis are exceptions; these occur in men either as often as or more often than in women (Rubtsov et al., 2010). Autoimmune diseases include many forms of arthritis that affect primarily

---

[21]Autoimmune diseases are a group of about 50 diseases in which the immune system abnormally recognizes self-tissues or proteins as foreign, turns on itself, and attacks an organ in the body (Palm and Medzhitov, 2009). The classification of autoimmune diseases has typically been dictated by the clinical presentation of the end organ that is being destroyed or injured. For instance, if the end organ is the pancreas, the disease is type 1 diabetes, and the patient will see an endocrinologist. If the immune system attacks the joints, the disease is rheumatoid arthritis, and the patient will see a rheumatologist. Any organ can be the subject of autoimmune attack, and the list of autoimmune diseases numbers more than 80 (Fairweather et al., 2008).

TABLE 3-1 Incidence Ratio of Autoimmunity Based on Sex

	Female:Male
Thyroid disease (Hashimoto's)	10:1
Graves disease	7:1
Sjogren's syndrome	9:1
Lupus	8:1
Rheumatoid arthritis	2.5:1
Scleroderma	3:1
Multiple sclerosis	3:1

SOURCE: AARDA (2010).

women—such as lupus, arthritis, fibromyalgia, and rheumatoid arthritis. Greater female vulnerability to autoimmunity is seen in animals. For instance, female mice are more prone to type 1 diabetes (in the nonobese diabetic [NOD] mouse model) and to Sjogren syndrome than male mice (Quintana and Cohen, 2001).

Autoimmune diseases affect women in the prime of their lives and can have a major impact on their quality of life (Gale and Gillespie, 2001); they are associated with high health-care costs and loss of productivity (Lau and Mak, 2009). The effects of autoimmune diseases were highlighted in a report to Congress that stated that "virtually all [autoimmune diseases] are debilitating, and require lifelong medical care. Although treatments exist for many autoimmune diseases, we do not yet have definitive cures for any of them. As a result, autoimmune diseases impose a heavy financial and emotional burden on patients and their families, and contribute significantly to our rising national health care costs" (HHS, 2005). There is evidence that the impact of rheumatoid arthritis on work disability is greater in women than in men (Wallenius et al., 2009).

Disparities Among Groups

Some autoimmune diseases are more common in black, American Indian, and Latina women than in white women (AARDA, 2010). For example, black women are 3 times more likely to have lupus than white women. In contrast, arthritis is most common in non-Hispanic white women (27.2%) followed by non-Hispanic black women (23.5%). Asian women (11.5%) had the lowest prevalence of arthritis (HRSA, 2008).

Research Advances in Knowledge of Biology

The 2001 IOM report *Exploring the Biological Contributions to Human Health: Does Sex Matter?* summarized potential environmental, hormonal, genetic, and life-stage causes of autoimmunity and evaluated the evidence that those causes would differ between the sexes. The report concluded that although environmental factors (for example, drug-induced cases of lupus and toxin-induced scleroderma-like disease), hormones, and genetics all affect the immune system and could play a role in some of the differences, none can fully account for sex differences in the more common, idiopathic autoimmune diseases (IOM, 2001b). With respect to life-stage causes of autoimmunity, the report stated that "most diseases that are predominantly in females cluster in the young-adult years, whereas autoimmune diseases that affect younger or older patients are more evenly divided between the sexes" (IOM, 2001b). Since that report, further work has explored the pathophysiology of autoimmunity and the underlying causes of sex differences in autoimmunity.

Over the last 20 years, research on autoimmune diseases has taken advantage of novel molecular-biology techniques, including transgenic and knockout mice that are susceptible to autoimmune diseases, to explore the genetic components of autoimmunity (see Alarcon-Riquelme, 2007, for review). Research has examined complement-system–related genetic differences in autoimmune diseases, and some data suggest a partial role of the complement system in susceptibility and disease severity (Murray et al., 2007; Yu and Whitacre, 2004). A role for micro-chimerism[22] has also been suggested (Ando and Davies, 2003; Sarkar and Miller, 2004). Because of the higher prevalence of autoimmune diseases in women, the role of the X chromosome in autoimmune diseases has been explored, especially its inactivation patterns (Invernizzi et al., 2008, 2009). No genetic difference has yet been identified to which any autoimmune disease or the predisposition of women to autoimmune diseases can be fully attributable. The etiology of auto-immune diseases is probably a complex interaction of more than one gene and environmental factors in the broad sense (Alarcon-Riquelme, 2007).

In both the NOD mouse model of autoimmunity and in humans who have Sjogren's syndrome, there is dysregulation at the level of translation of the LMP2 proteasome protein (Yan et al., 1997). Without a fully functional proteasome there is interruption in T-cell education to self-proteins expressed in the major histocompatibility complex (MHC) class I surface protein and interruption of the critical regulators of life and death balance for T-cell selection (Faustman et al., 1991; Hayashi and Faustman, 1999).

The role of hormones in sex differences in autoimmunity, especially the role of the ER, has also been studied (Ackerman, 2006). Until the late 1990s, only a single type of ER, ER-α, was thought to exist. That receptor is localized to the reproductive organs, mammary glands, bone, cardiovascular system, and some brain regions (Couse et al., 1997). The gene for a second type of ER, ER-β, has been identified, and research has demonstrated that it is distributed in a wide

---

[22]"Microchimerism is the presence of a low level of non-host stem cells or their progeny in an individual. The most common source of microchimerism is pregnancy" (Sarkar and Miller, 2004).

variety of tissues (Kuiper et al., 1996, 1997; Mosselman et al., 1996). With the discovery of that receptor has come the demonstration that estrogen can influence the development and function of CD4(+) T-helper immune cells (Pernis, 2007). Research in murine models of systemic lupus erythematosus (SLE) and other autoimmune diseases has also found differences in the ER between mice that get autoimmune diseases and mice that do not (Greenstein et al., 2001).

As reviewed by Invernizzi and colleagues (2008), research over the last 20 years has investigated whether X-chromosome inactivation could play a role in autoimmunity. For example, women who have primary billiary cirrhosis, systemic sclerosis, and autoimmune thyroid disease have enhanced X monosomy in blood lymphoctyes (Invernizzi et al., 2004, 2005). The potential role of X-chromosome inactivation, X-chromosome monosomy, and preferential loss of an X-chromosome in autoimmune diseases remains unclear (Invernizzi et al., 2009).

Differences have also been seen in risk of rejection of transplanted organs, depending on the sex of the donor and the sex of the recipient. Female recipients of male kidneys had greater risks of graft failure after transplantation, but not beyond the 10-year mark (Kim and Gill, 2009). H–Y antigen mismatch underlies the effect (Kim and Gill, 2009).

Research Advances in Prevention

Environment has always been considered a risk factor for autoimmunity, with gene–environment interactions thought to be potentially important (Cooper et al., 1999). For example, vitamin D has been proposed to play a role in autoimmune disease (Szodoray et al., 2008). People living in northern climates have a higher risk of autoimmunity, such as multiple sclerosis, than people of the same ethnicity living near the equator (Beretich and Beretich, 2009; Kulie et al., 2009; Kurtzke, 1975). Many have speculated that that could be related to vitamin D deficiencies in people who live in northern climates (Ascherio and Munger, 2007; Ebers, 2009). At the cellular level, vitamin D is obligatory for many steps in T-cell education, including steps related to the activation of NFkB, the main controlling protein for life–death decisions in T-cell education (Mahon et al., 2003).[23] It has been speculated that the exposure of the immune system to a broader range of parasites and infections is beneficial in shaping the immune system to prevent self-reactivity (Kaufman, 2010). Thus, the hygiene theory postulates that the cleanliness of civilization may contribute to the increasing incidence of autoimmunity and allergies. There are also intestinal forms of autoimmunity, such as celiac disease, that are triggered by wheat in food but for wheat to trigger or exacerbate the disease, a person must have an altered set point and predisposition for autoimmunity. Many clustered cases of autoimmunity have been considered to

---

[23]An IOM committee is currently updating the recommended dietary intake of vitamin D; that report will include an evaluation of the role of vitamin D in chronic diseases.

be secondary to viruses, although most of the evidence is circumstantial. Viruses can interfere with the MHC class I education pathway for self–non-self T-cell recognition (Cohn, 2008).

SLE is an autoimmune rheumatic disease that is often severe and is most commonly diagnosed in women in their childbearing years. Exposure of genetically predisposed people to one or more environmental triggers, such as Epstein-Barr virus, is thought to mediate the development of SLE (Simard and Costenbader, 2007). Stress caused by life events also may trigger or exacerbate autoimmunity, as is reported frequently in SLE patients (Karasawa et al., 2005).

Research Advances in Diagnosis

A survey commissioned by the American Autoimmune Related Diseases Association shows that it takes an average of 4 years for a correct diagnosis of an autoimmune disease to be made, an average of 4.04 physicians are seen before the diagnosis is made, and over 45% of the women who received a diagnosis of autoimmune diseases had been told that they were chronic complainers or were too concerned with their health (AARDA, 2010). Those statistics point to the need for more awareness of autoimmune diseases and for better training in medical school. There is no course syllabus for autoimmune diseases in general for physicians or nurses.

Research Advances in Treatment

Over the last 4 years, many new treatments for autoimmunity have emerged. Most of them work to suppress the immune system, because clinical therapies with more restricted targets have failed. However, lifelong and systemic immunosuppressive drugs are not only extremely expensive but associated with drug-induced complications—side effects on the normal parts of the immune system (Uetrecht, 2009).

Knowledge Gaps

Despite some progress in understanding the immune system and the pathophysiology of autoimmunity, there is no confirmed mechanism that explains why women are affected more than men by autoimmune disease, either for a single autoimmune disease or for them as a group. Furthermore, most medications used to treat people for these diseases are lifelong expensive treatments. Elucidation of the differences in the etiology and pathophysiology of these disorders is important because it might allow more to be done to protect women from autoimmune diseases, at least to the same degree as men.

Lessons Learned

The extensive morbidity and associated effects of autoimmune diseases on women's quality of life highlight the need to look beyond mortality as an end point in researching women's health. The importance of awareness among physicians of the signs, symptoms, and prevalence of diseases in women to improve the time between onset of symptoms and diagnosis is also evident from autoimmune disease.

Dementia of the Alzheimer Type and Other Dementias

Of all of the chronic, progressive age-associated diseases that threaten the lives, dignity, and independence of elderly women, perhaps none is more dreaded than dementia; dementia of the Alzheimer type (Alzheimer's disease) is the leading type of dementia (Golanska et al., 2009).

Incidence, Prevalence, and Mortality in Women

About 4.8% of women 71–79 years old have dementia, a figure that rises to 27.8% between 80–89 years old and 34.7% at or after the age of 90 years (Plassman et al., 2007). The overall age-adjusted risk is about 50% higher in women than in men (Bachman et al., 1992; Canadian Study of Health and Aging, 1994; Launer et al., 1999), but the sex difference appears to lie principally in the overall increased average longevity of women (Hebert et al., 2001; Plassman et al., 2007). That increased longevity also means that women often outlive their partners and therefore have a high probability of having lost a member of their family support network by the time their Alzheimer's disease is manifested. Research to delay or prevent dementia in aging women has high priority in women's health research.

Research Advances in Knowledge of Biology

An active field of research in Alzheimer's disease is the investigation of extracellular beta-amyloid plaques and neurofibrillary tangles—the pathologic findings used by Alzheimer over a century ago to characterize the disease (Lannfelt et al., 1995). Research includes their roles in the pathophysiology of Alzheimer's disease and how to modulate the rate of production, polymerization, solubility, and clearance of the beta-amyloid protein that accumulates in the plaques in the extracellular brain environment (Lannfelt et al., 1995). In vitro and animal experiments (including genetically engineered animal models) have examined the contributions of genetics, enzyme activities, apoptotosis, hormones, metabolism, and such other forces as the oxidative stress and inflammation that occur with aging to the clinical manifestations of Alzheimer's disease.

Researchers have investigated the role of sex hormones, especially estrogen, in women's susceptibility to Alzheimer's disease and dementia. Results of basic-science research, small clinical trials, and cohort studies of aging communities before the WHI suggested a potential role of post-menopausal estrogen therapy (estrogen or estrogen plus progestin) in attenuating the risk of cognitive dysfunction in older women (Ancelin and Ritchie, 2005). Therefore, a substudy of the WHI, the Women's Health Initiative Memory Study (WHIMS), was conducted; it specifically examined the effect of hormone therapy—combined conjugated equine estrogen (CEE) plus medroxyprogesterone acetate or CEE alone in women with prior hysterectomy—in 4,532 WHI participants over 65 years old who did not have cognitive impairment at baseline (Shumaker et al., 2004). Annual Mini-Mental Status Examinations (MMSE) conducted over an average of 4.2 years revealed not only revealed no tendency toward stabilization of cognitive function in participants on hormone replacement but some greater declines in MMSE results in women who had lower baseline scores and received CEE. Some current research on this issue is being conducted in women closer to the menopausal transition, examining whether there is a critical window for hormone therapy (Sherwin, 2003), but some researchers have little enthusiasm for female-hormone replacement in the prevention of dementia and Alzheimer's disease in aging post-menopausal women (Markou et al., 2005).

Studies of whether specific cognitive domains (for example, verbal abilities and memory) are differentially affected by sex have had mixed results. Genetic factors might confound the role of estrogen in Alzheimer's disease (MacLusky, 2004). For example, there could be interactions between estrogen and the apolipoprotein e4 phenotype (either heterozygous or homozygous) (MacLusky, 2004). Depression, a disease that is also more common in women than in men, is frequently associated with Alzheimer's disease, especially at its initial presentation and in early stages (Migliorelli et al., 1995). It is unknown, however, whether the etiology and pathophysiology of the two conditions are related.

Knowledge Gaps

There have been few major advances in the diagnosis and detection of or treatment for dementia and Alzheimer's disease. Early onset dementia, however, is often misdiagnosed as Alzheimer's disease rather than due to vascular dementias, frontotemporal lobar degenerations, traumatic head injury, or alcohol-related dementia, and that misdiagnosis can have adverse effects on outcomes (Mendez, 2006). A basic understanding of its pathogenesis is lacking, despite improved understanding of the role of plaques and tangles in Alzheimer's disease. Much work remains to identify risk factors, clarify any potential roles of hormones, and improve treatments. To make progress in Alzheimer's disease or dementia, a major scientific research thrust needs to occur, as has occurred for other diseases where progress has been made. Research needs to provide evidence on the natural history of the disease, identification of risk factors to lead to prevention efforts, biomarkers for diagnosis, and measurement of the efficacy of new treatments.

Lessons Learned

The severely debilitating effects of Alzheimer's disease and other dementias emphasize the importance of looking beyond mortality end points to improve quality of life and to consider health and prevention over the entire lifetime to identify ways earlier in life to prevent such conditions as Alzheimer's later in life.

Gynecologic Cancers Other Than Cervical Cancer

The committee considers gynecologic cancers other than cervical cancer— corpus and uterine cancer, as well as ovarian cancer—to be a category of diseases in which there has been little progress over the last 20 years. Few gains have been made on improving survival rates.

Incidence, Prevalence, and Mortality in Women

Corpus and uterine cancer, most of which is endometrial cancer and will be referred to as such here, are the most common cancers of the female reproductive organs. It is estimated that there will be 42,160 new cases of endometrial cancer in the United States in 2009 (ACS, 2009d; NCI, 2009b). Most cases occur in women over 55 years old; the median age at diagnosis was 62 years and the median age at death was 72 years of age in 2002–2006 (NCI, 2009b). The American Cancer Society (ACS, 2009d) estimates that about 7,780 women in the United States will have died from endometrial cancer during 2009.

Ovarian cancer is the ninth-most common cancer in women (not counting skin cancer) and the fifth-leading cause of cancer death in women in the United States. It is estimated that there will have been 21,880 new cases of ovarian cancer and 13,850 deaths from it in the United States in 2010 (ACS, 2010b). Most women who have ovarian cancer receive the diagnosis when they are 60 years old or older (ACS, 2010b). Only modest gains have been made in survival of ovarian cancer over the last few decades (Cho and Shih Ie, 2009). Although the 5-year survival rate of women who receive the diagnosis in early stages (localized) of the disease is > 93%, women who are in an advanced stage (distant, cancer has metastasized) have a 5-year survival rate of < 28% (NCI, 2010d).

Disparities Among Groups

Endometrial cancer is more common in white women than black women (incidence, 24.4 per 100,000 in white women and 20.6 per 100,000 in black women), but black women are more likely to die from it (mortality, 7.2 per 100,000 and 3.9 per 100,000 for black and white women, respectively) (NCI, 2010e). The incidence of and deaths from endometrial cancer are lower in Asian and Pacific Islander women, American Indian and Alaskan Native women, and Hispanic women (incidence rates 17.3, 16.8, and 17.6 per 100,000 respectively; mortality, 2.5, 2.9, and 3.0 per 100,000, respectively) (NCI, 2010e).

Research Advances in Knowledge of Biology

Research on endometrial cancer has investigated biomarkers on endometrial-cancer cells, including the progesterone receptor, IGFR I, retinaldehyde dehydrogenase type II, and secreted frizzled-related protein 4 (Boruban et al., 2008). Such biomarkers have not yet been adequately characterized for use in diagnosis or for the development of treatments.

Evidence indicates that there are genetic factors in ovarian cancer; risk is higher in women who have a history of ovarian or breast cancer in a first-degree relative (Clarke-Pearson, 2009). Ovarian cancers are classified by type and degree of differentiation, but their management is not targeted toward specific classes of these cancers. Recent data indicate that the different types of tumors might have different underlying pathology that could be considered in the development of targeted treatments (Cho and Shih Ie, 2009). The development of rapid phenotypic analyses through proteomics could lead to improved diagnostic, screening and therapeutic tools (Faca et al., 2009).

Research Advances in Prevention

Physical activity is associated with reduced risk of endometrial cancer; the risk in physically active women is 20–40% lower than in inactive women (Friedenreich et al., 2010). The greatest reduction in risk is among those who have the highest levels of physical activity (Kramer and Wells, 1996). Several of the studies, however, did not adjust for the postmenopausal use of unopposed estrogen, which increases endometrial cancer risk (NCI, 2009b). Physical activity may reduce risk through effects on hormones (Kramer and Wells, 1996) or by lowering body fat (AICR, 2007); a few studies have examined how body weight and physical activity interact to affect the incidence of endometrial cancer, but the findings have been too inconsistent to support conclusions (NCI, 2009b). Morbidly obese women who have endometrial cancer have a greater likelihood of dying from their comorbidities or their cancers than leaner women who have endometrial cancer (Fader et al., 2009).

The *BRCA2* gene mutation that greatly increases the risk of breast cancer also greatly increases the risk of ovarian cancer (Clarke-Pearson, 2009). Women who test positive for the *BRCA2* gene mutation, especially those who have had breast cancer, have the option of a bilateral oophorectomy to prevent ovarian cancer.

Studies of the role of physical activity in the prevention of ovarian cancer have yielded inconsistent results, ranging from a reduced risk of ovarian cancer with activity to no association or a slight increase in risk with greater activity (Bertone et al., 2001; Biesma et al., 2006; Mink et al., 1996). One study found that sedentary behavior increases risk, but it did not decrease with light or moderate physical activity (Patel et al., 2006a). Physical activity helps in managing weight, which may be a risk factor for ovarian cancer, but how weight is related to the development of ovarian cancer is not well understood (AICR, 2007).

There is "limited suggestive evidence" of an association between intake of nonstarchy vegetables and a decrease in ovarian cancer (AICR, 2007; IOM, 2003). A pooled analysis of 12 prospective studies, however, found only a nonsignificant decrease in risk in women who had the highest intake of nonstarchy vegetables (Koushik et al., 2005). Another review of 7 cohort and 27 case–control studies found some evidence that vegetable but not fruit consumption has beneficial effects on the risk of ovarian cancer. So far, evidence of a role of other dietary exposures in ovarian-cancer risk is largely inconclusive (AICR, 2007). A possible increased risk caused by high meat consumption has been observed (for example, Schulz et al., 2004). In the WHI dietary-modification trial, women randomized to a low-fat diet had a statistically significant 40% reduction in risk of ovarian cancer compared with women on a usual diet looking at the last 4.1 years of a 8.1-year followup (Prentice et al., 2007). Results did not appear to be affected by the weight loss experienced by the dietary-change group or by a family history of ovarian cancer (Prentice et al., 2007). The total number of ovarian-cancer cases was relatively small, however. Having low lifetime exposure to estrogen—including low exposure because of late menarche, bearing children, and early menopause—also reduces risk (ACS, 2009e; Barber, 1987; Gates et al., 2010; Hankinson et al., 1995; Jordan et al., 2005). Epidemiologic studies found that oral contraceptive use is protective against both endometrial and ovarian cancer (Deligeoroglou et al., 2003).

Research Advances in Diagnosis

Endometrial cancer is diagnosed histologically. Pathologists are sometimes inconsistent in their diagnosis of endometrial cancer (Boruban et al., 2008; Zaino et al., 2006).

Ovarian cancer is also diagnosed histologically (Cho and Shih Ie, 2009). Over two-thirds of ovarian-cancer cases have progressed to stage 3 or 4, which involves the peritoneal cavity or other organs, when diagnosed (Clarke-Pearson,

2009). There is no routine screening for ovarian cancer. Large randomized trials, such as the Prostate, Lung, Colon, and Ovarian Cancer Screening Trial (PLCO), give promise of determining the efficacy of ovarian-cancer screening for reducing mortality (Clarke-Pearson, 2009). Serum CA125 assay, physical examination, and imaging examination (transvaginal ultrasonography) have been used with differing schedules for followup of asymptomatic women who had a prior ovarian-cancer diagnosis, with increased CA125 indicative of relapse in 56–94% of cases (Gadducci and Cosio, 2009). However, transvaginal ultrasonography and measurement of serum antigen CA125 are not specific for ovarian cancer (Roett and Evans, 2009).

Research Advances in Treatment

Surgery followed by radiotherapy is the main treatment for localized endometrial cancer, the most common presentation of the disease (Deeks, 2007). The combination of chemotherapy and hormone therapy is standard for advanced and recurrent endometrial cancer (Chaudhry and Asselin, 2009). The development of minimally invasive surgical techniques has decreased morbidity and improved quality of life in women after hysterectomy (Fiorelli et al., 2008). Hogberg (2008) reviewed data from a phase III trial conducted by the Gynecologic Oncology Group that demonstrated improved survival but increased toxicity, depending on the treatment regimen used. Adjuvants have been shown to reduce locoregional recurrence in stage 1 disease but not the risk of death (Deeks, 2007).

Stage and histologic grade of cancer at diagnosis, presence or absence of residual disease at the completion of initial surgery, functional stage and age, and use or nonuse of platinum-based chemotherapy are all important prognostic factors for ovarian cancer (Clarke-Pearson, 2009). New surgery and treatments with combinations of cytotoxic drugs have improved 5-year survival rates, but the overall cure rate remains around 30% (Bast et al., 2009).

Knowledge Gaps

Despite the increased efficacy and decreased toxicity of treatments, few gains have been made over the last 20 years in survival rates of people who have advanced endometrial cancer. Most women who receive a diagnosis of ovarian cancer present with advanced disease, and their long-term survival remains low.

Lessons Learned

The lack of progress on gynecologic cancers highlights the need for continued research on women's health. The high mortality rate for some of these cancers that accompany a typical presentation with advanced-stage disease and poor prognosis highlight the disadvantages of not having a diagnostic test that allows early detection at a point in disease progression when therapy can save lives.

Gynecologic Disorders (Nonmalignant)

Nonmalignant gynecologic disorders are common in women. They include uterine fibroids, endometriosis, chronic pelvic pain, pelvic floor disorders (including pelvic organ prolapse), polycystic ovarian syndrome, and STIs.[24] These disorders cause morbidity in many women and greatly affect their quality of life. The committee considers there to have been little progress made against these conditions over the last 20 years, including in methods of detection and screening, as well as prognosis and therapy for those who develop the disease.

Incidence, Prevalence, and Mortality in Women

Uterine fibroids, or leiomyomas, are the most common solid pelvic tumors in women and cause symptoms in about 25% of women of reproductive age (Cramer and Patel, 1990). Data from several studies indicate that endometriosis affects up to 10% of women in the general population and up to 50% of premenopausal women, with a prevalence of 38% (range, 20–50%) in infertile women and in 71–87% in women who have chronic pelvic pain (Balasch et al., 1996; Carter, 1994; Koninckx et al., 1991; Ling, 1999). Of women of reproductive age, about 7% have hyperandrogenic chronic anovulation or polycystic ovarian syndrome (PCOS) (Azziz et al., 2004). An estimated one-third of all US women have some type of pelvic-floor disorder in their lifetimes. In a recent study, the weighted prevalence of at least one pelvic floor disorder was 23.7%, and 15.7% of these women experienced urinary incontinence (Nygaard et al., 2008). In a study of over 5,000 women 18–50 years old, about 15% had chronic pelvic pain in the last 3 months (Mathias et al., 1996). Finally, except for colds and influenza, STIs are the most common contagious diseases in the United States, and some are increasing in incidence, with millions of new cases of STIs each year (see Chapter 2).

Disparities Among Groups

Black women have an increased risk of uterine fibroids (Evans and Brunsell, 2007; Okolo, 2008) as well as a higher percentage of hysterectomies in women who are diagnosed with uterine fibroids (68% of black women diagnosed with uterine fibroids; 33% of white women) (Keshavarz et al., 2002). Black women have higher rates of chlamydiosis, gonorrhea, and primary and secondary syphilis than other racial or ethnic groups (CDC, 2008f). Those disparities are not ex-

---

[24]STIs other than HIV/AIDS are discussed in this section. HIV/AIDS is discussed earlier in this chapter.

plained by relationship and partner attributes (for example, marital history or sex with older, casual, and nonmonogamous partners (Harawa et al., 2003).

Research Advances in Knowledge of Biology

The primary cause and pathogenesis of uterine fibroids, and of racial dispari-ties in fibroid biology, remain largely unknown (Andersen, 1998; Chen et al., 2001). Endometriosis is understood to constitute a complex interaction between endometrial genes and hormones, but many questions remain. The etiology of PCOS, pelvic-floor disorders, and pelvic pain remains poorly understood, and there has been little advance in understanding the underlying biologic mecha-nisms of these conditions. Researchers have decoded the genetic makeup of several common STIs, and these may lead to new pathways for treatment and diagnosis and to a vaccine strategy (Carlton et al., 2007).

Research Advances in Prevention

No substantial advances have been made in preventing nonmalignant gyne-cologic disorders.

Research Advances in Diagnosis

There has been little advance in the diagnosis of many nonmalignant gyneco-logic conditions over the last 15 years. A detailed history, physical examination, and imaging studies remain the mainstay of diagnosis of gynecologic disorders. Genetic testing for nonmalignant gynecologic conditions has not been used because of a lack of understanding of potential targets. However, polymerase-chain-reaction testing has become more available for STIs and allow one-swab testing for multiple STIs.

Research Advances in Treatment

Although there has been very little advance in prevention, the treatment of gynecologic disorders has advanced. New medical and surgical treatments for uterine fibroids have evolved, although there is no defined gold standard on which to base practice (David and Ebert, 2005; Rougier-Chapman et al., 2001). A variety of grafts and meshes have recently been advocated for treatment for prolapse although a greater evidence base demonstrating the safety and effi-cacy of these products is needed (Silva and Karram, 2005). Pharmacologic and surgical treatment options are available for treatment for endometriosis, and new medical treatments—such as the levonorgestrel intrauterine device, selec-tive progesterone-receptor modulators, angiogenesis inhibitors, and aromatase inhibitors—have shown some promise in the last decade. A few options are available for treating PCOS and pelvic pain; treatment is largely symptom based and empirical (Chwalisz et al., 2004; Ferrero et al., 2009; Lockhat et al., 2004; Scarpellini et al., 2002).

Hysterectomy is an invasive procedure with complication rates (including infection, hemorrhage, thromboembolism, injury to adjacent organs, and death) of 17 to 23% (Makinen et al., 2001) and long-term effects on psychosexual health (McPherson et al., 2005). Despite those complications and new alternate options, about 600,000 hysterectomies are performed every year in the United States, making it the second most frequent major surgical procedure among reproductive-aged women (CDC, 2004); fibroid tumors, endometriosis, and uterine prolapse are the three conditions most associated with hysterectomies (CDC, 2004).

More progress has been made with STIs. Over the last decade, over 60 substances were identified as potential intravaginal or rectal microbicides, and about one-fourth of them have reached various stages of human testing (Fleck, 2004; Ramjee et al., 2000). A number of studies have examined the safety, efficacy, and tolerability of topical microbicides in preventing STIs, and new vaccine strategies have evolved (Harwell et al., 2003; Mayer et al., 2001).

Knowledge Gaps

Research on nonmalignant gynecologic conditions is sparse. Little is known about their underlying biology or prevention and treatment strategies. No methods controlled by women for preventing STIs are available. STI rates are increasing in high-risk populations, and a goal of eradication of STIs or a more aggressive targeting of STIs may be a potential public-health strategy.

Lung Cancer

Despite substantial research on lung and bronchial cancer,[25] including studies that analyze data on women separately, little progress has been made in decreasing lung-cancer mortality in women. It remains the leading cause of cancer death in women in the United States, and there are few diagnostic, screening, and treatment options. The committee, therefore, considers lung cancer a disease where research has led to little progress against the disease.

Incidence, Prevalence, and Mortality in Women

Changing patterns of cigarette use led to greater increases in rates of lung cancer in women than in men; the rate in women increased by a factor of 4 from

---

[25]The term *lung cancer* will be used in this report to refer to lung and bronchial cancer.

the early 1960s to 2000 (Thomas et al., 2005).[26] In 2007, about one-fifth of US women 18 years old or older were current smokers[27] (CDC, 2008g). Lung cancer accounted for only 3% of female cancer deaths in 1950 and 25% in 2000 (HHS, 2001), and the estimate in 2008 is 26% (HRSA, 2008). Recent data indicate that death rates from lung cancer in women have leveled off since 2003 in some states and regions (Jemal et al., 2008).

The incidence of lung cancer is the second highest cancer incidence in women; there were an estimated 105,770 new cases in 2010, and the median age at diagnosis was 71. An estimated 71,080 women will die from lung cancer in the United States in 2010 at a median age of 72 years (NCI, 2010f).

Women and men with less than a high school education had a higher risk of lung cancer compared to college-educated women and men (Clegg et al., 2009). Similarly, women and men with an annual family income less than $12,500 had a significantly higher incidence of lung cancer compared to women and men with an annual family income of $50,000 or more (Clegg et al., 2009).

Disparities Among Groups

The incidence of lung cancer is similar in white and black women (54.7 per 100,000 and 54.8 per 100,000, respectively), but it is lower in American Indian and Alaskan Native women (39.7 per 100,000), Asian and Pacific Islander (28.1 per 100,000), and Hispanic women (25.4 per 100,000) (NCI, 2010f). Some evidence suggests that among cigarette-smokers, black and native Hawaiian women are more susceptible to lung cancer than white, Japanese American, and Latina women (Haiman et al., 2006). Lung-cancer incidence is also greater in those who have lower income (Clegg et al., 2009).

Many studies have demonstrated differences between blacks and whites in the lung-cancer treatment received (Farjah et al., 2009; Hardy et al., 2009). There were also great disparities in treatment between people in the highest socioeconomic quartile and older patients, women, and those in lower socioeconomic quartiles. The disparity (between blacks and whites) in treatment did not narrow much in the last 12 years. Factors other than doctors' recommendations—such as distrust, beliefs and perceptions about lung cancer and treatment for it, and lower access to care despite insurance—might be involved in racial disparities (Farjah et al., 2009).

Socioeconomic status plays a large role in mortality from lung cancer in both men and women. Lower education levels are associated with higher lung-cancer

---

[26]Lung-cancer deaths in men decreased over the same period; this reflects the decrease in men's smoking, which in earlier periods had been much higher than women's, but which has been declining faster than women's (see Chapter 2 for discussion of smoking).

[27]Defined as "those who smoked more than 100 cigarettes in their lifetime and now smoke every day or some days" (CDC, 2008g).

incidence and mortality (Alberg and Nonemaker, 2008; Clegg et al., 2009; Kinsey et al., 2008). Mortality from lung cancer decreased from 1993 to 2001 in people who had at least 16 years of education in every sex and race stratum except black women, whose mortality was stable; it increased in white women who had less than 12 years of education (Kinsey et al., 2008).

Research Advances in Understanding of Underlying Biology

It is unknown whether there are sex differences in the susceptibility to lung cancer (Planchard et al., 2009). A number of studies have found that women have a higher risk of lung cancer than men (Brownson et al., 1992; Harris et al., 1993; Henschke and Miettinen, 2004; Henschke et al., 2006; McDuffie et al., 1987; Osann et al., 1993; Risch et al., 1993; Zang and Wynder, 1996), but other studies have found no difference (Bain et al., 2004; Freedman et al., 2008; Kreuzer et al., 2000; Thun et al., 2002, 2008). A meta-analysis of data from the Nurses' Health Study and the Health Professionals Follow-Up Study found no sex difference in lung-cancer rates in women and men with comparable smoking histories (Bain et al., 2004).

Research has looked at a number of genetic and cellular differences that might play a role in potential sex differences in the susceptibility to and survival of lung cancer. The data are not clear and seem to vary among lung-cancer types, but there is some evidence that oncogene activity could play a role (Ahrendt et al., 2001; D'Amico et al., 2000; Nelson et al., 1999). Research has also looked at differences in gastrin-releasing peptide receptor (Shriver et al., 2000), HER-2/neu (Negro et al., 2004; Vallbohmer et al., 2006), PTHrP (Montgrain et al., 2007), cytochrome p450 1A1 expression (Dresler et al., 2000; Mollerup et al., 1999), and DNA-repair capacity (Spitz et al., 2003; Wei et al., 2000). Estrogen could also be involved; there is a variant of ERα in lung cells (Mollerup et al., 2002), and non–small-cell lung carcinoma (NSCLC) responds to estrogen (Stabile et al., 2002).

Research Advances in Prevention

Smoking is estimated to cause about 95% of lung cancer cases, so understanding the reasons that women initiate and continue smoking is critical (see Chapter 2). Given the high incidence of lung cancer in women, the cases not related to smoking still constitute a substantial public-health problem. Little is known about other preventive measures for lung cancer. Some research has demonstrated that diet affects susceptibility to lung cancer, especially in women (Cranganu and Camporeale, 2009).

Research Advances in Diagnosis

Posttreatment survival of lung cancer is much higher if it is diagnosed at an earlier stage, when tumors are smaller (ACS, 2009f). Asymptomatic people are not screened routinely for lung cancer (Smith et al., 2009), and the data are mixed as to whether screening of them would be effective. Some data indicate that screening increases 10-year survival (with a survival rate of 88%) (Henschke et al., 2006); other data show an increase in the number of new cases of lung cancer and the number of resections in a trial of computer tomographic scanning but no concomitant decrease in advanced lung cancer or in lung-cancer deaths (Bach et al., 2007)—a suggestion of the importance of how a screening method is assessed (Black and Baron, 2007). Two large clinical trials—the National Lung Screening Trial and the PLCO Cancer Screening Trial—are underway and it is hoped that they will clarify whether screening results in decreased mortality from lung cancer. Computer-aided detection can detect about half the lesions that are overlooked by initial interpretation by a radiologist, so it holds promise for improving lung-cancer screening (White and Spitz, 1993).

Research Advances in Treatment

The rate of survival of lung cancer (measured as years of survival after diagnosis or treatment) is better in women than in men, and women typically live longer after treatment (Henschke et al., 2006; Ouellette et al., 1998). Some suggest that stage at diagnosis underlies the differences (Ferguson et al., 2000), but others have found better overall survival in women even if they have inoperable NSCLC (McGovern et al., 2009; Visbal et al., 2004). The longer survival in women does not appear to be treatment specific, having been seen after radiotherapy (Werner-Wasik et al., 1999), chemotherapy (Albain et al., 1991; Lord et al., 2002; Simon et al., 2008; Tsao et al., 2006; Wheatley-Price et al., 2009; Yamamoto et al., 2008), and surgery (Bouchardy et al., 1999; Keller et al., 2002). Although Wheatley-Price and colleagues (2009) and Yamamoto and colleagues (2008) observed better survival in women after chemotherapy, they also noted its greater toxicity in women, which would affect their quality of life. Prognostic markers may be sex specific (Dannenberg et al., 2003).

Knowledge Gaps

Despite a large amount of research, including research in women, lung cancer remains the leading cause of cancer deaths in women; the 5-year survival rate if it is detected at a late stage, which occurs in 45% of patients, is 15% (Pearman, 2008). Study results on what sex differences exist are at times contradictory.

Lessons Learned

The increase in survival observed after some treatments (for example, resection) and the contradictory results of screening programs highlight the importance of clinical trials of early detection of lung cancer. The fact that many cases of lung cancer are considered preventable, that is, they would not have occurred in the absence of smoking, highlights the need for effective public-health interventions.

CONCLUSIONS

- For those conditions where substantial progress has been made in improving women's health—breast cancer, cardiovascular disease, and cervical cancer—there is a large and diverse body of research from the last 20 years, including basic research at the molecular, cellular and organ level; animal studies; observational studies; and small and large randomized controlled clinical trials (for example, the WHI). That research led to advances in the understanding of the underlying biology and pathophysiology of the disease, which in turn led to advances in the prevention and diagnosis of and treatment for those conditions in women. Research has resulted in improved diagnostic tests and screening for diseases such as breast and cervical cancer; vaccines against a virus that causes cervical cancer, making prevention of cervical cancer possible; new treatments for cardiovascular disease; and targeted therapies for breast cancer. Although much work remains and the incidence and mortality for some of those diseases remains high, those advances have led to decreases in prevalence (for example, of cervical cancer) or in mortality (for example, from breast cancer and cardiovascular disease).
- Fewer gains, however, have been made in many other conditions that affect women's health.
- Even for conditions where research has led to progress and improved health outcomes for women in general, disparities or inequities in that progress remain among groups of women, with some populations carrying a much greater burden of disease.
- Even when great progress has been made through scientific advances, other factors in or determinants of health can present barriers to improving women's health, such as the effects of societal beliefs or morals on the use of the vaccine for cervical cancer, social acceptance of and stigmas attached to depression, and use of and compliance with use of contraceptives to prevent unintended pregnancy.
- Knowledge about differences in the manifestation of diseases is crucial for further studies to identify the underlying biology of disease in women vs men and to develop appropriate prevention, diagnosis, and treatment strategies for women.

REFERENCES

AARDA (American Autoimmune Related Diseases Association) 2010. *Autoimmunity: A Major Women's Health Issue.* http://www.aarda.org/women_and_autoimmunity.php (accessed May 25, 2010).

Abbott, T. A., 3rd, B. J. Lawrence, and S. Wallach. 1996. Osteoporosis: The need for comprehensive treatment guidelines. *Clinical Therapeutics* 18(1):127–149; discussion 126.

Ackerman, L. S. 2006. Sex hormones and the genesis of autoimmunity. *Archives of Dermatology* 142(3):371–376.

ACOG (American Congress of Obstetricions and Gynecologists). 2003. *Cervical Cancer Screening: Testing Can Start Later and Occur Less Often Under New ACOG Recommendations.* http://www.acog.org/from_home/publications/press_releases/nr07-31-03-1.cfm (accessed November 15, 2009).

———. 2009. ACOG practice bulletin no. 109: Cervical cytology screening. *Obstetrics and Gynecology* 114(6):1409–1420.

ACS (American Cancer Society). 2009a. *Detailed Guide: Breast Cancer What Are the Key Statistics for Breast Cancer?* http://www.cancer.org/docroot/cri/content/cri_2_4_1x_what_are_the_key_statistics_for_breast_cancer_5.asp (accessed May 3, 2010).

———. 2009b. *Detailed Guide: Cervical Cancer What Are the Key Statistics About Cervical Cancer?* http://www.cancer.org/docroot/CRI/content/CRI_2_4_1X_What_are_the_key_statistics_for_cervical_cancer_8.asp (accessed November 19, 2009).

———. 2009c. *American Cancer Society Guidelines for the Early Detection of Cancer.* http://www.cancer.org/docroot/ped/content/ped_2_3x_acs_cancer_detection_guidelines_36.asp (accessed November 17, 2009).

———. 2009d. *Overview: Endometrial Cancer: How Many Women Get Endometrial Cancer?* http://www.cancer.org/docroot/CRI/content/CRI_2_2_1x_How_Many_Women_Get_Endometrial_Cancer.asp?sitearea= (accessed 2009).

———. 2009e. *Detailed Guide: Ovarian Cancer. What Are the Risk Factors for Ovarian Cancer?* http://www.cancer.org/docroot/CRI/content/CRI_2_4_2X_What_are_the_risk_factors_for_ovarian_cancer_33.asp (accessed May 25, 2010).

———. 2009f. *Detailed Guide: Lung Cancer—Non-Small Cell How Is Non-Small Cell Lung Cancer Staged?* http://www.cancer.org/docroot/CRI/content/CRI_2_4_3x_How_Is_Non-Small_Cell_Lung_Cancer_Staged.asp (accessed December 14, 2009).

———. 2010a. *Breast Cancer Facts & Figures: 2009–2010.* Atlanta, GA:ACS, Inc..

———. 2010b. *Ovarian Cancer.* http://www.cancer.org/Cancer/OvarianCancer/DetailedGuide/ovarian-cancer-key-statistics (accessed August 10, 2010).

Ademuyiwa, F. O., and O. I. Olopade. 2003. Racial differences in genetic factors associated with breast cancer. *Cancer and Metastasis Reviews* 22(1):47–53.

AHA (American Heart Association). 2009. *Women and Cardiovascular Diseases—Statistics 2009.* http://www.americanheart.org/downloadable/heart/1236184538758WOMEN.pdf (accessed December 1, 2009).

———. 2010. *Heart Attack Symptoms and Warning Signs.* http://www.americanheart.org/presenter.jhtml?identifier=4595 (accessed May 24, 2010).

Ahmed, B., C. N. Bairey Merz, B. D. Johnson, V. Bittner, S. L. Berga, G. D. Braunstein, T. K. Hodgson, K. Smith, L. Shaw, S. F. Kelsey, and G. Sopko. 2008. Diabetes mellitus, hypothalamic hypoestrogenemia, and coronary artery disease in premenopausal women (from the National Heart, Lung, and Blood Institute sponsored WISE study). *American Journal of Cardiology* 102(2):150–154.

Ahrendt, S. A., P. A. Decker, E. A. Alawi, Y. R. Zhu Yr, M. Sanchez-Cespedes, S. C. Yang, G. B. Haasler, A. Kajdacsy-Balla, M. J. Demeure, and D. Sidransky. 2001. Cigarette smoking is strongly associated with mutation of the k-ras gene in patients with primary adenocarcinoma of the lung. *Cancer* 92(6):1525–1530.

AHRQ (Agency for Healthcare Research and Quality). 2009. *Cardiovascular Disease and Other Chronic Conditions in Women: Recent Findings*. Rockville, MD: AHRQ.

AICR (American Institute for Cancer Research). 2007. *Food, Nutrition, Physical Activity, and the Prevention of Cancer: A Global Perspective*. Washington, DC: AICR.

Aitken, R. J., M. A. Baker, G. F. Doncel, M. M. Matzuk, C. K. Mauck, and M. J. Harper. 2008. As the world grows: Contraception in the 21st century. *Journal of Clinical Investigation* 118(4):1330–1343.

Alarcon-Riquelme, M. E. 2007. Recent advances in the genetics of autoimmune diseases. *Annals of the New York Academy of Sciences* 1110:1–9.

Albain, K. S., J. J. Crowley, M. LeBlanc, and R. B. Livingston. 1991. Survival determinants in extensive-stage non–small-cell lung cancer: The Southwest Oncology Group experience. *Journal Clinical Oncology* 9(9):1618–1626.

Albain, K. S., W. E. Barlow, S. Shak, G. N. Hortobagyi, R. B. Livingston, I. T. Yeh, P. Ravdin, R. Bugarini, F. L. Baehner, N. E. Davidson, G. W. Sledge, E. P. Winer, C. Hudis, J. N. Ingle, E. A. Perez, K. I. Pritchard, L. Shepherd, J. R. Gralow, C. Yoshizawa, D. C. Allred, C. K. Osborne, and D. F. Hayes. 2010. Prognostic and predictive value of the 21-gene recurrence score assay in postmenopausal women with node-positive, oestrogen-receptor-positive breast cancer on chemotherapy: A retrospective analysis of a randomised trial. *Lancet Oncology* 11(1):55–65.

Alberg, A. J., and J. Nonemaker. 2008. Who is at high risk for lung cancer? Population-level and individual-level perspectives. *Seminars in Respiratory and Critical Care Medicine* 29(3): 223–232.

Alberts, D. S., and N. Mason-Liddil. 1989. The role of cisplatin in the management of advanced squamous cell cancer of the cervix. *Seminars in Oncology* 16(4 Suppl. 6):66–78.

Alegría, M., G. Canino, P. E. Shrout, M. Woo, N. Duan, D. Vila, M. Torres, C. N. Chen, and X. L. Meng. 2008. Prevalence of mental illness in immigrant and non-immigrant US Latino groups. *American Journal of Psychiatry* 165(3):359–369.

Alexander, F. E., T. J. Anderson, H. K. Brown, A. P. Forrest, W. Hepburn, A. E. Kirkpatrick, B. B. Muir, R. J. Prescott, and A. Smith. 1999. 14 years of follow-up from the Edinburgh randomised trial of breast-cancer screening. *Lancet* 353(9168):1903–1908.

Alexander, K. P., A. Y. Chen, L. K. Newby, J. B. Schwartz, R. F. Redberg, J. S. Hochman, M. T. Roe, W. B. Gibler, E. M. Ohman, and E. D. Peterson. 2006. Sex differences in major bleeding with glycoprotein IIB/IIIA inhibitors: Results from the CRUSADE (Can Rapid risk stratification of Unstable angina patients Suppress ADverse outcomes with Early implementation of the ACC/ AHA guidelines) initiative. *Circulation* 114(13):1380–1387.

Alliegro, M. B., M. Dorrucci, A. N. Phillips, P. Pezzotti, S. Boros, M. Zaccarelli, R. Pristera, and G. Rezza. 1997. Incidence and consequences of pregnancy in women with known duration of HIV infection. Italian Seroconversion Study Group. *Archives of Internal Medicine* 157(22): 2585–2590.

Ancelin, M. L., and K. Ritchie. 2005. Lifelong endocrine fluctuations and related cognitive disorders. *Current Pharmaceutical Design* 11(32):4229–4252.

Andersen, J. 1998. Factors in fibroid growth. *Baillière's Clinical Obstetrics and Gynaecology* 12(2): 225–243.

Anderson, R. J., K. E. Freedland, R. E. Clouse, and P. J. Lustman. 2001. The prevalence of comorbid depression in adults with diabetes: A meta-analysis. *Diabetes Care* 24(6):1069–1078.

Andersson, I., and L. Janzon. 1997. Reduced breast cancer mortality in women under age 50: Updated results from the Malmo Mammographic Screening Program. *Journal of the National Cancer Institute Monographs* (22):63–67.

Ando, T., and T. F. Davies. 2003. Postpartum autoimmune thyroid disease: The potential role of fetal microchimerism. *Journal of Clinical Endocrinology and Metabolism* 88(7):2965–2971.

Angold, A., E. J. Costello, and C. M. Worthman. 1998. Puberty and depression: The roles of age, pubertal status and pubertal timing. *Psychological Medicine* 28(1):51–61.

Antinori, A., F. Baldini, E. Girardi, A. Cingolani, M. Zaccarelli, S. Di Giambenedetto, A. Barracchini, P. De Longis, R. Murri, V. Tozzi, A. Ammassari, M. G. Rizzo, G. Ippolito, and A. De Luca. 2001. Female sex and the use of anti-allergic agents increase the risk of developing cutaneous rash associated with nevirapine therapy. *AIDS* 15(12):1579–1581.

Antithrombotic Trialists Collaboration. 2002. Collaborative meta-analysis of randomised trials of antiplatelet therapy for prevention of death, myocardial infarction, and stroke in high risk patients. *British Medical Journal* 324(7329):71–86.

Antoniou, A. C., A. P. Cunningham, J. Peto, D. G. Evans, F. Lalloo, S. A. Narod, H. A. Risch, J. E. Eyfjord, J. L. Hopper, M. C. Southey, H. Olsson, O. Johannsson, A. Borg, B. Pasini, P. Radice, S. Manoukian, D. M. Eccles, N. Tang, E. Olah, H. Anton-Culver, E. Warner, J. Lubinski, J. Gronwald, B. Gorski, L. Tryggvadottir, K. Syrjakoski, O. P. Kallioniemi, H. Eerola, H. Nevanlinna, P. D. Pharoah, and D. F. Easton. 2008. The BOADICEA model of genetic susceptibility to breast and ovarian cancers: Updates and extensions. *British Journal of Cancer* 98(8):1457–1466.

Arbyn, M., C. Bergeron, P. Klinkhamer, P. Martin-Hirsch, A. G. Siebers, and J. Bulten. 2008. Liquid compared with conventional cervical cytology: A systematic review and meta-analysis. *Obstetrics and Gynecology* 111(1):167–177.

Asarnow, J. R., L. H. Jaycox, N. Duan, A. P. LaBorde, M. M. Rea, P. Murray, M. Anderson, C. Landon, L. Tang, and K. B. Wells. 2005. Effectiveness of a quality improvement intervention for adolescent depression in primary care clinics: A randomized controlled trial. *Journal of the American Medical Association* 293(3):311–319.

Ascherio, A., and K. L. Munger. 2007. Environmental risk factors for multiple sclerosis. Part II: Noninfectious factors. *Annals of Neurology* 61(6):504–513.

Austin, R. M., and I. Ramzy. 1998. Increased detection of epithelial cell abnormalities by liquid-based gynecologic cytology preparations. A review of accumulated data. *Acta Cytologica* 42(1):178–184.

Azziz, R., K. S. Woods, R. Reyna, T. J. Key, E. S. Knochenhauer, and B. O. Yildiz. 2004. The prevalence and features of the polycystic ovary syndrome in an unselected population. *Journal of Clinical Endocrinology and Metabolism* 89(6):2745–2749.

Bach, P. B., J. R. Jett, U. Pastorino, M. S. Tockman, S. J. Swensen, and C. B. Begg. 2007. Computed tomography screening and lung cancer outcomes. *Journal of the American Medical Association* 297(9):953–961.

Bachman, D. L., P. A. Wolf, R. Linn, J. E. Knoefel, J. Cobb, A. Belanger, R. B. D'Agostino, and L. R. White. 1992. Prevalence of dementia and probable senile dementia of the Alzheimer type in the Framingham Study. *Neurology* 42(1):115–119.

Bae, S., and L. Zhang. 2005. Gender differences in cardioprotection against ischemia/reperfusion injury in adult rat hearts: Focus on Akt and protein kinase C signaling. *Journal of Pharmacology and Experimental Therapeutics* 315(3):1125–1135.

Bailey, A. C., and M. Fisher. 2008. Current use of antiretroviral treatment. *British Medical Bulletin* 87:175–192.

Bailey, A. L., C. L. Campbell, and S. S. Smyth. 2010. Aspirin for the primary prevention of cardiovascular disease in women. *Current Cardiovascular Risk Reports* 4:209–215.

Bain, C., D. Feskanich, F. E. Speizer, M. Thun, E. Hertzmark, B. A. Rosner, and G. A. Colditz. 2004. Lung cancer rates in men and women with comparable histories of smoking. *Journal of the National Cancer Institute* 96(11):826–834.

Bairey Merz, C. N., L. J. Shaw, S. E. Reis, V. Bittner, S. F. Kelsey, M. Olson, B. D. Johnson, C. J. Pepine, S. Mankad, B. L. Sharaf, W. J. Rogers, G. M. Pohost, A. Lerman, A. A. Quyyumi, and G. Sopko. 2006. Insights from the NHLBI-sponsored Women's Ischemia Syndrome Evaluation (WISE) Study: Part II: Gender differences in presentation, diagnosis, and outcome with regard to gender-based pathophysiology of atherosclerosis and macrovascular and microvascular coronary disease. *Journal of the American College of Cardiology* 47(3 Suppl.):S21–S29.

Balasch, J., M. Creus, F. Fabregues, F. Carmona, J. Ordi, S. Martinez-Roman, and J. A. Vanrell. 1996. Visible and non-visible endometriosis at laparoscopy in fertile and infertile women and in patients with chronic pelvic pain: A prospective study. *Human Reproduction* 11(2):387–391.

Baquet, C. R., S. I. Mishra, P. Commiskey, G. L. Ellison, and M. DeShields. 2008. Breast cancer epidemiology in blacks and whites: Disparities in incidence, mortality, survival rates and histology. *Journal of the National Medical Association* 100(5):480–488.

Baraona, E., C. S. Abittan, K. Dohmen, M. Moretti, G. Pozzato, Z. W. Chayes, C. Schaefer, and C. S. Lieber. 2001. Gender differences in pharmacokinetics of alcohol. *Alcoholism—Clinical and Experimental Research* 25(4):502–507.

Barber, H. R. 1987. Ovarian cancer: Cause, diagnosis, and treatment. *Comprehensive Therapy* 13(6): 25–33.

Barkan, S. E., S. L. Melnick, S. Preston-Martin, K. Weber, L. A. Kalish, P. Miotti, M. Young, R. Greenblatt, H. Sacks, and J. Feldman. 1998. The Women's Interagency HIV Study. *Epidemiology* 9(2):117–125.

Barnholtz-Sloan, J., N. Patel, D. Rollison, K. Kortepeter, J. MacKinnon, and A. Giuliano. 2009. Incidence trends of invasive cervical cancer in the United States by combined race and ethnicity. *Cancer Causes and Control* 20(7):1129–1138.

Barre-Sinoussi, F., J. C. Chermann, F. Rey, M. T. Nugeyre, S. Chamaret, J. Gruest, C. Dauguet, C. Axler-Blin, F. Vezinet-Brun, C. Rouzioux, W. Rozenbaum, and L. Montagnier. 2004. Isolation of a t-lymphotropic retrovirus from a patient at risk for acquired immune deficiency syndrome (AIDS). 1983. *Revista de Investigación Clínica* 56(2):126–129.

Bartella, L., S. B. Thakur, E. A. Morris, D. D. Dershaw, W. Huang, E. Chough, M. C. Cruz, and L. Liberman. 2007. Enhancing nonmass lesions in the breast: Evaluation with proton (1H) MR spectroscopy. *Radiology* 245(1):80–87.

Bast, R. C., Jr., B. Hennessy, and G. B. Mills. 2009. The biology of ovarian cancer: New opportunities for translation. *Nature Reviews. Cancer* 9(6):415–428.

Batur, P., J. Elder, and M. Mayer. 2003. Update on contraception: Benefits and risks of the new formulations. *Cleveland Clinic Journal of Medicine* 70(8):681–682, 685–686, 668–690 passim.

Beals, J., D. K. Novins, P. Spicer, C. M. Mitchell, and S. M. Manson. 2005. Prevalence of mental disorders and utilization of mental health services in two American Indian reservation populations: Mental health disparities in a national context. *American Journal of Psychiatry* 162:1723–1732.

Beatson, G. W. 1896. On the treatment of inoperable cases of carcinoma of the mamma: Suggestions for a new method of treatment with illustrative cases. *Lancet* 148(3802):104–107.

Becker, D. F., and C. M. Grilo. 2006. Prediction of drug and alcohol abuse in hospitalized adolescents: Comparisons by gender and substance type. *Behaviour Research and Therapy* 44(10): 1431–1440.

Belle, D., and J. Doucet. 2003. Poverty, inequality, and discrimination as sources of depression among US women. *Psychology of Women Quarterly* 27(2):101–113.

Benagiano, G., C. Bastianelli, and M. Farris. 2007. Hormonal contraception: State of the art and future perspectives. *Minerva Ginecologica* 59(3):241–270.

Beral, V., C. Hermon, C. Kay, P. Hannaford, S. Darby, and G. Reeves. 1999. Mortality associated with oral contraceptive use: 25 year follow up of cohort of 46 000 women from Royal College of General Practitioners' Oral Contraception Study. *British Medical Journal* 318(7176):96–100.

Beretich, B. D., and T. M. Beretich. 2009. Explaining multiple sclerosis prevalence by ultraviolet exposure: A geospatial analysis. *Multiple Sclerosis* 15(8):891–898.

Berg, C. J., J. Chang, W. M. Callaghan, and S. J. Whitehead. 2003. Pregnancy-related mortality in the United States, 1991–1997. *Obstetrics and Gynecology* 101(2):289–296.

Berg, C. J., A. P. Mackay, C. Qin, and W. M. Callaghan. 2009. Overview of maternal morbidity during hospitalization for labor and delivery in the United States: 1993–1997 and 2001–2005. *Obstetrics and Gynecology* 113(5):1075–1081.

Berg, W. A. 2009. Tailored supplemental screening for breast cancer: What now and what next? *American Journal of Roentgeneology* 192(2):390–399.

Berg, W. A., I. N. Weinberg, D. Narayanan, M. E. Lobrano, E. Ross, L. Amodei, L. Tafra, L. P. Adler, J. Uddo, W. Stein, 3rd, and E. A. Levine. 2006. High-resolution fluorodeoxyglucose positron emission tomography with compression ("positron emission mammography") is highly accurate in depicting primary breast cancer. *Breast Journal* 12(4):309–323.

Berg, W. A., J. D. Blume, J. B. Cormack, E. B. Mendelson, D. Lehrer, M. Bohm-Velez, E. D. Pisano, R. A. Jong, W. P. Evans, M. J. Morton, M. C. Mahoney, L. Hovanessian Larsen, R. G. Barr, D. M. Farria, H. S. Marques, K. Boparai, and for the ACRIN 6666 Investigators. 2008. Combined screening with ultrasound and mammography vs mammography alone in women at elevated risk of breast cancer. *Journal of the American Medical Association* 299(18):2151–2163.

Berger, J. S., M. J. Krantz, J. M. Kittelson, and W. R. Hiatt. 2009. Aspirin for the prevention of cardiovascular events in patients with peripheral artery disease: A meta-analysis of randomized trials. *Journal of the American Medical Association* 301(18):1909–1919.

Bermejo-Pérez, M. J., S. Márquez-Calderón, and A. Llanos-Méndez. 2007. Effectiveness of preventive interventions in *BRCA1/2* gene mutation carriers: A systematic review. *International Journal of Cancer* 121(2):225–231.

Berndt, E. R., L. M. Koran, S. N. Finkelstein, A. J. Gelenberg, S. G. Kornstein, I. M. Miller, M. E. Thase, G. A. Trapp, and M. B. Keller. 2000. Lost human capital from early-onset chronic depression. *American Journal of Psychiatry* 157(6):940–947.

Bernstein, L. 2008. Identifying population-based approaches to lower breast cancer risk. *Oncogene* 27(S2):S3–S8.

Berry, D. A., E. S. Iversen, Jr., D. F. Gudbjartsson, E. H. Hiller, J. E. Garber, B. N. Peshkin, C. Lerman, P. Watson, H. T. Lynch, S. G. Hilsenbeck, W. S. Rubinstein, K. S. Hughes, and G. Parmigiani. 2002. BRCAPRO validation, sensitivity of genetic testing of *BRCA1/BRCA2*, and prevalence of other breast cancer susceptibility genes. *Journal Clinical Oncology* 20(11):2701–2712.

Berry, D. A., K. A. Cronin, S. K. Plevritis, D. G. Fryback, L. Clarke, M. Zelen, J. S. Mandelblatt, A. Y. Yakovlev, J. D. F. Habbema, E. J. Feuer, T. C. Intervention, and Surveillance Modeling Network Collaborators. 2005. Effect of screening and adjuvant therapy on mortality from breast cancer. *New England Journal of Medicine* 353(17):1784–1792.

Bersoff-Matcha, S. J., W. C. Miller, J. A. Aberg, C. van Der Horst, H. J. Hamrick, Jr., W. G. Powderly, and L. M. Mundy. 2001. Sex differences in nevirapine rash. *Clinical Infectious Diseases* 32(1):124–129.

Bertone, E. R., W. C. Willett, B. A. Rosner, D. J. Hunter, C. S. Fuchs, F. E. Speizer, G. A. Colditz, and S. E. Hankinson. 2001. Prospective study of recreational physical activity and ovarian cancer. *Journal of the National Cancer Institute* 93(12):942–948.

Biesma, R. G., L. J. Schouten, M. J. Dirx, R. A. Goldbohm, and P. A. van den Brandt. 2006. Physical activity and risk of ovarian cancer: Results from the Netherlands Cohort Study (The Netherlands). *Cancer Causes & Control* 17(1):109–115.

Bing, E. G., M. A. Burnam, D. Longshore, J. A. Fleishman, C. D. Sherbourne, A. S. London, B. J. Turner, F. Eggan, B. Beckman, B. Vitiello, S. C. Morton, M. Orlando, S. A. Bozzette, L. Ortiz-Barron, and M. Shapiro. 2001. Psychiatric disorders and drug use among human immunodeficiency virus-infected adults in the United States. *Archives of General Psychiatry* 58(8):721–728.

Birnbaum, C. S., L. S. Cohen, J. W. Bailey, L. R. Grush, L. M. Robertson, and Z. N. Stowe. 1999. Serum concentrations of antidepressants and benzodiazepines in nursing infants: A case series. *Pediatrics* 104(1):e11.

Bischoff-Ferrari, H. A., B. Dawson-Hughes, J. A. Baron, P. Burckhardt, R. Li, D. Spiegelman, B. Specker, J. E. Orav, J. B. Wong, H. B. Staehelin, E. O'Reilly, D. P. Kiel, and W. C. Willett. 2007. Calcium intake and hip fracture risk in men and women: A meta-analysis of prospective cohort studies and randomized controlled trials. *American Journal of Clinical Nutrition* 86(6): 1780–1790.

Bischoff-Ferrari, H. A., W. C. Willett, J. B. Wong, A. E. Stuck, H. B. Staehelin, E. J. Orav, A. Thoma, D. P. Kiel, and J. Henschkowski. 2009. Prevention of nonvertebral fractures with oral vitamin D and dose dependency: A meta-analysis of randomized controlled trials. *Archives of Internal Medicine* 169(6):551–561.

Bishop, J. W., S. H. Bigner, T. J. Colgan, M. Husain, L. P. Howell, K. M. McIntosh, D. A. Taylor, and M. H. Sadeghi. 1998. Multicenter masked evaluation of autocyte prep thin layers with matched conventional smears. Including initial biopsy results. *Acta Cytologica* 42(1):189–197.

Bjurstam, N., L. Bjorneld, J. Warwick, E. Sala, S. W. Duffy, L. Nystrom, N. Walker, E. Cahlin, O. Eriksson, L. O. Hafstrom, H. Lingaas, J. Mattsson, S. Persson, C. M. Rudenstam, H. Salander, J. Save-Soderbergh, and T. Wahlin. 2003. The Gothenburg Breast Screening Trial. *Cancer* 97(10):2387–2396.

Black, W. C., and J. A. Baron. 2007. CT screening for lung cancer: Spiraling into confusion? *Journal of the American Medical Association* 297(9):995–997.

Blake, S. M., H. Amaro, P. M. Schwartz, and L. J. Flinchbaugh. 2001. A review of substance abuse prevention interventions for young adolescent girls. *Journal of Early Adolescence* 21(3): 294–324.

Blauwet, L. A., and R. F. Redberg. 2007. The role of sex-specific results reporting in cardiovascular disease. *Cardiology in Review* 15(6):275–278.

Blauwet, L. A., S. N. Hayes, D. McManus, R. F. Redberg, and M. N. Walsh. 2007. Low rate of sex-specific result reporting in cardiovascular trials. *Mayo Clinic Proceedings* 82(2):166–170.

Blumsohn, A. 2003. Bone remodeling markers: Assessment of fracture risk and fracture risk reduction. *Current Osteoporosis Reports* 1(3):91–97.

Bonfanti, P., C. Gulisano, E. Ricci, L. Timillero, L. Valsecchi, S. Carradori, L. Pusterla, P. Fortuna, S. Miccolis, C. Magnani, A. Gabbuti, F. Parazzini, C. Martinelli, I. Faggion, S. Landonio, T. Quirino, and G. Vigevani. 2003. Risk factors for lipodystrophy in the CISAI cohort. *Biomedicine and Pharmacotherapy* 57(9):422–427.

Boone, J., T. R. Nelson, K. K. Lindfors, and J. A. Seibert. 2001. Dedicated breast CT: Radiation dose and image quality evaluation. *Radiology* 221(3):657–667.

Boone, J., A. Kwan, K. Yang, G. Burkett, K. Lindfors, and T. Nelson. 2006. Computed tomography for imaging the breast. *Journal of Mammary Gland Biology and Neoplasia* 11(2):103–111.

Boonen, S., P. Lips, R. Bouillon, H. A. Bischoff-Ferrari, D. Vanderschueren, and P. Haentjens. 2007. Need for additional calcium to reduce the risk of hip fracture with vitamin D supplementation: Evidence from a comparative metaanalysis of randomized controlled trials. *Journal of Clinical Endocrinology and Metabolism* 92(4):1415–1423.

Bordeleau, L., S. Panchal, and P. Goodwin. 2010. Prognosis of BRCA-associated breast cancer: A summary of evidence. *Breast Cancer Research and Treatment* 119(1):13–24.

Borer, K. T. 2005. Physical activity in the prevention and amelioration of osteoporosis in women— Interaction of mechanical, hormonal and dietary factors. *Sports Medicine* 35(9):779–830.

Boruban, M. C., K. Altundag, G. S. Kilic, and J. Blankstein. 2008. From endometrial hyperplasia to endometrial cancer: Insight into the biology and possible medical preventive measures. *European Journal of Cancer Prevention* 17(2):133–138.

Bosch, F. X., A. Lorincz, N. Munoz, C. J. Meijer, and K. V. Shah. 2002. The causal relation between human papillomavirus and cervical cancer. *Journal of Clinical Pathology* 55(4):244–265.

Bouchardy, C., G. Fioretta, M. De Perrot, M. Obradovic, and A. Spiliopoulos. 1999. Determinants of long term survival after surgery for cancer of the lung: A population-based study. *Cancer* 86(11):2229–2237.

Bower, J. E. 2008. Behavioral symptoms in patients with breast cancer and survivors. *Journal of Clinical Oncology* 26(5):768–777.

Brady, K. T., D. E. Grice, L. Dustan, and C. Randall. 1993. Gender differences in substance use disorders. *American Journal of Psychiatry* 150(11):1707–1711.

Brady, K. T., S. E. Back, and S. F. Greenfield. 2009. *Women and Addiction: A Comprehensive Handbook.* New York: The Guilford Press.

Braithwaite, R. S., N. F. Col, and J. B. Wong. 2003. Estimating hip fracture morbidity, mortality and costs. *Journal of the American Geriatrics Society* 51(3):364–370.

Brauer, C. A., M. Coca-Perraillon, D. M. Cutler, and A. B. Rosen. 2009. Incidence and mortality of hip fractures in the United States. *Journal of the American Medical Association* 302(14): 1573–1579.

Braunwald, E., E. M. Antman, J. W. Beasley, R. M. Califf, M. D. Cheitlin, J. S. Hochman, R. H. Jones, D. Kereiakes, J. Kupersmith, T. N. Levin, C. J. Pepine, J. W. Schaeffer, E. E. Smith, III, D. E. Steward, P. Theroux, R. J. Gibbons, J. S. Alpert, D. P. Faxon, V. Fuster, G. Gregoratos, L. F. Hiratzka, A. K. Jacobs, and S. C. Smith, Jr. 2002. ACC/AHA 2002 guideline update for the management of patients with unstable angina and non-ST-segment elevation myocardial infarction—summary article: A report of the American College of Cardiology/American Heart Association task force on practice guidelines (Committee on the Management of Patients With Unstable Angina). *Journal of the American College of Cardiology* 40(7):1366–1374.

Breitburd, F., R. Kirnbauer, N. Hubbert, B. Nonnenmacher, C. Trin-Dinh-Desmarquet, G. Orth, J. Schiller, and D. Lowy. 1995. Immunization with viruslike particles from cottontail rabbit papillomavirus (CRPV) can protect against experimental CRPV infection. *Journal of Virology* 69(6):3959–3963.

Brieger, D., K. A. Eagle, S. G. Goodman, P. G. Steg, A. Budaj, K. White, and G. Montalescot. 2004. Acute coronary syndromes without chest pain, an underdiagnosed and undertreated high-risk group. *Chest* 126(2):461–469.

Briel, M., G. G. Schwartz, P. L. Thompson, J. A. de Lemos, M. A. Blazing, G. A. van Es, M. Kayikcioglu, H. R. Arntz, F. R. den Hartog, N. J. Veeger, F. Colivicchi, J. Dupuis, S. Okazaki, R. S. Wright, H. C. Bucher, and A. J. Nordmann. 2006. Effects of early treatment with statins on short-term clinical outcomes in acute coronary syndromes: A meta-analysis of randomized controlled trials. *Journal of the American Medical Association* 295(17):2046–2056.

Britt, K., A. Ashworth, and M. Smalley. 2007. Pregnancy and the risk of breast cancer. *Endocrine-Related Cancer* 14(4):907–933.

Brown, K. A., and E. R. Simpson. 2010. Obesity and breast cancer: Progress to understanding the relationship. *Cancer Research* 70(1):4–7.

Brownson, R. C., M. C. Alavanja, E. T. Hock, and T. S. Loy. 1992. Passive smoking and lung cancer in nonsmoking women. *American Journal of Public Health* 82(11):1525–1530.

Brugts, J. J., T. Yetgin, S. E. Hoeks, A. M. Gotto, J. Shepherd, R. G. Westendorp, A. J. de Craen, R. H. Knopp, H. Nakamura, P. Ridker, R. van Domburg, and J. W. Deckers. 2009. The benefits of statins in people without established cardiovascular disease but with cardiovascular risk factors: Meta-analysis of randomised controlled trials. *British Medical Journal* 338:b2376.

Buchberger, W., A. Niehoff, P. Obrist, P. DeKoekkoek-Doll, and M. Dunser. 2000. Clinically and mammographically occult breast lesions: Detection and classification with high-resolution sonography. *Seminars in Ultrasound, CT and MRI* 21(4):325–336.

Buchbinder, S. 2009. The epidemiology of new HIV infections and interventions to limit HIV transmission. *Topics in HIV Medicine* 17(2):37–43.

Buckley, D. I., R. Fu, M. Freeman, K. Rogers, and M. Helfand. 2009. C-reactive protein as a risk factor for coronary heart disease: A systematic review and meta-analyses for the US Preventive Services Task Force. *Annals of Internal Medicine* 151(7):483–495.

Buencamino, M. C., A. L. Sikon, A. Jain, and H. L. Thacker. 2009. An observational study on the adherence to treatment guidelines of osteopenia. *Journal of Women's Health* 18(6):873–881.

Bukstein, O. G., L. J. Glancy, and Y. Kaminer. 1992. Patterns of affective comorbidity in a clinical population of dually diagnosed adolescent substance abusers. *Journal of the American Academy of Child and Adolescent Psychiatry* 31(6):1041–1045.

Buzdar, A. U., G. N. Hortobagyi, T. L. Smith, S. Kau, C. Marcus, F. A. Holmes, V. Hug, G. Fraschini, F. C. Ames, and R. G. Martin. 1988. Adjuvant therapy of breast cancer with or without additional treatment with alternate drugs. *Cancer* 62(10):2098–2104.

Cal EPA (California Environmental Protection Agency). 2005. *Proposed Identification of Environmental Tobacco Smoke as a Toxic Air Contaminant. Part B: Health Effects.* Sacramento: California Environmental Protection Agency.

Campo, M. S. 2002. Animal models of papillomavirus pathogenesis. *Virus Research* 89(2): 249–261.

Campos-Outcalt, D. 2009. The case for HPV immunization. *Journal of Family Practice* 58(12): 660–664.

Canadian Study of Health and Aging. 1994. Canadian Study of Health and Aging: Study methods and prevalence of dementia. *Canadian Medical Association Journal* 150(6):899–913.

Canto, J. G., R. J. Goldberg, M. M. Hand, R. O. Bonow, G. Sopko, C. J. Pepine, and T. Long. 2007. Symptom presentation of women with acute coronary syndromes: Myth vs reality. *Archives of Internal Medicine* 167(22):2405–2413.

Carey, L. A., C. M. Perou, C. A. Livasy, L. G. Dressler, D. Cowan, K. Conway, G. Karaca, M. A. Troester, C. K. Tse, S. Edmiston, S. L. Deming, J. Geradts, M. C. U. Cheang, T. O. Nielsen, P. G. Moorman, H. S. Earp, and R. C. Millikan. 2006. Race, breast cancer subtypes, and survival in the Carolina Breast Cancer Study. *Journal of the American Medical Association* 295(21):2492–2502.

Carlton, J. M., R. P. Hirt, J. C. Silva, A. L. Delcher, M. Schatz, Q. Zhao, J. R. Wortman, S. L. Bidwell, U. C. M. Alsmark, S. Besteiro, T. Sicheritz-Ponten, C. J. Noel, J. B. Dacks, P. G. Foster, C. Simillion, Y. Van de Peer, D. Miranda-Saavedra, G. J. Barton, G. D. Westrop, S. Muller, D. Dessi, P. L. Fiori, Q. Ren, I. Paulsen, H. Zhang, F. D. Bastida-Corcuera, A. Simoes-Barbosa, M. T. Brown, R. D. Hayes, M. Mukherjee, C. Y. Okumura, R. Schneider, A. J. Smith, S. Vanacova, M. Villalvazo, B. J. Haas, M. Pertea, T. V. Feldblyum, T. R. Utterback, C-L. Shu, K. Osoegawa, P. J. de Jong, I. Hrdy, L. Horvathova, Z. Zubacova, P. Dolezal, S-B. Malik, J. M. Logsdon, Jr., K. Henze, A. Gupta, C. C. Wang, R. L. Dunne, J. A. Upcroft, P. Upcroft, O. White, S. L. Salzberg, P. Tang, C-H. Chiu, Y-S. Lee, T. M. Embley, G. H. Coombs, J. C. Mottram, J. Tachezy, C. M. Fraser-Liggett, and P. J. Johnson. 2007. Draft genome sequence of the sexually transmitted pathogen trichomonas vaginalis. *Science* 315(5809):207–212.

Carter, J. E. 1994. Combined hysteroscopic and laparoscopic findings in patients with chronic pelvic pain. *Journal of the American Association of Gynecologic Laparoscopists* 2(1):43–47.

Carter, J. J., L. A. Koutsky, J. P. Hughes, S. K. Lee, J. Kuypers, N. Kiviat, and D. A. Galloway. 2000. Comparison of human papillomavirus types 16, 18, and 6 capsid antibody responses following incident infection. *Journal of Infectious Diseases* 181(6):1911–1919.

Cauley, J. A., D. E. Thompson, K. C. Ensrud, J. C. Scott, and D. Black. 2000. Risk of mortality following clinical fractures. *Osteoporosis International* 11(7):556–561.

CDC (Centers for Disease Control and Prevention). 1999. Ten great public health achievements—United States, 1900–1999. *Morbidity and Mortality Weekly Report* 48(12):241–243.

———. 2001. Mortality from coronary heart disease and acute myocardial infarction—United States, 1998. *Morbidity and Mortality Weekly Report* 50(06):90–93.

———. 2002a. *Women and Smoking: A report of the Surgeon General.* http://www.cdc.gov/mmwr/preview/mmwrhtml/rr5112a4.htm (accessed August 17, 2009).

———. 2002b. *Drug-Associated HIV Transmission Continues in the United States.* CDC. http://www.cdc.gov/hiv/resources/factsheets/idu.htm (accessed May 14, 2010).

———. 2002c. US Public Health Service Task Force recommendations for use of antiretroviral drugs in pregnant HIV-1–infected women for maternal health and interventions to reduce perinatal HIV-1 transmission in the United States. *Morbidity and Mortality Weekly Report,* http://www.cdc.gov/mmwr/preview/mmwrhtml/rr5118a1.htm (accessed May 17, 2010).

———. 2003. Late versus early testing of HIV—16 sites, United States, 2000–2003. *Morbidity and Mortality Weekly Report* 52(26):581–586.

————. 2004. Hysterectomy in the United States, 2000–2004. In *Women's Reproductive Health: Hysterectomy Fact Sheet.* Atlanta, GA: CDC.

————. 2006. Revised recommendations for HIV testing of adults, adolescents, and pregnant women in health-care settings. *Morbidity and Mortality Weekly Report* 55(RR14), http://www.cdc. gov/mmwr/preview/mmwrhtml/rr5514a1.htm (accessed May 14, 2010).

————. 2008a. *HIV/AIDS in the United States: An Update.* Atlanta, GA:CDC.

————. 2008b. Subpopulation estimates from the HIV incidence surveillance system—United States, 2006. *Morbidity and Mortality Weekly Report* 57(36):985–989.

————. 2008c. *CDC HIV/AIDS Fact Sheet: HIV/AIDS Among Women.* http://www.cdc.gov/hiv/ topics/women/resources/factsheets/pdf/women.pdf (accessed June 29, 2009).

————. 2008d. HIV prevalence estimates—United States, 2006. *Morbidity and Mortality Weekly Report* 57(39):1073–1076.

————. 2008e. *Safe Motherhood Promoting Health for Women Before, During, and After Pregnancy.* http://www.cdc.gov/nccdphp/publications/aag/pdf/drh.pdf (accessed May 3, 2010)

————. 2008f. *Sexually Transmitted Disease Surveillance 2007.* http://www.cdc.gov/std/stats07/ Surv2007FINAL.pdf (accessed May 4, 2009).

————. 2008g. *Current Smoking.* http://www.cdc.gov/nchs/data/nhis/earlyrelease/200812_08.pdf (accessed August 17, 2009).

————. 2010. *Breast Cancer Statistics.* Division of Cancer Prevention and Control, National Center for Chronic Disease Prevention and Health Promotion, http://www.cdc.gov/cancer/breast/sta-tistics/ (accessed May 3, 2010).

Chan, K. K., and R. Naik. 2008. Advances in surgical treatment of cervical cancer. *Women's Health* 4(3):245–256.

Chasan-Taber, L., and M. J. Stampfer. 1998. Epidemiology of oral contraceptives and cardiovascular disease. *Annals of Internal Medicine* 128(6):467–477.

Chatham, L. R., M. L. Hiller, G. A. Rowan-Szal, G. W. Joe, and D. D. Simpson. 1999. Gender dif-ferences at admission and follow-up in a sample of methadone maintenance clients. *Substance Use and Misuse* 34(8):1137–1165.

Chaudhry, P., and E. Asselin. 2009. Resistance to chemotherapy and hormone therapy in endometrial cancer. *Endocrine-Related Cancer* 16(2):363–380.

Chauhan, M. S., K. K. Ho, D. S. Baim, R. E. Kuntz, and D. E. Cutlip. 2005. Effect of gender on in-hospital and one-year outcomes after contemporary coronary artery stenting. *American Journal of Cardiology* 95(1):101–104.

Chen, C-R., G. M. Buck, N. G. Courey, K. M. Perez, and J. Wactawski-Wende. 2001. Risk factors for uterine fibroids among women undergoing tubal sterilization. *American Journal of Epidemiol-ogy* 153(1):20–26.

Chesnut, C. H., 3rd, S. Silverman, K. Andriano, H. Genant, A. Gimona, S. Harris, D. Kiel, M. LeBoff, M. Maricic, P. Miller, C. Moniz, M. Peacock, P. Richardson, N. Watts, and D. Baylink. 2000. A randomized trial of nasal spray salmon calcitonin in postmenopausal women with established osteoporosis: The prevent recurrence of osteoporotic fractures study. PROOF study group. *American Journal of Medicine* 109(4):267–276.

Chia, S. K., C. H. Speers, Y. D'yachkova, A. Kang, S. Malfair-Taylor, J. Barnett, A. Coldman, K. A. Gelmon, S. E. O'Reilly, and I. A. Olivotto. 2007. The impact of new chemotherapeutic and hormone agents on survival in a population-based cohort of women with metastatic breast cancer. *Cancer* 110(5):973–979.

Chlebowski, R. T., S. L. Hendrix, R. D. Langer, M. L. Stefanick, M. Gass, D. Lane, R. J. Rodabough, M. A. Gilligan, M. G. Cyr, C. A. Thomson, J. Khandekar, H. Petrovitch, and A. McTiernan. 2003. Influence of estrogen plus progestin on breast cancer and mammography in healthy post-menopausal women: The Women's Health Initiative Randomized Trial. *Journal of the American Medical Association* 289(24):3243–3253.

Chlebowski, R. T., L. H. Kuller, R. L. Prentice, M. L. Stefanick, J. E. Manson, M. Gass, A. K. Aragaki, J. K. Ockene, D. S. Lane, G. E. Sarto, A. Rajkovic, R. Schenken, S. L. Hendrix, P. M. Ravdin, T. E. Rohan, S. Yasmeen, G. Anderson, and the WHI Investigators. 2009. Breast cancer after use of estrogen plus progestin in postmenopausal women. *New England Journal of Medicine* 360(6):573–587.

Cho, K. R., and M. Shih Ie. 2009. Ovarian cancer. *Annual Review of Pathology* 4:287–313.

Chou, A. F., S. H. Scholle, C. S. Weisman, A. S. Bierman, R. Correa-de-Araujo, and L. Mosca. 2007a. Gender disparities in the quality of cardiovascular disease care in private managed care plans. *Women's Health Issues* 17(3):120–130.

Chou, A. F., L. Wong, C. S. Weisman, S. Chan, A. S. Bierman, R. Correa-de-Araujo, and S. H. Scholle. 2007b. Gender disparities in cardiovascular disease care among commercial and medicare managed care plans. *Women's Health Issues* 17(3):139–149.

Christian, A. H., W. Rosamond, A. R. White, and L. Mosca. 2007. Nine-year trends and racial and ethnic disparities in women's awareness of heart disease and stroke: An American Heart Association national study. *Journal of Women's Health* 16(1):68–81.

Chwalisz, K., L. Larsen, K. McCrary, and A. Edmonds. 2004. Effects of the novel selective progesterone receptor modulator (SPRM) asoprisnil on selected hormonal parameters in subjects with leiomyomata. *Fertility and Sterility* 82(Suppl. 2):S306.

Clark, D. A., A. T. Beck, and G. K. Brown. 1992. Sociotropy, autonomy, and life event perceptions in dysphoric and nondysphoric individuals. *Cognitive Therapy and Research* 16(6):635–652.

Clarke-Pearson, D. L. 2009. Clinical practice. Screening for ovarian cancer. *New England Journal of Medicine* 361(2):170–177.

Claus, E. B., J. Schildkraut, E. S. Iversen, Jr., D. Berry, and G. Parmigiani. 1998. Effect of *BRCA1* and *BRCA2* on the association between breast cancer risk and family history. *Journal of the National Cancer Institute* 90(23):1824–1829.

Cleary, M. P., M. E. Grossmann, and A. Ray. 2010. Effect of obesity on breast cancer development. *Veterinary Pathology* 47(2):202–213.

Clegg, L. X., M. E. Reichman, B. A. Miller, B. F. Hankey, G. K. Singh, Y. D. Lin, M. T. Goodman, C. F. Lynch, S. M. Schwartz, V. W. Chen, L. Bernstein, S. L. Gomez, J. J. Graff, C. C. Lin, N. J. Johnson, and B. K. Edwards. 2009. Impact of socioeconomic status on cancer incidence and stage at diagnosis: Selected findings from the Surveillance, Epidemiology, and End Results: National Longitudinal Mortality Study. *Cancer Causes and Control* 20(4):417–435.

Clemons, M., and P. Goss. 2001. Estrogen and the risk of breast cancer. *New England Journal of Medicine* 344(4):276–285.

Close, P., A. Neuprez, and J. Y. Reginster. 2006. Developments in the pharmacotherapeutic management of osteoporosis. *Expert Opinion on Pharmacotherapy* 7(12):1603–1615.

Cohen, S., D. Janicki-Deverts, and G. E. Miller. 2007. Psychological stress and disease. *Journal of the American Medical Association* 298(14):1685–1687.

Cohn, M. 2008. What roles do regulatory T cells play in the control of the adaptive immune response? *International Immunology* 20(9):11.

Cohn, S. E., J. G. Park, D. H. Watts, A. Stek, J. Hitti, P. A. Clax, S. Yu, J. J. Lertora, and ACTG A5093 Protocol Team. 2007. Depo-medroxyprogesterone in women on antiretroviral therapy: Effective contraception and lack of clinically significant interactions. *Clinical Pharmacology and Therapeutics* 81(2):222–227.

Collins, N., R. McManus, R. Wooster, J. Mangion, S. Seal, S. R. Lakhani, W. Ormiston, P. A. Daly, D. Ford, D. F. Easton, et al. 1995. Consistent loss of the wild type allele in breast cancers from a family linked to the BRCA2 gene on chromosome 13q12–13. *Oncogene* 10(8):1673–1675.

Compton, S. N., J. S. March, D. Brent, A. M. Albano, R. Weersing, and J. Curry. 2004. Cognitive-behavioral psychotherapy for anxiety and depressive disorders in children and adolescents: An evidence-based medicine review. *Journal of the American Academy of Child and Adolescent Psychiatry* 43(8):930–959.

Cook, N. R., J. E. Buring, and P. M. Ridker. 2006. The effect of including C-reactive protein in cardiovascular risk prediction models for women. *Annals of Internal Medicine* 145(1):21–29.

Cooke, T., J. Reeves, A. Lannigan, and P. Stanton. 2001. The value of the human epidermal growth factor receptor-2 (HER2) as a prognostic marker. *European Journal of Cancer* 37(Suppl. 1):3–10.

Cooper, C., and L. J. Melton, 3rd. 1992. Epidemiology of osteoporosis. *Trends in Endocrinology and Metabolism* 3(6):224–229.

Cooper, C., S. Westlake, N. Harvey, K. Javaid, E. Dennison, and M. Hanson. 2006. Review: Developmental origins of osteoporotic fracture. *Osteoporosis International* 17(3):337–347.

Cooper, E. R., M. Charurat, L. Mofenson, I. C. Hanson, J. Pitt, C. Diaz, K. Hayani, E. Handelsman, V. Smeriglio, R. Hoff, and W. Blattner. 2002. Combination antiretroviral strategies for the treatment of pregnant HIV-1-infected women and prevention of perinatal HIV-1 transmission. *Journal of Acquired Immune Deficiency Syndromes* 29(5):484–494.

Cooper, G. S., F. W. Miller, and J. P. Pandey. 1999. The role of genetic factors in autoimmune disease: Implications for environmental research. *Environmental Health Perspectives* 107 (Suppl. 5): 693–700.

Correa-de-Araujo, R. 2006. Serious gaps: How the lack of sex/gender-based research impairs health. *Journal of Women's Health* 15(10):1116–1122.

Correa-de-Araujo, R., and C. M. Clancy. 2006. Catalyzing quality of care improvements for women. *Women's Health Issues* 16(2):41–43.

Corsetti, V., N. Houssami, A. Ferrari, M. Ghirardi, S. Bellarosa, O. Angelini, C. Bani, P. Sardo, G. Remida, E. Galligioni, and S. Ciatto. 2008. Breast screening with ultrasound in women with mammography-negative dense breasts: Evidence on incremental cancer detection and false positives, and associated cost. *European Journal of Cancer* 44(4):539–544.

Couse, J. F., J. Lindzey, K. Grandien, J. A. Gustafsson, and K. S. Korach. 1997. Tissue distribution and quantitative analysis of estrogen receptor-alpha (ERALPHA) and estrogen receptor-beta (ERBETA) messenger ribonucleic acid in the wild-type and eralpha-knockout mouse. *Endocrinology* 138(11):4613–4621.

Coyle, Y. M. 2009. Lifestyle, genes, and cancer. *Methods in Molecular Biology* 472:25–56.

Cramer, J. A., and S. Silverman. 2006. Persistence with bisphosphonate treatment for osteoporosis: Finding the root of the problem. *American Journal of Medicine* 119(4 Suppl. 1):S12–S17.

Cramer, S. F., and A. Patel. 1990. The frequency of uterine leiomyomas. *American Journal of Clinical Pathology* 94(4):435–438.

Cranganu, A., and J. Camporeale. 2009. Nutrition aspects of lung cancer. *Nutrition in Clinical Practice* 24(6):688–700.

Cranney, A., T. Horsley, S. O'Donnell, H. A. Weiler, L. Puil, D. S. Ooi, S.A. Atkinson, L.M. Ward, D. Moher, D. A. Hanley, M. Fang, F. Yazd, C. Garritty, M. Sampson, N. Barrowman, A. Tsertsvadze, and V. Mamaladze. 2007. *Effectiveness and Safety of Vitamin D in Relation to Bone Health. Evidence Report/Technology Assessment No. 158. Prepared by the University of Ottawa Evidence-Based Practice Center (UO-EPC) Under Contract No. 290-02-0021.* AHRQ Publication No. 07-E013. Rockville, MD: Agency for Healthcare Research and Quality.

Creinin, M. D., E. Vittinghoff, E. Schaff, C. Klaisle, P. D. Darney, and C. Dean. 1997. Medical abortion with oral methotrexate and vaginal misoprostol. *Obstetrics and Gynecology* 90(4):611–616.

Crystal, P., S. D. Strano, S. Shcharynski, and M. J. Koretz. 2003. Using sonography to screen women with mammographically dense breasts. *American Journal of Roentgenology* 181(1):177–182.

Cuijpers, P., A. van Straten, F. Smit, C. Mihalopoulos, and A. Beekman. 2008. Preventing the onset of depressive disorders: A meta-analytic review of psychological interventions. *American Journal of Psychiatry* 165(10):1272–1280.

Cummings, S. M., B. Bride, K. M. Cassie, and A. Rawlins-Shaw. 2008. Substance abuse. *Journal of Gerontological Social Work* 50(Suppl. 1):215–241.

Cummings, S. R., and D. Black. 1995. Bone mass measurements and risk of fracture in Caucasian women: A review of findings from prospective studies. *American Journal of Medicine* 98(2A):24S–28S.

Cunningham, M., and L. H. Zayas. 2002. Reducing depression in pregnancy: Designing multimodal interventions. *Social Work* 47:114–123.

Cuschieri, K. 2009. Should boys receive the human papillomavirus vaccine? No. *British Medical Journal* 339:b4921.

Cuzick, J., T. Powles, U. Veronesi, J. Forbes, R. Edwards, S. Ashley, and P. Boyle. 2003. Overview of the main outcomes in breast-cancer prevention trials. *Lancet* 361(9354):296–300.

D'Amico, T. A., T. A. Aloia, M-B. H. Moore, J. E. Herndon, II, K. R. Brooks, C. L. Lau, and D. H. Harpole, Jr. 2000. Molecular biologic substaging of stage I lung cancer according to gender and histology. *Annals of Thoracic Surgery* 69(3):882–886.

Dannenberg, H., P. Komminoth, W. N. M. Dinjens, E. J. M. Speel, and R. R. de Krijger. 2003. Molecular genetic alterations in adrenal and extra-adrenal pheochromocytomas and paragangliomas. *Endocrine Pathology* 14(4):329–350.

Davey, E., A. Barratt, L. Irwig, S. F. Chan, P. Macaskill, P. Mannes, and A. M. Saville. 2006. Effect of study design and quality on unsatisfactory rates, cytology classifications, and accuracy in liquid-based versus conventional cervical cytology: A systematic review. *Lancet* 367(9505):122–132.

David, M., and A. D. Ebert. 2005. Treatment of uterine fibroids by embolization: Advantages, disadvantages, and pitfalls. *European Journal of Obstetrics, Gynecology, and Reproductive Biology* 123(2):131–138.

De Clercq, E. 2007. The design of drugs for HIV and HCV. *Nature Reviews Drug Discovery* 6(12):1001–1018.

De Groot, A. S. 2000. HIV infection among incarcerated women: Epidemic behind bars. *AIDS Reader* 10(5):287–295.

De Laet, C., J. A. Kanis, A. Oden, H. Johanson, O. Johnell, P. Delmas, J. A. Eisman, H. Kroger, S. Fujiwara, P. Garnero, E. V. McCloskey, D. Mellstrom, L. J. Melton, 3rd, P. J. Meunier, H. A. Pols, J. Reeve, A. Silman, and A. Tenenhouse. 2005. Body mass index as a predictor of fracture risk: A meta-analysis. *Osteoporosis International* 16(11):1330–1338.

Dean-Gaitor, H. D., and P. L. Fleming. 1999. Epidemiology of AIDS in incarcerated persons in the United States, 1994–1996. *AIDS* 13(17):2429–2435.

DeCara, J. M. 2003. Noninvasive cardiac testing in women. *Journal of the American Medical Women's Association* 58(4):254–263.

Deeks, E. 2007. Local therapy in endometrial cancer: Evidence based review. *Current Opinion in Oncology* 19(5):512–515.

Deligeoroglou, E., E. Michailidis, and G. Creatsas. 2003. Oral contraceptives and reproductive system cancer. In *Women's Health and Disease: Gynecologic and Reproductive Issues*. Vol. 997, Annals of the New York Academy of Sciences, edited by G. Creatsas, G. Mastorakos and G. P. Chrousos. New York: New York Academy of Sciences. Pp. 199–208.

DeMeo, M. T., E. A. Mutlu, A. Keshavarzian, and M. C. Tobin. 2002. Intestinal permeation and gastrointestinal disease. *Journal of Clinical Gastroenterology* 34(4):385–396.

Dennison, E., Z. Cole, and C. Cooper. 2005. Diagnosis and epidemiology of osteoporosis. *Current Opinion in Rheumatology* 17(4):456–461.

DeRubeis, R. J., L. A. Gelfand, T. Z. Tang, and A. D. Simons. 1999. Medications versus cognitive behavior therapy for severely depressed outpatients: Mega-analysis of four randomized comparisons. *American Journal of Psychiatry* 156(7):1007–1013.

DeSantis, C., A. Jemal, E. Ward, and M. J. Thun. 2008. Temporal trends in breast cancer mortality by state and race. *Cancer Causes and Control* 19(5):537–545.

Desta, Z., B. A. Ward, N. V. Soukhova, and D. A. Flockhart. 2004. Comprehensive evaluation of tamoxifen sequential biotransformation by the human cytochrome P450 system in vitro: Prominent roles for CYP3A and CYP2D6. *Journal of Pharmacology and Experimental Therapeutics* 310(3):1062–1075.

Devesa, S. S., E. S. Pollack, and J. L. Young, Jr. 1984. Assessing the validity of observed cancer incidence trends. *American Journal of Epidemiology* 119(2):274–291.

Di Leo, A., H. L. Gomez, Z. Aziz, Z. Zvirbule, J. Bines, M. C. Arbushites, S. F. Guerrera, M. Koehler, C. Oliva, S. H. Stein, L. S. Williams, J. Dering, R. S. Finn, and M. F. Press. 2008. Phase III, double-blind, randomized study comparing lapatinib plus paclitaxel with placebo plus paclitaxel as first-line treatment for metastatic breast cancer. *Journal Clinical Oncology* 26(34):5544–5552.

Diehl, A., B. Croissant, A. Batra, G. Mundle, H. Nakovics, and K. Mann. 2007. Alcoholism in women: Is it different in onset and outcome compared to men? *European Archives of Psychiatry and Clinical Neuroscience* 257(6):344–351.

Diekmann, F., S. Diekmann, F. Jeunehomme, S. Muller, B. Hamm, and U. Bick. 2005. Digital mammography using iodine-based contrast media: Initial clinical experience with dynamic contrast medium enhancement. *Investigative Radiology* 40(7):397–404.

Dolan, S. E., J. S. Huang, K. M. Killilea, M. P. Sullivan, N. Aliabadi, and S. Grinspoon. 2004. Reduced bone density in HIV-infected women. *AIDS* 18(3):475–483.

Dracup, K. 2007. The challenge of women and heart disease. *Archives of Internal Medicine* 167(22): 2396.

Dresler, C. M., C. Fratelli, J. Babb, L. Everley, A. A. Evans, and M. L. Clapper. 2000. Gender differences in genetic susceptibility for lung cancer. *Lung Cancer* 30(3):153–160.

Dromain, C., C. Balleyguier, S. Muller, M-C. Mathieu, F. Rochard, P. Opolon, and R. Sigal. 2006. Evaluation of tumor angiogenesis of breast carcinoma using contrast-enhanced digital mammography. *American Journal of Roentgenology* 187(5):W528–W537.

Dube, M. P., and F. R. Sattler. 2010. Inflammation and complications of HIV disease. *Journal of Infectious Diseases* 201(12):1783–1785.

Dürst, M., L. Gissmann, H. Ikenberg, and H. zur Hausen. 1983. A papillomavirus DNA from a cervical carcinoma and its prevalence in cancer biopsy samples from different geographic regions. *Proceedings of the National Academy of Sciences of the United States of America* 80(12):3812–3815.

Dürst, M., R. T. Dzarlieva-Petrusevska, P. Boukamp, N. E. Fusenig, and L. Gissmann. 1987. Molecular and cytogenetic analysis of immortalized human primary keratinocytes obtained after transfection with human papillomavirus type 16 DNA. *Oncogene* 1(3):251–256.

Dwight-Johnson, M., C. D. Sherbourne, D. Liao, and K. B. Wells. 2000. Treatment preferences among depressed primary care patients. *Journal of General Internal Medicine* 15(8):527–534.

Early Breast Cancer Trialists' Collaborative Group. 2005. Effects of chemotherapy and hormonal therapy for early breast cancer on recurrence and 15-year survival: An overview of the randomised trials. *Lancet* 365(9472):1687–1717.

Easton, D. F., D. T. Bishop, D. Ford, and G. P. Crockford. 1993. Genetic linkage analysis in familial breast and ovarian cancer: Results from 214 families. The breast cancer linkage consortium. *American Journal of Human Genetics* 52(4):678–701.

Ebers, G. C. 2009. Editorial regarding "Explaining Multiple Sclerosis Prevalence by Ultraviolet Exposure: A Geospatial Analysis," by Beretich and Beretich. *Multiple Sclerosis* 15(8):889–890.

Eifel, P. J. 2006. Concurrent chemotherapy and radiation therapy as the standard of care for cervical cancer. *Nature Clinical Practice. Oncology* 3(5):248–255.

Elhwuegi, A. S. 2004. Central monoamines and their role in major depression. *Progress in Neuropsychopharmacology and Biolical Psychiatry* 28(3):435–451.

Elsasser, A., K. Suzuki, and J. Schaper. 2000. Unresolved issues regarding the role of apoptosis in the pathogenesis of ischemic injury and heart failure. *Journal of Molecular and Cellular Cardiology* 32(5):711–724.

Emkey, R. D., and M. Ettinger. 2006. Improving compliance and persistence with bisphosphonate therapy for osteoporosis. *American Journal of Medicine* 119(4 Suppl. 1):S18–S24.

Ensrud, K. E., D. E. Thompson, J. A. Cauley, M. C. Nevitt, D. M. Kado, M. C. Hochberg, A. C. Santora, 2nd, and D. M. Black. 2000. Prevalent vertebral deformities predict mortality and hospitalization in older women with low bone mass. Fracture Intervention Trial Research Group. *Journal of the American Geriatrics Society* 48(3):241–249.

Erblich, J., D. H. Bovbjerg, C. Norman, H. B. Valdimarsdottir, and G. H. Montgomery. 2000. It won't happen to me: Lower perception of heart disease risk among women with family histories of breast cancer. *Preventive Medicine* 31(6):714–721.

Esserman, L., Y. Shieh, and I. Thompson. 2009. Rethinking screening for breast cancer and prostate cancer. *Journal of the American Medical Association* 302(15):1685–1692.

Essex, M., M. F. McLane, T. H. Lee, N. Tachibana, J. I. Mullins, J. Kreiss, C. K. Kasper, M. C. Poon, A. Landay, S. F. Stein, D. P. Francis, C. Cabradilla, D. N. Lawrence, and B. L. Evatt. 1983. Antibodies to human T-cell leukemia virus membrane antigens (HTLV-MA) in hemophiliacs. *Science* 221(4615):1061–1064.

Ettinger, B., S. T. Harris, D. Kendler, B. Kessel, M. R. McClung, G. I. Gorodeski, M. L. Rothert, V. W. Henderson, M. K. Richardson, R. R. Freedman, J. C. Gallagher, S. R. Goldstein, J. V. Pinkerton, N. K. Reame, L. Speroff, C. A. Stuenkel, I. Schiff, W. H. Utian, I. D. Graham, P. K. Lammers, P. P. Boggs, and The North American Menopause Society. 2006. Management of osteoporosis in postmenopausal women: 2006 position statement of the North American Menopause Society. *Menopause* 13(3):340–367.

European Study Group on Heterosexual Transmission of HIV. 1992. Comparison of female to male and male to female transmission of HIV in 563 stable couples. European Study Group on Heterosexual Transmission of HIV. *British Medical Journal* 304(6830):809–813.

Evangelista, O., and M. A. McLaughlin. 2009. Review of cardiovascular risk factors in women. *Gender Medicine* 6(Pt. 1):17–36.

Evans, P., and S. Brunsell. 2007. Uterine fibroid tumors: Diagnosis and treatment. *American Family Physician* 75(10):1503–1508.

Faca, V., H. Wang, and S. Hanash. 2009. Proteomic global profiling for cancer biomarker discovery. *Methods in Molecular Biology* 492:309–320.

Fader, A. N., L. N. Arriba, H. E. Frasure, and V. E. von Gruenigen. 2009. Endometrial cancer and obesity: Epidemiology, biomarkers, prevention and survivorship. *Gynecologic Oncology* 114(1):121–127.

Fairweather, D., S. Frisancho-Kiss, and N. R. Rose. 2008. Sex differences in autoimmune disease from a pathological perspective. *American Journal of Pathology* 173(3):600–609.

Fallowfield, L. 2005. Acceptance of adjuvant therapy and quality of life issues. *Breast* 14(6):612–616.

Farjah, F., D. E. Wood, N. D. Yanez, 3rd, T. L. Vaughan, R. G. Symons, B. Krishnadasan, and D. R. Flum. 2009. Racial disparities among patients with lung cancer who were recommended operative therapy. *Archives of Surgery* 144(1):14–18.

Farquhar, C., R. Basser, S. Hetrick, A. Lethaby, and J. Marjoribanks. 2003. High dose chemotherapy and autologous bone marrow or stem cell transplantation versus conventional chemotherapy for women with metastatic breast cancer. *Cochrane Database of Systematic Reviews* 1:CD003142.

Farzadegan, H., D. R. Hoover, J. Astemborski, C. M. Lyles, J. B. Margolick, R. B. Markham, T. C. Quinn, and D. Vlahov. 1998. Sex differences in HIV-1 viral load and progression to AIDS. *Lancet* 352(9139):1510–1514.

Faustman, D., X. P. Li, H. Y. Lin, Y. E. Fu, G. Eisenbarth, J. Avruch, and J. Guo. 1991. Linkage of faulty major histocompatibility complex class I to autoimmune diabetes. *Science* 254(5039):1756–1761.

Fawzi, W. W., G. I. Msamanga, D. Spiegelman, E. J. Urassa, N. McGrath, D. Mwakagile, G. Antelman, R. Mbise, G. Herrera, S. Kapiga, W. Willett, and D. J. Hunter. 1998. Randomised trial of effects of vitamin supplements on pregnancy outcomes and T cell counts in HIV-1-infected women in Tanzania. *Lancet* 351(9114):1477–1482.

FDA (US Food and Drug Administration). 2008. *FDA Licenses New Vaccine for Prevention of Cervical Cancer and Other Diseases in Females Caused by Human Papillomavirus.* http://www.fda. gov/NewsEvents/Newsroom/PressAnnouncements/2006/ucm108666.htm (accessed November 16, 2009).

———. 2009a. *FDA Approves New Vaccine for Prevention of Cervical Cancer.* US Department of Health and Human Services. http://www.fda.gov/NewsEvents/Newsroom/PressAnnouncements /ucm187048.htm (accessed April 14, 2010).

———. 2009b. *HIV/AIDS Historical Time Line 1981–1990.* http://www.fda.gov/ForConsumers/ ByAudience/ForPatientAdvocates/HIVandAIDSActivities/ucm151074.htm (accessed May 14, 2010).

———. 2010. *MQSA National Statistics.* http://www.fda.gov/Radiation-EmittingProducts/Mammog raphyQualityStandardsActandProgram/FacilityScorecard/ucm113858.htm (accessed August 7, 2010).

Ferenczy, A., and E. Franco. 2002. Persistent human papillomavirus infection and cervical neoplasia. *Lancet Oncology* 3(1):11–16.

Ferguson, M. K., J. Wang, P. C. Hoffman, D. J. Haraf, J. Olak, G. A. Masters, and E. E. Vokes. 2000. Sex-associated differences in survival of patients undergoing resection for lung cancer. *Annals of Thoracic Surgery* 69(1):245–249; discussion 249–250.

Fernandes, L. S., J. E. Tcheng, J. C. O'Shea, B. Weiner, T. J. Lorenz, C. Pacchiana, L. G. Berdan, K. J. Maresh, D. Joseph, M. Madan, T. Mann, R. Kiluru, J. S. Hochman, N. S. Kleiman, and ESPRIT Investigators. 2002. Is glycoprotein IIB/IIIA antagonism as effective in women as in men following percutaneous coronary intervention?: Lessons from the ESPRIT study. *Journal of the American College of Cardiology* 40(6):1085–1091.

Ferrero, S., P. L. Venturini, N. Ragni, G. Camerini, and V. Remorgida. 2009. Pharmacological treatment of endometriosis: Experience with aromatase inhibitors. *Drugs* 69:943–952.

Finer, L. B., and S. K. Henshaw. 2006. Disparities in rates of unintended pregnancy in the United States, 1994 and 2001. *Perspectives on Sexual and Reproductive Health* 38(2):90–96.

Fiorelli, J. L., T. J. Herzog, and J. D. Wright. 2008. Current treatment strategies for endometrial cancer. *Expert Review of Anticancer Therapy* 8(7):1149–1157.

Fisher, B., J. P. Costantino, D. L. Wickerham, C. K. Redmond, M. Kavanah, W. M. Cronin, V. Vogel, A. Robidoux, N. Dimitrov, J. Atkins, M. Daly, S. Wieand, E. Tan-Chiu, L. Ford, and N. Wolmark. 1998. Tamoxifen for prevention of breast cancer: Report of the National Surgical Adjuvant Breast and Bowel Project P-1 Study. *Journal of the National Cancer Institute* 90(18):1371–1388.

Fleck, F. 2004. Microbicides preventing HIV infection could be available by 2010. *Bulletin of the World Health Organization* 82(5):393–394.

Fletcher, S. W., and J. G. Elmore. 2003. Mammographic screening for breast cancer. *New England Journal of Medicine* 348(17):1672–1680.

Flexner, C. 2007. HIV drug development: The next 25 years. *Nature Reviews Drug Discovery* 6(12):959–966.

Fogel, C. I., and M. Belyea. 1999. The lives of incarcerated women: Violence, substance abuse, and at risk for HIV. *Journal of the Association of Nurses in AIDS Care* 10(6):66–74.

Fong, P. C., D. S. Boss, T. A. Yap, A. Tutt, P. Wu, M. Mergui-Roelvink, P. Mortimer, H. Swaisland, A. Lau, M. J. O'Connor, A. Ashworth, J. Carmichael, S. B. Kaye, J. H. M. Schellens, and J. S. de Bono. 2009. Inhibition of poly(ADP-ribose) polymerase in tumors from BRCA mutation carriers. *New England Journal of Medicine.*

Ford, E. S., U. A. Ajani, J. B. Croft, J. A. Critchley, D. R. Labarthe, T. E. Kottke, W. H. Giles, and S. Capewell. 2007. Explaining the decrease in U. S. deaths from coronary disease, 1980–2000. *New England Journal of Medicine* 356(23):2388–2398.

Fournier, J. C., R. J. DeRubeis, S. D. Hollon, S. Dimidjian, J. D. Amsterdam, R. C. Shelton, and J. Fawcett. 2010. Antidepressant drug effects and depression severity: A patient-level meta-analysis. *Journal of the American Medical Association* 303(1):47–53.

Fox, H. C., M. Talih, R. Malison, G. M. Anderson, M. J. Kreek, and R. Sinha. 2005. Frequency of recent cocaine and alcohol use affects drug craving and associated responses to stress and drug-related cues. *Psychoneuroendocrinology* 30(9):880–891.

Fox, H. C., K. A. Hong, P. Paliwal, P. T. Morgan, and R. Sinha. 2008. Altered levels of sex and stress steroid hormones assessed daily over a 28-day cycle in early abstinent cocaine-dependent females. *Psychopharmacology* 195(4):527–536.

Francis, R. M. 2008. Fracture risk assessment. *Current Orthopaedics* 22(5):322–327.

Franco, E. L., E. Duarte-Franco, and A. Ferenczy. 2001. Cervical cancer: Epidemiology, prevention and the role of human papillomavirus infection. *Canadian Medical Association Journal* 164(7):1017–1025.

Frank, E., D. J. Kupfer, J. M. Perel, C. Cornes, D. B. Jarrett, A. G. Mallinger, M. E. Thase, A. B. McEachran, and V. J. Grochocinski. 1990. Three-year outcomes for maintenance therapies in recurrent depression. *Archives of General Psychiatry* 47(12):1093–1099.

Frank, E., D. Novick, and D. J. Kupfer. 2005. Antidepressants and psychotherapy: A clinical research review. *Dialogues in Clinical Neuroscience* 7(3):263–272.

Frank, T., S. Manley, O. Olopade, S. Cummings, J. Garber, B. Bernhardt, K. Antman, D. Russo, M. Wood, L. Mullineau, C. Isaacs, B. Peshkin, S. Buys, V. Venne, P. Rowley, S. Loader, K. Offit, M. Robson, H. Hampel, D. Brener, E. Winer, S. Clark, B. Weber, L. Strong, and A. Thomas. 1998. Sequence analysis of *BRCA1* and *BRCA2*: Correlation of mutations with family history and ovarian cancer risk. *Journal Clinical Oncology* 16(7):2417–2425.

Freedman, N. D., M. F. Leitzmann, A. R. Hollenbeck, A. Schatzkin, and C. C. Abnet. 2008. Cigarette smoking and subsequent risk of lung cancer in men and women: Analysis of a prospective cohort study. *Lancet Oncology* 9(7):649–656.

French, R., and P. Brocklehurst. 1998. The effect of pregnancy on survival in women infected with HIV: A systematic review of the literature and meta-analysis. *British Journal of Obstetrics and Gynaecology* 105(8):827–835.

Friedenreich, C. M., L. S. Cook, A. M. Magliocco, M. A. Duggan, and K. S. Courneya. 2010. Case–control study of lifetime total physical activity and endometrial cancer risk. *Cancer Causes and Control* 21(7):1105–1116.

Frisell, J., and E. Lidbrink. 1997. The Stockholm mammographic screening trial: Risks and benefits in age group 40–49 years. *Journal of the National Cancer Institute Monographs* (22):49–51.

Frost, J. J., J. E. Darroch, and L. Remez. 2008. Improving contraceptive use in the United States. *Issues Brief (Alan Guttmacher Institute)* 1:1–8.

FUTURE II Study Group. 2007. Quadrivalent vaccine against human papillomavirus to prevent high-grade cervical lesions. *New England Journal of Medicine* 356(19):1915–1927.

Gadducci, A., and S. Cosio. 2009. Surveillance of patients after initial treatment of ovarian cancer. *Critical Reviews in Oncology/Hematology* 71(1):43–52.

Gale, E. A. M., and K. M. Gillespie. 2001. Diabetes and gender. *Diabetologia* 44(1):3–15.

Gallagher, J. C. 2007. Effect of early menopause on bone mineral density and fractures. *Menopause—the Journal of the North American Menopause Society* 14(3):567–571.

Gallo, J. J., S. D. Ryan, and D. E. Ford. 1999. Attitudes, knowledge, and behavior of family physicians regarding depression in late life. *Archives of Family Medicine* 8(3):249–256.

Gallo, R. C., P. S. Sarin, E. P. Gelmann, M. Robert-Guroff, E. Richardson, V. S. Kalyanaraman, D. Mann, G. D. Sidhu, R. E. Stahl, S. Zolla-Pazner, J. Leibowitch, and M. Popovic. 1983. Isolation of human t-cell leukemia virus in acquired immune deficiency syndrome (AIDS). *Science* 220(4599):865–867.

Garcia, P. M., L. A. Kalish, J. Pitt, H. Minkoff, T. C. Quinn, S. K. Burchett, J. Kornegay, B. Jackson, J. Moye, C. Hanson, C. Zorrilla, and J. F. Lew. 1999. Maternal levels of plasma human immunodeficiency virus type 1 RNA and the risk of perinatal transmission. Women and Infants Transmission Study group. *New England Journal of Medicine* 341(6):394–402.

Garcia-Closas, M., and S. Chanock. 2008. Genetic susceptibility loci for breast cancer by estrogen receptor status. *Clinical Cancer Research* 14(24):8000–8009.

Garfinkel, L., C. C. Boring, and C. W. Heath, Jr. 1994. Changing trends. An overview of breast cancer incidence and mortality. *Cancer* 74(1 Suppl):222–227.

Garland, S. M., M. Hernandez-Avila, C. M. Wheeler, G. Perez, D. M. Harper, S. Leodolter, G. W. K. Tang, D. G. Ferris, M. Steben, J. Bryan, F. J. Taddeo, R. Railkar, M. T. Esser, H. L. Sings, M. Nelson, J. Boslego, C. Sattler, E. Barr, L. A. Koutsky, and the Females United to Unilaterally Reduce Endo/Ectocervical Disease I Investigators. 2007. Quadrivalent vaccine against human papillomavirus to prevent anogenital diseases. *New England Journal of Medicine* 356(19): 1928–1943.

Garnero, P., E. Sornay-Rendu, M. C. Chapuy, and P. D. Delmas. 1996. Increased bone turnover in late postmenopausal women is a major determinant of osteoporosis. *Journal of Bone and Mineral Research* 11(3):337–349.

Gates, M. A., B. A. Rosner, J. L. Hecht, and S. S. Tworoger. 2010. Risk factors for epithelial ovarian cancer by histologic subtype. *American Journal of Epidemiology* 171(1):45–53.

Gehlbach, S. H., J. S. Avrunin, E. Puleo, and R. Spaeth. 2007. Fracture risk and antiresorptive medication use in older women in the USA. *Osteoporosis International* 18(6):805–810.

Gelmann, E. P., M. Popovic, D. Blayney, H. Masur, G. Sidhu, R. E. Stahl, and R. C. Gallo. 1983. Proviral DNA of a retrovirus, human T-cell leukemia virus, in two patients with AIDS. *Science* 220(4599):862–865.

Genant, H. K., K. Engelke, and S. Prevrhal. 2008. Advanced CT bone imaging in osteoporosis. *Rheumatology* 47 (Suppl. 4):iv9–iv16.

Gensichen, J., M. Beyerm, C. Muth, F. M. Gerlach, M. Von Koff, and J. Ormel. 2006. Case management to improve major depression in primary health care: A systematic review. *Psychological Medicine* 36(01):7–14.

Geusens, P., P. Autier, S. Boonen, J. Vanhoof, K. Declerck, and J. Raus. 2002. The relationship among history of falls, osteoporosis, and fractures in postmenopausal women. *Archives of Physical Medicine and Rehabilitation* 83(7):903–906.

Geyer, C. E., J. Forster, D. Lindquist, S. Chan, C. G. Romieu, T. Pienkowski, A. Jagiello-Gruszfeld, J. Crown, A. Chan, B. Kaufman, D. Skarlos, M. Campone, N. Davidson, M. Berger, C. Oliva, S. D. Rubin, S. Stein, and D. Cameron. 2006. Lapatinib plus capecitabine for HER2-positive advanced breast cancer. *New England Journal of Medicine* 355(26):2733–2743.

Ghafoor, A., A. Jemal, E. Ward, V. Cokkinides, R. Smith, and M. Thun. 2003. Trends in breast cancer by race and ethnicity. *CA: A Cancer Journal for Clinicians* 53(6):342–355.

Gibbons, S. K., and H. M. Keys. 2000. Advanced cervical cancer. *Current Treatment Options in Oncology* 1(2):157–160.

Ginsburg, E. S., N. K. Mello, J. H. Mendelson, R. L. Barbieri, S. K. Teoh, M. Rothman, X. Gao, and J. W. Sholar. 1996. Effects of alcohol ingestion on estrogens in postmenopausal women. *Journal of the American Medical Association* 276(21):1747–1751.

Giuliano, A. R., M. Papenfuss, M. Nour, L. M. Canfield, A. Schneider, and K. Hatch. 1997. Antioxidant nutrients: Associations with persistent human papillomavirus infection. *Cancer Epidemiology Biomarkers & Prevention* 6(11):917–923.

Giuliano, A. R., E. M. Siegel, D. J. Roe, S. Ferreira, M. L. Baggio, L. Galan, E. Duarte-Franco, L. L. Villa, T. E. Rohan, J. R. Marshall, and E. L. Franco. 2003. Dietary intake and risk of persistent human papillomavirus (HPV) infection: The Ludwig-Mcgill HPV Natural History Study. *Journal of Infectious Diseases* 188(10):1508–1516.

Golanska, E., K. Hulas-Bigoszewska, M. Sieruta, I. Zawlik, M. Witusik, S. M. Gresner, T. Sobow, M. Styczynska, B. Peplonska, M. Barcikowska, P. P. Liberski, and E. H. Corder. 2009. Earlier onset of Alzheimer's disease: Risk polymorphisms within PRNP, PRND, CYP46, and APOE genes. *Journal of Alzheimer's Disease* 17(2):359–368.

Goldberg, R. J. 1981. Management of depression in the patient with advanced cancer. *Journal of the American Medical Association* 246(4):373–376.

Goldhahn, J., B. Mitlak, P. Aspenberg, J. A. Kanis, R. Rizzoli, and J. Y. Reginster. 2008. Critical issues in translational and clinical research for the study of new technologies to enhance bone repair. *Journal of Bone and Joint Surgery—Series A* 90(Suppl. 1):43–47.

Goldman, L. S., N. H. Nielsen, and H. C. Champion. 1999. Awareness, diagnosis, and treatment of depression. *Journal of General Internal Medicine* 14(9):569–580.

Goldstein, J. M., L. J. Seidman, L. M. O'Brien, N. J. Horton, D. N. Kennedy, N. Makris, V. S. Caviness, Jr., S. V. Faraone, and M. T. Tsuang. 2002. Impact of normal sexual dimorphisms on sex differences in structural brain abnormalities in schizophrenia assessed by magnetic resonance imaging. *Archives of General Psychiatry* 59(2):154–164.

Gordon, P. B., and L. S. Goldenberg. 1995. Malignant breast masses detected only by ultrasound. A retrospective review. *Cancer* 76(4):626–630.

Goss, P. E., J. N. Ingle, S. Martino, N. J. Robert, H. B. Muss, M. J. Piccart, M. Castiglione, D. Tu, L. E. Shepherd, K. I. Pritchard, R. B. Livingston, N. E. Davidson, L. Norton, E. A. Perez, J. S. Abrams, P. Therasse, M. J. Palmer, and J. L. Pater. 2003. A randomized trial of letrozole in postmenopausal women after five years of tamoxifen therapy for early-stage breast cancer. *New England Journal of Medicine* 349(19):1793–1802.

Gotlib, I. H., V. E. Whiffen, J. H. Mount, K. Milne, and N. I. Cordy. 1989. Prevalence rates and demographic characteristics associated with depression in pregnancy and the postpartum. *Journal of Consulting and Clinical Psychology* 57(2):269–274.

Gotzsche, P. C., and O. Olsen. 2000. Is screening for breast cancer with mammography justifiable? *Lancet* 355(9198):129–134.

Grady, D., L. Chaput, and M. Kristof. 2003. *Diagnosis and Treatment of Coronary Heart Disease in Women: Systematic Reviews of Evidence on Selected Topics.* Evidence Report/Technology Assessment No. 81. (Prepared by the University of California, San Francisco-Stanford Evidence-based Practice Center under Contract No 290-97-0013.) AHRQ Publication No. 03-E037. Rockville, MD: Agency for Healthcare Research and Quality.

Grann, V., A. B. Troxel, N. Zojwalla, D. Hershman, S. A. Glied, and J. S. Jacobson. 2006. Regional and racial disparities in breast cancer-specific mortality. *Social Science and Medicine* 62(2):337–347.

Grant, B. F., D. A. Dawson, F. S. Stinson, S. P. Chou, M. C. Dufour, and R. P. Pickering. 2004. The 12-month prevalence and trends in DSM-IV alcohol abuse and dependence: United States, 1991–1992 and 2001–2002. *Drug and Alcohol Dependence* 74(3):223–234.

Greenblatt, R. M., S. A. Lukehart, F. A. Plummer, T. C. Quinn, C. W. Critchlow, R. L. Ashley, L. J. D'Costa, J. O. Ndinya-Achola, L. Corey, A. R. Ronald, and K. K. Holmes. 1988. Genital ulceration as a risk factor for human immunodeficiency virus infection. *AIDS* 2(1):47–50.

Greenfield, S. F. 2002. Women and alcohol use disorders. *Harvard Review of Psychiatry* 10(2):76–85.

Greenfield, S. F., and S. Pirard. 2009. Gender-specific treatment for women with substance use disorders. In *Women and Addiction: A Comprehensive Handbook*, edited by K. Brady, S. E. Back and S. F. Greenfield. New York: Guilford Press. Pp. 289–306.

Greenstein, B., R. Roa, Y. Dhaher, E. Nunn, A. Greenstein, M. Khamashta, and G. R. Hughes. 2001. Estrogen and progesterone receptors in murine models of systemic lupus erythematosus. *International Immunopharmacology* 1(6):1025–1035.

Gregg, E. W., M. A. Pereira, and C. J. Caspersen. 2000. Physical activity, falls, and fractures among older adults: A review of the epidemiologic evidence. *Journal of the American Geriatrics Society* 48(8):883–893.

Grella, C. E. 2008. From generic to gender-responsive treatment: Changes in social policies, treatment services, and outcomes of women in substance abuse treatment. *Journal of Psychoactive Drugs* (Suppl. 5):327–343.

Grella, C. E., and V. Joshi. 1999. Gender differences in drug treatment careers among clients in the National Drug Abuse Treatment Outcome Study. *American Journal of Drug and Alcohol Abuse* 25(3):385–406.

Grigoriadis, S., and G. E. Robinson. 2007. Gender issues in depression. *Annals of Clinical Psychiatry* 19(4):247–255.

Groginsky, E., N. Bowdler, and J. Yankowitz. 1998. Update on vertical HIV transmission. *Journal of Reproductive Medicine* 43(8):637–646.

Guarneri, V., and P. Conte. 2009. Metastatic breast cancer: Therapeutic options according to molecular subtypes and prior adjuvant therapy. *Oncologist* 14(7):645–656.

Guidos, B. J., and S. M. Selvaggi. 1999. Use of the thin prep pap test in clinical practice. *Diagnostic Cytopathology* 20(2):70–73.

Gulati, M., H. R. Black, L. J. Shaw, M. F. Arnsdorf, C. N. Merz, M. S. Lauer, T. H. Marwick, D. K. Pandey, R. H. Wicklund, and R. A. Thisted. 2005. The prognostic value of a nomogram for exercise capacity in women. *New England Journal of Medicine* 353(5):468–475.

Gulati, M., R. M. Cooper-DeHoff, C. McClure, B. D. Johnson, L. J. Shaw, E. M. Handberg, I. Zineh, S. F. Kelsey, M. F. Arnsdorf, H. R. Black, C. J. Pepine, and C. N. Merz. 2009. Adverse cardiovascular outcomes in women with nonobstructive coronary artery disease: A report from the Women's Ischemia Syndrome Evaluation Study and the St. James Women Take Heart Project. *Archives of Internal Medicine* 169(9):843–850.

Gur, D., G. S. Abrams, D. M. Chough, M. A. Ganott, C. M. Hakim, R. L. Perrin, G. Y. Rathfon, J. H. Sumkin, M. L. Zuley, and A. I. Bandos. 2009. Digital breast tomosynthesis: Observer performance study. *American Journal of Roentgeneology* 193(2):586–591.

Guthrie, B. J., and L. J. Flinchbaugh. 2001. Gender-specific substance prevention programming: Going beyond just focusing on girls. *Journal of Early Adolescence* 21(3):354–372.

Haas, J., C. Kaplan, E. Gerstenberger, and K. Kerlikowske. 2004. Changes in the use of postmenopausal hormone therapy after the publication of clinical trial results. *Annals of Internal Medicine* 140:184–188.

Hackley, B. 2010. Antidepressant medication use in pregnancy: Safety of antidepressants in pregnancy. *Journal of Midwifery and Women's Health* 55(2):90–100.

Hader, S. L., D. K. Smith, J. S. Moore, and S. D. Holmberg. 2001. HIV infection in women in the United States: Status at the millennium. *Journal of the American Medical Association* 285(9): 1186–1192.

Hagen, A. I., K. A. Kvistad, L. Maehle, M. M. Holmen, H. Aase, B. Styr, A. Vabo, J. Apold, P. Skaane, and P. Moller. 2007. Sensitivity of MRI versus conventional screening in the diagnosis of BRCA-associated breast cancer in a national prospective series. *Breast Journal* 16(4):367–374.

Haiman, C. A., D. O. Stram, L. R. Wilkens, M. C. Pike, L. N. Kolonel, B. E. Henderson, and L. Le Marchand. 2006. Ethnic and racial differences in the smoking-related risk of lung cancer. *New England Journal of Medicine* 354(4):333–342.

Hakim-Elahi, E., H. M. Tovell, and M. S. Burnhill. 1990. Complications of first-trimester abortion: A report of 170,000 cases. *Obstetrics and Gynecology* 76(1):129–135.

Hall, H. I., R. Song, P. Rhodes, J. Prejean, Q. An, L. M. Lee, J. Karon, R. Brookmeyer, E. H. Kaplan, M. T. McKenna, and R. S. Janssen. 2008. Estimation of HIV incidence in the United States. *Journal of the American Medical Association* 300(5):520–529.

Hall, J. M., and D. P. McDonnell. 2005. Coregulators in nuclear estrogen receptor action: From concept to therapeutic targeting. *Molecular Interventions* 5(6):343–357.

Hall, J. M., M. K. Lee, B. Newman, J. E. Morrow, L. A. Anderson, B. Huey, and M. C. King. 1990. Linkage of early-onset familial breast cancer to chromosome 17q21. *Science* 250(4988):1684–1689.

Hammen, C. 1999. The emergence of an interpersonal approach to depression. In *The Interactional Nature of Depression: Advances In Interpersonal Approaches*, edited by T. Joiner and J. Coyne. Washington, DC: American Psychological Association.

Hankinson, S. E., G. A. Colditz, D. J. Hunter, W. C. Willett, M. J. Stampfer, B. Rosner, C. H. Hennekens, and F. E. Speizer. 1995. A prospective study of reproductive factors and risk of epithelial ovarian cancer. *Cancer* 76(2):284–290.

Hannan, M. T., D. T. Felson, B. Dawson-Hughes, K. L. Tucker, L. A. Cupples, P. W. Wilson, and D. P. Kiel. 2000. Risk factors for longitudinal bone loss in elderly men and women: The Framingham Osteoporosis Study. *Journal of Bone and Mineral Research* 15(4):710–720.

Harawa, N. T., S. Greenland, S. D. Cochran, W. E. Cunningham, and B. Visscher. 2003. Do differences in relationship and partner attributes explain disparities in sexually transmitted disease among young white and black women? *Journal of Adolescent Health* 32(3):187–191.

Hardy, D., C. C. Liu, R. Xia, J. N. Cormier, W. Chan, A. White, K. Burau, and X. L. Du. 2009. Racial disparities and treatment trends in a large cohort of elderly black and white patients with nonsmall cell lung cancer. *Cancer* 115(10):2199–2211.

Harlow, S. D., P. Schuman, M. Cohen, S. E. Ohmit, S. Cu-Uvin, X. H. Lin, K. Anastos, D. Burns, R. Greenblatt, H. Minkoff, L. Muderspach, A. Rompalo, D. Warren, M. A. Young, and R. S. Klein. 2000. Effect of HIV infection on menstrual cycle length. *Journal of Acquired Immune Deficiency Syndromes* 24(1):68–75.

Harper, D. M., E. L. Franco, C. Wheeler, D. G. Ferris, D. Jenkins, A. Schuind, T. Zahaf, B. Innis, P. Naud, N. S. De Carvalho, C. M. Roteli-Martins, J. Teixeira, M. M. Blatter, A. P. Korn, W. Quint, and G. Dubin. 2004. Efficacy of a bivalent L1 virus-like particle vaccine in prevention of infection with human papillomavirus types 16 and 18 in young women: A randomised controlled trial. *Lancet* 364(9447):1757–1765.

Harris, R. E., E. A. Zang, J. I. Anderson, and E. L. Wynder. 1993. Race and sex differences in lung cancer risk associated with cigarette smoking. *International Journal of Epidemiology* 22(4):592–599.

Harro, C. D., Y. Y. Pang, R. B. Roden, A. Hildesheim, Z. Wang, M. J. Reynolds, T. C. Mast, R. Robinson, B. R. Murphy, R. A. Karron, J. Dillner, J. T. Schiller, and D. R. Lowy. 2001. Safety and immunogenicity trial in adult volunteers of a human papillomavirus 16 L1 virus-like particle vaccine. *Journal of the National Cancer Institute* 93(4):284–292.

Hartman, A. R., B. L. Daniel, A. W. Kurian, M. A. Mills, K. W. Nowels, F. M. Dirbas, K. E. Kingham, N. M. Chun, R. J. Herfkens, J. M. Ford, and S. K. Plevritis. 2004. Breast magnetic resonance image screening and ductal lavage in women at high genetic risk for breast carcinoma. *Cancer* 100(3):479–489.

Harwell, J. I., T. Moench, K. H. Mayer, S. Chapman, I. Rodriguez, and S. Cu-Uvin. 2003. A pilot study of treatment of bacterial vaginosis with a buffering vaginal microbicide. *Journal of Women's Health* 12(3):255–259.

Haus, A. G. 1990. Technologic improvements in screen-film mammography. *Radiology* 174(3): 628–637.

Hausauer, A., T. Keegan, E. Chang, and C. Clarke. 2007. Recent breast cancer trends among Asian/ Pacific Islander, Hispanic, and African–American women in the US: Changes by tumor subtype. *Breast Cancer Research* 9:R90.

Hausauer, A., T. Keegan, E. Chang, S. Glaser, H. Howe, and C. Clarke. 2009. Recent trends in breast cancer incidence in US white women by county-level urban/rural and poverty status. *BMC Medicine* 7(1):31.

Hayashi, T., and D. Faustman. 1999. NOD mice are defective in proteasome production and activation of NF-kappaB. *Molecular Cell Biology* 19(12):8646–8659.

Health Council of the Netherlands. 2002. *The Benefit of Population Screening for Breast Cancer with Mammography*. http://www.gezondheidsraad.nl/en/publications/benefit-population-screening-breast-cancer-mammography (accessed November 16, 2009).

Heath, K. V., K. J. Chan, J. Singer, M. V. O'Shaughnessy, J. S. Montaner, and R. S. Hogg. 2002. Incidence of morphological and lipid abnormalities: Gender and treatment differentials after initiation of first antiretroviral therapy. *International Journal of Epidemiology* 31(5):1016–1020.

Hebert, R., M. F. Dubois, C. Wolfson, L. Chambers, and C. Cohen. 2001. Factors associated with long-term institutionalization of older people with dementia: Data from the Canadian Study of Health and Aging. *Journals of Gerontology. Series A, Biological Sciences and Medical Sciences* 56(11):M693–M699.

Henderson, I. C., D. A. Berry, G. D. Demetri, C. T. Cirrincione, L. J. Goldstein, S. Martino, J. N. Ingle, M. R. Cooper, D. F. Hayes, K. H. Tkaczuk, G. Fleming, J. F. Holland, D. B. Duggan, J. T. Carpenter, E. Frei, III, R. L. Schilsky, W. C. Wood, H. B. Muss, and L. Norton. 2003. Improved outcomes from adding sequential Paclitaxel but not from escalating Doxorubicin dose in an adjuvant chemotherapy regimen for patients with node-positive primary breast cancer. *Journal Clinical Oncology* 21(6):976–983.

Hendrick, R. E., R. A. Smith, J. H. Rutledge, 3rd, and C. R. Smart. 1997. Benefit of screening mammography in women aged 40–49: A new meta-analysis of randomized controlled trials. *Journal of the National Cancer Institute Monographs* (22):87–92.

Henschke, C. I., and O. S. Miettinen. 2004. Women's susceptibility to tobacco carcinogens. *Lung Cancer* 43(1):1–5.

Henschke, C. I., D. F. Yankelevitz, D. M. Libby, M. W. Pasmantier, J. P. Smith, and O. S. Miettinen. 2006. Survival of patients with stage 1 lung cancer detected on CT screening. *The New England Journal of Medicine* 355(17):1763–1771.

Herrera, F. G., L. Vidal, A. Oza, M. Milosevic, and A. Fyles. 2008. Molecular targeted agents combined with chemo-radiation in the treatment of locally advanced cervix cancer. *Reviews on Recent Clinical Trials* 3:111–120.

Hersh, A. L., M. L. Stefanick, and R. S. Stafford. 2004. National use of postmenopausal hormone therapy: Annual trends and response to recent evidence. *Journal of the American Medical Association* 291(1):47–53.

HHS (US Department of Health and Human Services). 1999. *Mental Health: A Report of the Surgeon General*. Rockville, MD: US Department of Health and Human Services, Substance Abuse and Mental Health Services Administration, Center for Mental Health Services, National Institutes of Health, National Institute of Mental Health.

———. 2000. *Healthy People 2010: Understanding and Improving Health*. Washington, DC: US Government Printing Office.

———. 2001. *Women and Smoking: A Report of the Surgeon General*. http://www.surgeongeneral. gov/library/womenandtobacco/index.html (accessed January 13, 2010).

———. 2003. *Drug Use Among Racial/Ethnic Minorities*. Washington, DC: US Department of Health and Human Services.

———. 2005. *Progress in Autoimmune Diseases Research*. Washington, DC: US Department of Health and Human Services.

———. 2007. *ATHENA (Athletes Targeting Healthy Exercise and Nutrition Alternatives)*. http://www. nrepp.samhsa.gov/listofprograms.asp?textsearch=alcohol&ShowHide=1&Sort=1&N1=1&A3= 3&G2=2 (accessed February 22, 2010).

———. 2008. *Substance Abuse and HIV/AIDS*. US Department of Health and Human Services.

———. 2009. *FDA Approves New Indication for Gardasil to Prevent Genital Warts in Men and Boys*. http://www.fda.gov/NewsEvents/Newsroom/PressAnnouncements/ucm187003.htm (accessed June 12, 2010).

———. 2010. *FDA Drug Safety Communication: Ongoing Safety Review of Oral Bisphosphonates and Atypical Subtrochanteric Femur Fractures*. http://www.fda.gov/Drugs/DrugSafety/ PostmarketDrugSafetyInformationforPatientsandProviders/ucm203891.htm (accessed July 7, 2010).

Hibbitts, S. 2009. Should boys receive the human papillomavirus vaccine? Yes. *British Medical Journal* 339:b4928.

Hillier, T. A., K. L. Stone, D. C. Bauer, J. H. Rizzo, K. L. Pedula, J. A. Cauley, K. E. Ensrud, M. C. Hochberg, and S. R. Cummings. 2007. Evaluating the value of repeat bone mineral density measurement and prediction of fractures in older women: The study of osteoporotic fractures. *Archives of Internal Medicine* 167(2):155–160.

Hindmarch, I. 2002. Beyond the monoamine hypothesis: Mechanisms, molecules and methods. *European Psychiatry* 17(Suppl. 3):294–299.

Hippisley-Cox, J., and C. Coupland. 2010. Individualising the risks of statins in men and women in England and Wales: Population-based cohort study. *Heart* 96(12):939–947.

Hirose, K., N. Hamajima, T. Takezaki, T. Kuroishi, K. Kuzuya, S. Sasaki, S. Tokudome, and K. Tajima. 1998. Smoking and dietary risk factors for cervical cancer at different age group in Japan. *Journal of Epidemiology* 8(1):6–14.

Hitti, J., L. M. Frenkel, A. M. Stek, S. A. Nachman, D. Baker, A. Gonzalez-Garcia, A. Provisor, E. M. Thorpe, M. E. Paul, M. Foca, J. Gandia, S. Huang, L. J. Wei, L. M. Stevens, D. H. Watts, and J. McNamara. 2004. Maternal toxicity with continuous nevirapine in pregnancy: Results from PACTG 1022. *Journal of Acquired Immune Deficiency Syndromes* 36(3):772–776.

Hogan, M. F. 2003. The President's New Freedom Commission: Recommendations to transform mental health care in America. *Psychiatric Services* 54(11):1467–1474.

Hogberg, T. 2008. Adjuvant chemotherapy in endometrial carcinoma: Overview of randomised trials. *Clinical Oncology* 20(6):463–469.

Holdcraft, L. C., and W. G. Iacono. 2004. Cross-generational effects on gender differences in psychoactive drug abuse and dependence. *Drug and Alcohol Dependence* 74(2):147–158.

Hollon, S. D., R. B. Jarrett, A. A. Nierenberg, M. E. Thase, M. Trivedi, and A. J. Rush. 2005. Psychotherapy and medication in the treatment of adult and geriatric depression: Which monotherapy or combined treatment? *Journal of Clinical Psychiatry* 66(4):455–468.

Hoyert, D. L. 2007. Maternal mortality and related concepts. *Vital Health Statistics* 3(33):1–13.

HRSA (Health Resources and Services Agency). 2008. *Women's Health USA 2008.* Rockville, MD: US Department of Health and Human Services.

Hser, Y. I., M. D. Anglin, and M. W. Booth. 1987. Sex differences in addict careers. 3. Addiction. *American Journal of Drug and Alcohol Abuse* 13(3):231–251.

Hua, S., C. B. Kallen, R. Dhar, M. T. Baquero, C. E. Mason, B. A. Russell, P. K. Shah, J. Liu, A. Khramtsov, M. S. Tretiakova, T. N. Krausz, O. I. Olopade, D. L. Rimm, and K. P. White. 2008. Genomic analysis of estrogen cascade reveals histone variant H2A.Z associated with breast cancer progression. *Molecular Systems Biology* 4:188.

Huang, C. Q., B. R. Dong, Z. C. Lu, J. R. Yue, and Q. X. Liu. 2010. Chronic diseases and risk for depression in old age: A meta-analysis of published literature. *Ageing Research Reviews* 9(2):131–141.

Huang, Q. Y., and A. W. C. Kung. 2006. Genetics of osteoporosis. *Molecular Genetics and Metabolism* 88:295–306.

Huang, W., P. R. Fisher, K. Dulaimy, L. A. Tudorica, B. O'Shea, and T. M. Button. 2004. Detection of breast malignancy: Diagnostic MR protocol for improved specificity1. *Radiology* 232(2):585–591.

Hull, S. C., and A. L. Caplan. 2009. The case for vaccinating boys against human papillomavirus. *Public Health Genomics* 12(5-6):362–367.

Hung, C-F., B. Ma, A. Monie, S-W. Tsen, and T-C. Wu. 2008. Therapeutic human papillomavirus vaccines: Current clinical trials and future directions. *Expert Opinion on Biological Therapy* 8(4):421–439.

Hung, J., B. Chaitman, J. Lam, J. Lesperance, G. Dupras, P. Fines, and M. Bourassa. 1984. Noninvasive diagnostic test choices for the evaluation of coronary artery disease in women: A multivariate comparison of cardiac fluoroscopy, exercise electrocardiography and exercise thallium myocardial perfusion scintigraphy. *Journal of the American College of Cardiology* 4(1):8–16.

Ikeda, K. 2008. Osteocytes in the pathogenesis of osteoporosis. *Geriatrics and Gerontology International* 8(4):213–217.

Innes, K. E., and T. E. Byers. 2001. Smoking during pregnancy and breast cancer risk in very young women (United States). *Cancer Causes and Control* 12(2):179–185.

The International Perinatal HIV Group. 1999. The mode of delivery and the risk of vertical transmission of human immunodeficiency virus type 1: A meta analysis of 15 prospective cohort studies. *New England Journal of Medicine* 340:977–987.

Invernizzi, P., M. Miozzo, P. M. Battezzati, I. Bianchi, F. R. Grati, G. Simoni, C. Selmi, M. Watnik, M. E. Gershwin, and M. Podda. 2004. Frequency of monosomy X in women with primary biliary cirrhosis. *Lancet* 363(9408):533–535.

Invernizzi, P., M. Miozzo, C. Selmi, L. Persani, P. M. Battezzati, M. Zuin, S. Lucchi, P. L. Meroni, B. Marasini, S. Zeni, M. Watnik, F. R. Grati, G. Simoni, M. E. Gershwin, and M. Podda. 2005. X chromosome monosomy: A common mechanism for autoimmune diseases. *Journal of Immunology* 175(1):575–578.

Invernizzi, P., S. Pasini, and M. Podda. 2008. X chromosome in autoimmune diseases. *Expert Review of Clinical Immunology* 4(5):591–597.

Invernizzi, P., S. Pasini, C. Selmi, M. E. Gershwin, and M. Podda. 2009. Female predominance and X chromosome defects in autoimmune diseases. *Journal of Autoimmunity* 33(1):12–16.

IOM. 1993. *Clinical Applications of Mifepristone (RU486) and Other Antiprogestins: Assessing the Science and Recommending a Research Agenda.* Washington, DC: National Academy Press.

———. 1995. *The Best Intentions: Unintended Pregnancy and the Well-Being of Children and Families.* Washington, DC: National Academy Press.

———. 2001a. *No Time to Lose: Getting More from HIV Prevention.* Washington, DC: National Academy Press.

———. 2001b. *Exploring the Biological Contributions to Human Health: Does Sex Matter?* Washington, DC: National Academy Press.

———. 2003. *Fulfilling the Potential for Cancer Prevention and Early Detection.* Washington, DC: The National Academies Press.

———. 2004a. *Strategies to Leverage Research Funding: Guiding DoD's Peer Reviewed Medical Research Programs.* Washington, DC: The National Academies Press.

———. 2004b. *Frontiers in Contraceptive Research.* Washington, DC: The National Academies Press.

———. 2005. *Complementary and Alternative Medicine in the United States.* Washington, DC: National Academies Press.

———. 2006. *From Cancer Patient to Cancer Survivor—Lost in Transition: An American Society of Clinical Oncology and Institute of Medicine Symposium.* Edited by M. Hewitt and P. A. Ganz. Washington, DC: The National Academies Press.

———. 2008. *Cancer Care for the Whole Patient: Meeting Psychosocial Health Needs.* Edited by N. E. Adler and A. Page. Washington, DC: The National Academies Press.

———. 2009. *A Review of the HHS Family Planning Program: Mission, Management, and Measurement of Results.* Washington, DC: The National Academies Press.

Iwamoto, J., T. Takeda, and Y. Sato. 2005. Effect of treadmill exercise on bone mass in female rats. *Experimental Animals* 54(1):1–6.

Jackson, R. D., A. Z. LaCroix, M. Gass, R. B. Wallace, J. Robbins, C. E. Lewis, T. Bassford, S. A. Beresford, H. R. Black, P. Blanchette, D. E. Bonds, R. L. Brunner, R. G. Brzyski, B. Caan, J. A. Cauley, R. T. Chlebowski, S. R. Cummings, I. Granek, J. Hays, G. Heiss, S. L. Hendrix, B. V. Howard, J. Hsia, F. A. Hubbell, K. C. Johnson, H. Judd, J. M. Kotchen, L. H. Kuller, R. D. Langer, N. L. Lasser, M. C. Limacher, S. Ludlam, J. E. Manson, K. L. Margolis, J. McGowan, J. K. Ockene, M. J. O'Sullivan, L. Phillips, R. L. Prentice, G. E. Sarto, M. L. Stefanick, L. Van Horn, J. Wactawski-Wende, E. Whitlock, G. L. Anderson, A. R. Assaf, and D. Barad. 2006. Calcium plus vitamin D supplementation and the risk of fractures. *New England Journal of Medicine* 354(7):669–683.

Jansson, A., M. Gustafsson, and E. Wilander. 1998. Efficiency of cytological screening for detection of cervical squamous carcinoma. A study in the county of Uppsala 1991–1994. *Upsala Journal of Medical Sciences* 103(2):147–154.

Jemal, A., E. Ward, and M. J. Thun. 2007. Recent trends in breast cancer incidence rates by age and tumor characteristics among US women. *Breast Cancer Research* 9(3):R28.

Jemal, A., M. J. Thun, L. A. Ries, H. L. Howe, H. K. Weir, M. M. Center, E. Ward, X. C. Wu, C. Eheman, R. Anderson, U. A. Ajani, B. Kohler, and B. K. Edwards. 2008. Annual report to the nation on the status of cancer, 1975–2005, featuring trends in lung cancer, tobacco use, and tobacco control. *Journal of the National Cancer Institute* 100(23):1672–1694.

Jemal, A., R. Siegel, E. Xu, and E. Ward. 2010. Cancer Statistics, 2010. *CA: A Cancer Journal for Clinicians* 60(5):277–300.

Jong, R. A., M. J. Yaffe, M. Skarpathiotakis, R. S. Shumak, N. M. Danjoux, A. Gunesekara, and D. B. Plewes. 2003. Contrast-enhanced digital mammography: Initial clinical experience. *Radiology* 228(3):842–850.

Jordan, S. J., P. M. Webb, and A. C. Green. 2005. Height, age at menarche, and risk of epithelial ovarian cancer. *Cancer Epidemiology Biomarkers and Prevention* 14(8):2045–2048.

Juethner, S. N., C. Williamson, M. B. Ristig, P. Tebas, W. Seyfried, and J. A. Aberg. 2003. Nonnucleoside reverse transcriptase inhibitor resistance among antiretroviral-naive HIV-positive pregnant women. *Journal of Acquired Immune Deficiency Syndromes* 32(2):153–156.

Kaas, R., S. Verhoef, J. Wesseling, M. A. Rookus, H. S. A. Oldenburg, M-J. V. Peeters, and E. J. T. Rutgers. 2010. Prophylactic mastectomy in *BRCA1* and *BRCA2* mutation carriers: Very low risk for subsequent breast cancer. *Annals of Surgery* 251(3):488–492.

Kado, D. M., W. S. Browner, L. Palermo, M. C. Nevitt, H. K. Genant, and S. R. Cummings. 1999. Vertebral fractures and mortality in older women—A prospective study. Study of Osteoporotic Fractures Research Group. *Archives of Internal Medicine* 159(11):1215–1220.

Kaiser Family Foundation. 2009. *HIV/AIDS Policy Fact Sheet. The HIV/AIDS Epidemic in the United States*. Menlo Park, CA: Kaiser Family Foundation.

Källén, B. 2007. The safety of antidepressant drugs during pregnancy. *Expert Opinion on Drug Safety* 6(4):357–370.

Kanis, J. A. 2002. Diagnosis of osteoporosis and assessment of fracture risk. *Lancet* 359(9321): 1929–1936.

Kanis, J. A., F. Borgstrom, C. De Laet, H. Johansson, O. Johnell, B. Jonsson, A. Oden, N. Zethraeus, B. Pfleger, and N. Khaltaev. 2005. Assessment of fracture risk. *Osteoporosis International* 16(6):581–589.

Kaplan, S. S. 2001. Clinical utility of bilateral whole-breast US in the evaluation of women with dense breast tissue. *Radiology* 221(3):641–649.

Karasawa, R., S. Ozaki, K. Nishioka, and T. Kato. 2005. Autoantibodies to peroxiredoxin I and IV in patients with systemic autoimmune diseases. *Microbiology and Immunology* 49(1):57–65.

Karellas, A., and S. Vedantham. 2008. Breast cancer imaging: A perspective for the next decade. *Medical Physics* 35(11):4878–4897.

Katon, W., M. Von Korff, E. Lin, G. Simon, E. Walker, J. Unutzer, T. Bush, J. Russo, and E. Ludman. 1999. Stepped collaborative care for primary care patients with persistent symptoms of depression: A randomized trial. *Archives of General Psychiatry* 56(12):1109–1115.

Kaufman, J. 2010. Evolution and immunity. *Immunology* 130:459–462.

Kell, M. R., and M. J. Kerin. 2004. Sentinel lymph node biopsy. *British Medical Journal* 328(7452): 1330–1331.

Keller, S. M., M. G. Vangel, S. Adak, H. Wagner, J. H. Schiller, A. Herskovic, R. Komaki, M. C. Perry, R. S. Marks, R. B. Livingston, and D. H. Johnson. 2002. The influence of gender on survival and tumor recurrence following adjuvant therapy of completely resected stages II and IIIA non-small cell lung cancer. *Lung Cancer* 37(3):303–309.

Kelly, K., J. Dean, W. Comulada, and S-J. Lee. 2009. Breast cancer detection using automated whole breast ultrasound and mammography in radiographically dense breasts. *European Radiology* 20(3):734–742.

Keshavarz, H., S. D. Hillis, B. A. Kieke, and P. A. Marchbanks. 2002. Hysterectomy surveillance— United States, 1994–1999. *Morbidity and Mortality Weekly Report* 51(SS-5).

Kessler, R. C. 2003. Epidemiology of women and depression. *Journal of Affective Disorders* 74(1): 5–13.

Kessler, R. C., and J. McLeod. 1984. Sex differences in vulnerability to undesirable life events *American Sociological Review* 49:620–631.

Kessler, R. C., P. Berglund, O. Demler, R. Jin, D. Koretz, K. R. Merikangas, A. J. Rush, E. E. Walters, and P. S. Wang. 2003. The epidemiology of major depressive disorder: Results from the National Comorbidity Survey Replication (NCS-R). *Journal of the American Medical Association* 289(23):3095–3105.

Keyes, K. M., B. F. Grant, and D. S. Hasin. 2008. Evidence for a closing gender gap in alcohol use, abuse, and dependence in the United States population. *Drug and Alcohol Dependence* 93(1-2):21–29.

Khalkhali, I., J. Villanueva-Meyer, S. L. Edell, J. L. Connolly, S. J. Schnitt, J. K. Baum, M. J. Houlihan, R. M. Jenkins, and S. B. Haber. 2000. Diagnostic accuracy of 99mTc-sestamibi breast imaging: Multicenter trial results. *Journal of Nuclear Medicine* 41(12):1973–1979.

Khawam, E. A., G. Laurencic, and D. A. Malone, Jr. 2006. Side effects of antidepressants: An overview. *Cleveland Clinic Journal of Medicine* 73(4):351–353, 356–361.

Kiel, D. P., D. T. Felson, J. J. Anderson, P. W. Wilson, and M. A. Moskowitz. 1987. Hip fracture and the use of estrogens in postmenopausal women. The Framingham Study. *New England Journal of Medicine* 317(19):1169–1174.

Kilts, C. D., R. E. Gross, T. D. Ely, and K. P. G. Drexler. 2004. The neural correlates of cue-induced craving in cocaine-dependent women. *American Journal of Psychiatry* 161(2):233–241.

Kim, C., Y. S. Kwok, P. Heagerty, and R. Redberg. 2001. Pharmacologic stress testing for coronary disease diagnosis: A meta-analysis. *American Heart Journal* 142(6):934–944.

Kim, C., R. F. Redberg, T. Pavlic, and K. A. Eagle. 2007. A systematic review of gender differences in mortality after coronary artery bypass graft surgery and percutaneous coronary interventions. *Clinical Cardiology* 30(10):491–495.

Kim, E. S., and V. Menon. 2009. Status of women in cardiovascular clinical trials. *Arteriosclerosis, Thrombosis, and Vascular Biology* 29(3):279–283.

Kim, S. J., and J. S. Gill. 2009. H-Y incompatibility predicts short-term outcomes for kidney transplant recipients. *Journal of the American Society of Nephrology* 20(9):2025–2033.

Kinsey, T., A. Jemal, J. Liff, E. Ward, and M. Thun. 2008. Secular trends in mortality from common cancers in the United States by educational attainment, 1993–2001. *Journal of the National Cancer Institute* 100(14):1003–1012.

Kirnbauer, R., F. Booy, N. Cheng, D. R. Lowy, and J. T. Schiller. 1992. Papillomavirus L1 major capsid protein self-assembles into virus-like particles that are highly immunogenic. *Proceedings of the National Academy of Sciences of the United States of America* 89(24):12180–12184.

Kirnbauer, R., J. Taub, H. Greenstone, R. Roden, M. Durst, L. Gissmann, D. R. Lowy, and J. T. Schiller. 1993. Efficient self-assembly of human papillomavirus type 16 L1 and L1-l2 into virus-like particles. *Journal of Virology* 67(12):6929–6936.

Kiyotani, K., T. Mushiroda, C. K. Imamura, N. Hosono, T. Tsunoda, M. Kubo, Y. Tanigawara, D. A. Flockhart, Z. Desta, T. C. Skaar, F. Aki, K. Hirata, Y. Takatsuka, M. Okazaki, S. Ohsumi, T. Yamakawa, M. Sasa, Y. Nakamura, and H. Zembutsu. 2010. Significant effect of polymorphisms in CYP2D6 and ABCC2 on clinical outcomes of adjuvant tamoxifen therapy for breast cancer patients. *Journal Clinical Oncology* 28(8):1287–1293.

Klerman, L. V. 2000. The intendedness of pregnancy: A concept in transition. *Maternal and Child Health Journal* 4(3):155–162.

Klinkhamer, P. J., W. J. Meerding, P. F. Rosier, and A. G. Hanselaar. 2003. Liquid-based cervical cytology. *Cancer* 99(5):263–271.

Kojic, E. M., and S. Cu-Uvin. 2007. Special care issues of women living with HIV-AIDS. *Infectious Disease Clinics of North America* 21(1): ix, 133–148.

Kolb, T. M., J. Lichy, and J. H. Newhouse. 2002. Comparison of the performance of screening mammography, physical examination, and breast US and evaluation of factors that influence them: An analysis of 27,825 patient evaluations. *Radiology* 225(1):165–175.

Komaki, R., J. D. Cox, S. J. Kister, F. E. Gump, and A. Estabrook. 1990. Stage I and II breast carcinoma: Treatment with limited surgery and radiation therapy versus mastectomy. *Radiology* 174(1):255–257.

Kong, D. F., V. Hasselblad, D. E. Kandzari, L. K. Newby, and R. M. Califf. 2002. Seeking the optimal aspirin dose in acute coronary syndromes. *American Journal of Cardiology* 90(6):622–625.

Koninckx, P. R., C. Meuleman, S. Demeyere, E. Lesaffre, and F. J. Cornillie. 1991. Suggestive evidence that pelvic endometriosis is a progressive disease, whereas deeply infiltrating endometriosis is associated with pelvic pain. *Fertility and Sterility* 55(4):759–765.

Kornstein, S. G., and R. K. Schneider. 2001. Clinical features of treatment-resistant depression. *Journal of Clinical Psychiatry* 62 (Suppl. 16):18–25.

Koss, M. P., J. A. Bailey, N. P. Yuan, V. M. Herrera, and E. L. Lichter. 2003. Depression and PTSD in survivors of male violence: Research and training initiatives to facilitate recovery. *Psychology of Women Quarterly* 27(2):130–142.

Koushik, A., D. J. Hunter, D. Spiegelman, K. E. Anderson, A. A. Arslan, W. L. Beeson, P. A. van den Brandt, J. E. Buring, J. R. Cerhan, G. A. Colditz, G. E. Fraser, J. L. Freudenheim, J. M. Genkinger, R. A. Goldbohm, S. E. Hankinson, K. L. Koenig, S. C. Larsson, M. Leitzmann, M. L. McCullough, A. B. Miller, A. Patel, T. E. Rohan, A. Schatzkin, E. Smit, W. C. Willett, A. Wolk, S. M. Zhang, and S. A. Smith-Warner. 2005. Fruits and vegetables and ovarian cancer risk in a pooled analysis of 12 cohort studies. *Cancer Epidemiology, Biomarkers and Prevention* 14(9):2160–2167.

Koutsky, L. A., K. A. Ault, C. M. Wheeler, D. R. Brown, E. Barr, F. B. Alvarez, L. M. Chiacchierini, K. U. Jansen, and the Proof of Principle Study Investigators. 2002. A controlled trial of a human papillomavirus type 16 vaccine. *New England Journal of Medicine* 347(21):1645–1651.

Krainer, M., S. Silva-Arrieta, M. G. FitzGerald, A. Shimada, C. Ishioka, R. Kanamaru, D. J. MacDonald, H. Unsal, D. M. Finkelstein, A. Bowcock, K. J. Isselbacher, and D. A. Haber. 1997. Differential contributions of *BRCA1* and *BRCA2* to early-onset breast cancer. *New England Journal of Medicine* 336(20):1416–1421.

Kramer, M. M., and C. L. Wells. 1996. Does physical activity reduce risk of estrogen dependent cancer in women? *Medicine & Science in Sports & Exercise* 28(3):322–334.

Kreuzer, M., P. Boffetta, E. Whitley, W. Ahrens, V. Gaborieau, J. Heinrich, K. H. Jockel, L. Kreienbrock, S. Mallone, F. Merletti, F. Roesch, P. Zambon, and L. Simonato. 2000. Gender differences in lung cancer risk by smoking: A multicentre case–control study in Germany and Italy. *British Journal of Cancer* 82(1):227–233.

Kriege, M., C. T. Brekelmans, C. Boetes, P. E. Besnard, H. M. Zonderland, I. M. Obdeijn, R. A. Manoliu, T. Kok, H. Peterse, M. M. Tilanus-Linthorst, S. H. Muller, S. Meijer, J. C. Oosterwijk, L. V. Beex, R. A. Tollenaar, H. J. de Koning, E. J. Rutgers, J. G. Klijn, and the Magnetic Resonance Imaging Screening Study Group. 2004. Efficacy of MRI and mammography for breast-cancer screening in women with a familial or genetic predisposition. *New England Journal of Medicine* 351(5):427–437.

Kriege, M., C. T. Brekelmans, C. Boetes, S. H. Muller, H. M. Zonderland, I. M. Obdeijn, R. A. Manoliu, T. Kok, E. J. Rutgers, H. J. Koning, J. G. Klijn, and Dutch MRI Screening (MRISC) Study Group. 2006. Differences between first and subsequent rounds of the MRISC breast cancer screening program for women with a familial or genetic predisposition. *Cancer* 106(11):2318–2326.

Krieger, N., J. T. Chen, and P. D. Waterman. 2010. Decline in US breast cancer rates after the Women's Health Initiative: Socioeconomic and racial/ethnic differentials. *American Journal of Public Health* 100(S1):S132–S139.

Kudenchuk, P. J., C. Maynard, J. S. Martin, M. Wirkus, and W. D. Weaver. 1996. Comparison of presentation, treatment, and outcome of acute myocardial infarction in men versus women (The Myocardial Infarction Triage and Intervention Registry). *American Journal of Cardiology* 78(1):9–14.

Kugaya, A., and G. Sanacora. 2005. Beyond monoamines: Glutamatergic function in mood disorders. *CNS Spectrums* 10(10):808–819.

Kuhl, C. K., S. Schrading, C. C. Leutner, N. Morakkabati-Spitz, E. Wardelmann, R. Fimmers, W. Kuhn, and H. H. Schild. 2005. Mammography, breast ultrasound, and magnetic resonance imaging for surveillance of women at high familial risk for breast cancer. *Journal of Clinical Oncology* 23(33):8469–8476.

Kuiper, G. G., E. Enmark, M. Pelto-Huikko, S. Nilsson, and J. A. Gustafsson. 1996. Cloning of a novel receptor expressed in rat prostate and ovary. *Proceedings of the National Academy of Sciences of the United States of America* 93(12):5925–5930.

Kuiper, G. G., B. Carlsson, K. Grandien, E. Enmark, J. Haggblad, S. Nilsson, and J. A. Gustafsson. 1997. Comparison of the ligand binding specificity and transcript tissue distribution of estrogen receptors alpha and beta. *Endocrinology* 138(3):863–870.

Kulie, T., A. Groff, J. Redmer, J. Hounshell, and S. Schrager. 2009. Vitamin D: An evidence-based review. *Journal of the American Board of Family Medicine* 22(6):698–706.

Kulski, J. K., J. W. Sadleir, S. R. Kelsall, M. S. Cicchini, G. Shellam, S. W. Peng, Y. M. Qi, D. A. Galloway, J. Zhou, and I. H. Frazer. 1998. Type specific and genotype cross reactive B epitopes of the L1 protein of HPV16 defined by a panel of monoclonal antibodies. *Virology* 243(2):275–282.

Kumpfer, K. L., P. Smith, and J. F. Summerhays. 2008. A wakeup call to the prevention field: Are prevention programs for substance use effective for girls? *Substance Use and Misuse* 43(8-9):978–1001.

Kurtzke, J. F. 1975. A reassessment of the distribution of multiple sclerosis. *Acta Neurologica Scandinavica* 51(2):137–157.

La Vecchia, C., A. Decarli, M. Fasoli, F. Parazzini, S. Franceschi, A. Gentile, and E. Negri. 1988. Dietary vitamin A and the risk of intraepithelial and invasive cervical neoplasia. *Gynecologic Oncology* 30(2):187–195.

Landesman, S. H., L. A. Kalish, D. N. Burns, H. Minkoff, H. E. Fox, C. Zorrilla, P. Garcia, M. G. Fowler, L. Mofenson, and R. Tuomala. 1996. Obstetrical factors and the transmission of human immunodeficiency virus type 1 from mother to child. The Women and Infants Transmission Study. *New England Journal of Medicine* 334(25):1617–1623.

Lang, J., and L. McCullough. 2008. Pathways to ischemic neuronal cell death: Are sex differences relevant? *Journal of Translational Medicine* 6(1):33.

Langan, N. P., and B. M. M. Pelissier. 2001. Gender differences among prisoners in drug treatment. *Journal of Substance Abuse* 13(3):291–301.

Lannfelt, L., H. Basun, L. O. Wahlund, B. A. Rowe, and S. L. Wagner. 1995. Decreased alpha-secretase-cleaved amyloid precursor protein as a diagnostic marker for Alzheimers disease. *Nature Medicine* 1(8):829–832.

Lansky, A. J., J. S. Hochman, P. A. Ward, G. S. Mintz, R. Fabunmi, P. B. Berger, G. New, C. L. Grines, C. G. Pietras, M. J. Kern, M. Ferrell, M. B. Leon, R. Mehran, C. White, J. H. Mieres, J. W. Moses, G. W. Stone, and A. K. Jacobs. 2005. Percutaneous coronary intervention and adjunctive pharmacotherapy in women: A statement for healthcare professionals from the American Heart Association. *Circulation* 111(7):940–953.

LaRosa, J. C., J. He, and S. Vupputuri. 1999. Effect of statins on risk of coronary disease: A meta-analysis of randomized controlled trials. *Journal of the American Medical Association* 282(24): 2340–2346.

Latka, M. H., F. Kapadia, and P. Fortin. 2008. The female condom: Effectiveness and convenience, not "female control," valued by US urban adolescents. *AIDs Education and Prevention* 20(2): 160–170.

Lau, C. S., and A. Mak. 2009. The socioeconomic burden of SLE. *Nature Reviews Rheumatology* 5(7):400–404.

Launer, L. J., K. Andersen, M. E. Dewey, L. Letenneur, A. Ott, L. A. Amaducci, C. Brayne, J. R. Copeland, J. F. Dartigues, P. Kragh-Sorensen, A. Lobo, J. M. Martinez-Lage, T. Stijnen, and A. Hofman. 1999. Rates and risk factors for dementia and Alzheimer's disease: Results from EURODEM pooled analyses. EURODEM Incidence Research Group and Work Groups. European Studies of Dementia. *Neurology* 52(1):78–84.

Leach, M. O., C. R. Boggis, A. K. Dixon, D. F. Easton, R. A. Eeles, D. G. Evans, F. J. Gilbert, I. Griebsch, R. J. Hoff, P. Kessar, S. R. Lakhani, S. M. Moss, A. Nerurkar, A. R. Padhani, L. J. Pointon, D. Thompson, and R. M. Warren. 2005. Screening with magnetic resonance imaging and mammography of a UK population at high familial risk of breast cancer: A prospective multicentre cohort study (MARIBS). *Lancet* 365(9473):1769–1778.

Leconte, I., C. Feger, C. Galant, M. Berliere, B. V. Berg, W. D'Hoore, and B. Maldague. 2003. Mammography and subsequent whole-breast sonography of nonpalpable breast cancers: The importance of radiologic breast density. *American Journal of Roentgeneology* 180(6):1675–1679.

Lee, A. V., J. G. Jackson, J. L. Gooch, S. G. Hilsenbeck, E. Coronado-Heinsohn, C. K. Osborne, and D. Yee. 1999. Enhancement of insulin-like growth factor signaling in human breast cancer: Estrogen regulation of insulin receptor substrate-1 expression in vitro and in vivo. *Molecular Endocrinology* 13(5):787–796.

Lee, J. R., F. Paultre, and L. Mosca. 2005. The association between educational level and risk of cardiovascular disease fatality among women with cardiovascular disease. *Women's Health Issues* 15(2):80–88.

Lehman, C. D., J. D. Blume, P. Weatherall, D. Thickman, N. Hylton, E. Warner, E. Pisano, S. J. Schnitt, C. Gatsonis, M. Schnall, G. A. DeAngelis, P. Stomper, E. L. Rosen, M. O'Loughlin, S. Harms, and D. A. Bluemke. 2005. Screening women at high risk for breast cancer with mammography and magnetic resonance imaging. *Cancer* 103(9):1898–1905.

Lehman, C. D., C. Isaacs, M. D. Schnall, E. D. Pisano, S. M. Ascher, P. T. Weatherall, D. A. Bluemke, D. J. Bowen, P. K. Marcom, D. K. Armstrong, S. M. Domchek, G. Tomlinson, S. J. Skates, and C. Gatsonis. 2007. Cancer yield of mammography, MR, and US in high-risk women: Prospective multi-institution breast cancer screening study. *Radiology* 244(2):381–388.

Lehtinen, M., and J. Paavonen. 2004. Vaccination against human papillomaviruses shows great promise. *Lancet* 364(9447):1731–1732.

Lenderink, T., E. Boersma, W. Ruzyllo, P. Widimsky, E. M. Ohman, P. W. Armstrong, L. Wallentin, and M. L. Simoons. 2004. Bleeding events with abciximab in acute coronary syndromes without early revascularization: An analysis of GUSTO IV-ACS. *American Heart Journal* 147(5):865–873.

Leslie, W. D., and Manitoba Bone Density Program. 2006. The impact of bone area on short-term bone density precision. *Journal of Clinical Densitometry* 9(2):150–153.

Leslie, W. D., S. O'Donnell, S. Jean, C. Lagace, P. Walsh, C. Bancej, S. Morin, D. A. Hanley, and A. Papaioannou. 2009. Trends in hip fracture rates in Canada. *Journal of the American Medical Association* 302(8):883–889.

Lewin, J. M., C. J. D'Orsi, R. E. Hendrick, L. J. Moss, P. K. Isaacs, A. Karellas, and G. R. Cutter. 2002. Clinical comparison of full-field digital mammography and screen-film mammography for detection of breast cancer. *American Journal of Roentgeneology* 179(3):671–677.

Lewis, J. P. 2007. An interpretation of the EBCTCG data. *Oncologist* 12(5):505–509.

Lewis-Fernandez, R., A. K. Das, C. Alfonso, M. M. Weissman, and M. Olfson. 2005. Depression in US Hispanics: Diagnostic and management considerations in family practice. *Journal of the American Board of Family Practice* 18(4):282–296.

Liberman, M., F. Sampalis, D. S. Mulder, and J. S. Sampalis. 2003. Breast cancer diagnosis by scintimammography: A meta-analysis and review of the literature. *Breast Cancer Research and Treatment* 80(1):115–126.

Linder, J. 1998. Recent advances in thin-layer cytology. *Diagnostic Cytopathology* 18(1):24–32.

Ling, F. W. 1999. Randomized controlled trial of depot leuprolide in patients with chronic pelvic pain and clinically suspected endometriosis. Pelvic Pain Study Group. *Obstetrics and Gynecology* 93(1):51–58.

Lloyd, T., V. M. Chinchilli, N. Johnson-Rollings, K. Kieselhorst, D. F. Eggli, and R. Marcus. 2000. Adult female hip bone density reflects teenage sports-exercise patterns but not teenage calcium intake. *Pediatrics* 106(1):40–44.

Lloyd-Jones, D., R. Adams, M. Carnethon, G. De Simone, T. B. Ferguson, K. Flegal, E. Ford, K. Furie, A. Go, K. Greenlund, N. Haase, S. Hailpern, M. Ho, V. Howard, B. Kissela, S. Kittner, D. Lackland, L. Lisabeth, A. Marelli, M. McDermott, J. Meigs, D. Mozaffarian, G. Nichol, C. O'Donnell, V. Roger, W. Rosamond, R. Sacco, P. Sorlie, R. Stafford, J. Steinberger, T. Thom, S. Wasserthiel-Smoller, N. Wong, J. Wylie-Rosett, and Y. Hong. 2009. Heart disease and stroke statistics—2009 update: A report from the American Heart Association Statistics Committee and Stroke Statistics Subcommittee. *Circulation* 119(3):480–486.

Lockhat, F. B., J. O. Emembolu, and J. C. Konje. 2004. The evaluation of the effectiveness of an intrauterine-administered progestogen (levonorgestrel) in the symptomatic treatment of endometriosis and in the staging of the disease. *Human Reproduction* 19(1):179–184.

Loizzi, V., G. Cormio, M. Vicino, and L. Selvaggi. 2008. Neoadjuvant chemotherapy: An alternative option of treatment for locally advanced cervical cancer. *Gynecologic and Obstetric Investigation* 65(2):96–103.

Longshore, D., P. L. Ellickson, D. F. McCaffrey, and P. A. St Clair. 2007. School-based drug prevention among at-risk adolescents: Effects of ALERT Plus. *Health Education and Behavior* 34(4):651–668.

Lord, R. V., J. Brabender, D. Gandara, V. Alberola, C. Camps, M. Domine, F. Cardenal, J. M. Sanchez, P. H. Gumerlock, M. Taron, J. J. Sanchez, K. D. Danenberg, P. V. Danenberg, and R. Rosell. 2002. Low ERCC1 expression correlates with prolonged survival after cisplatin plus gemcitabine chemotherapy in non-small cell lung cancer. *Clinical Cancer Research* 8(7):2286–2291.

Lukka, H., H. Hirte, A. Fyles, G. Thomas, L. Elit, M. Johnston, M. Fung Kee Fung, and G. Browman. 2002. Concurrent cisplatin-based chemotherapy plus radiotherapy for cervical cancer—A meta-analysis. *Clinical Oncology* 14(3):203–212.

Luppino, F. S., L. M. de Wit, P. F. Bouvy, T. Stijnen, P. Cuijpers, B. W. Penninx, and F. G. Zitman. 2010. Overweight, obesity, and depression: A systematic review and meta-analysis of longitudinal studies. *Archives of General Psychiatry* 67(3):220–229.

Lyman, G. H., A. E. Giuliano, M. R. Somerfield, A. B. Benson, 3rd, D. C. Bodurka, H. J. Burstein, A. J. Cochran, H. S. Cody, 3rd, S. B. Edge, S. Galper, J. A. Hayman, T. Y. Kim, C. L. Perkins, D. A. Podoloff, V. H. Sivasubramaniam, R. R. Turner, R. Wahl, D. L. Weaver, A. C. Wolff, and E. P. Winer. 2005. American Society of Clinical Oncology guideline recommendations for sentinel lymph node biopsy in early-stage breast cancer. *Journal of Clinical Oncology* 23(30):7703–7720.

Lyons, F., S. Hopkins, B. Kelleher, A. McGeary, G. Sheehan, J. Geoghegan, C. Bergin, F. M. Mulcahy, and P. A. McCormick. 2006. Maternal hepatotoxicity with nevirapine as part of combination antiretroviral therapy in pregnancy. *HIV Medicine* 7(4):255–260.

MacLusky, N. 2004. Estrogen and Alzheimer's disease: The apolipoprotein connection. *Endocrinology* 145(7):3062–3064.

Mahon, B. D., A. Wittke, V. Weaver, and M. T. Cantorna. 2003. The targets of vitamin D depend on the differentiation and activation status of CD4 positive T cells. *Journal of Cellular Biochemistry* 89(5):922–932.

Makinen, J., J. Johansson, C. Tomas, E. Tomas, P. K. Heinonen, T. Laatikainen, M. Kauko, A. M. Heikkinen, and J. Sjoberg. 2001. Morbidity of 10 110 hysterectomies by type of approach. *Human Reproduction* 16(7):1473–1478.

Malberg, J. E., and L. M. Monteggia. 2008. VGF, a new player in antidepressant action? *Science Signaling* 1(18):pe19.

Mandelbrot, L., J. Le Chenadec, A. Berrebi, A. Bongain, J. L. Benifla, J. F. Delfraissy, S. Blanche, and M. J. Mayaux. 1998. Perinatal HIV-1 transmission: Interaction between zidovudine prophylaxis and mode of delivery in the French Perinatal Cohort. *Journal of the American Medical Association* 280(1):55–60.

Manfredi, R., L. Calza, D. Cocchi, and F. Chiodo. 2003. Antiretroviral treatment and advanced age: Epidemiologic, laboratory, and clinical features in the elderly. *Journal of Acquired Immune Deficiency Syndromes* 33(1):112–114.

Marcus, S. M., E. A. Young, K. B. Kerber, S. Kornstein, A. H. Farabaugh, J. Mitchell, S. R. Wisniewski, G. K. Balasubramani, M. H. Trivedi, and A. J. Rush. 2005. Gender differences in depression: Findings from the STAR*D study. *Journal of Affective Disorders* 87(2-3):141–150.

Mariani, G., A. Fasolo, E. De Benedictis, and L. Gianni. 2009. Trastuzumab as adjuvant systemic therapy for HER2-positive breast cancer. *Nature Clinical Practice Oncology* 6(2):93–104.

Markou, A., T. Duka, and G. M. Prelevic. 2005. Estrogens and brain function. *Hormones* 4(1): 9–17.

Marsh, J. C., D. Cao, and T. D'Aunno. 2004. Gender differences in the impact of comprehensive services in substance abuse treatment. *Journal of Substance Abuse Treatment* 27(4):289–300.

Martin, M., T. Pienkowski, J. Mackey, M. Pawlicki, J-P. Guastalla, C. Weaver, E. Tomiak, T. Al-Tweigeri, L. Chap, E. Juhos, R. Guevin, A. Howell, T. Fornander, J. Hainsworth, R. Coleman, J. Vinholes, M. Modiano, T. Pinter, S. C. Tang, B. Colwell, C. Prady, L. Provencher, D. Walde, A. Rodriguez-Lescure, J. Hugh, C. Loret, M. Rupin, S. Blitz, P. Jacobs, M. Murawsky, A. Riva, C. Vogel, and the Breast Cancer International Research Group 001 Investigators. 2005. Adjuvant docetaxel for node-positive breast cancer. *New England Journal of Medicine* 352(22):2302–2313.

Mathew, A., and P. S. George. 2009. Trends in incidence and mortality rates of squamous cell carcinoma and adenocarcinoma of cervix—worldwide. *Asian Pacific Journal of Cancer Prevention* 10(4):645–650.

Mathias, S. D., M. Kuppermann, R. F. Liberman, R. C. Lipschutz, and J. F. Steege. 1996. Chronic pelvic pain: Prevalence, health-related quality of life, and economic correlates. *Obstetrics and Gynecology* 87(3):321–327.

Mayer, K. H., J. Peipert, T. Fleming, A. Fullem, T. Moench, S. Cu-Uvin, M. Bentley, M. Chesney, and Z. Rosenberg. 2001. Safety and tolerability of buffergel, a novel vaginal microbicide, in women in the United States. *Clinical Infectious Diseases* 32(3):476–482.

Mazhude, C., S. Jones, S. Murad, C. Taylor, and P. Easterbrook. 2002. Female sex but not ethnicity is a strong predictor of non-nucleoside reverse transcriptase inhibitor-induced rash. *AIDS* 16(11):1566–1568.

Mazure, C. 1998. Life stressors as risk factors in depression. *Clinical Psychology: Science and Practice* 5:291–313.

Mazure, C. M., M. L. Bruce, P. K. Maciejewski, and S. C. Jacobs. 2000. Adverse life events and cognitive-personality characteristics in the prediction of major depression and antidepressant response. *American Journal of Psychiatry* 157(6):896–903.

McDuffie, H. H., D. J. Klaassen, and J. A. Dosman. 1987. Female-male differences in patients with primary lung cancer. *Cancer* 59(10):1825–1830.

McGovern, S. L., Z. Liao, M. K. Bucci, M. F. McAleer, M. D. Jeter, J. Y. Chang, M. S. O'Reilly, J. D. Cox, P. K. Allen, and R. Komaki. 2009. Is sex associated with the outcome of patients treated with radiation for nonsmall cell lung cancer? *Cancer* 115(14):3233–3242.

McGuire, W., J. Blessing, D. Moore, S. Lentz, and G. Photopulos. 1996. Paclitaxel has moderate activity in squamous cervix cancer. A Gynecologic Oncology Group Study. *Journal Clinical Oncology* 14(3):792–795.

McPherson, K., A. Herbert, A. Judge, A. Clarke, S. Bridgman, M. Maresh, and C. Overton. 2005. Psychosexual health 5 years after hysterectomy: Population-based comparison with endometrial ablation for dysfunctional uterine bleeding. *Health Expectations* 8(3):234–243.

McQuellon, R. P., H. T. Thaler, D. Cella, and D. H. Moore. 2006. Quality of life (QOL) outcomes from a randomized trial of cisplatin versus cisplatin plus paclitaxel in advanced cervical cancer: A Gynecologic Oncology Group Study. *Gynecologic Oncology* 101(2):296–304.

Mehilli, J., A. Kastrati, J. Dirschinger, H. Bollwein, F-J. Neumann, and A. Schomig. 2000. Differences in prognostic factors and outcomes between women and men undergoing coronary artery stenting. *Journal of the American Medical Association* 284(14):1799–1805.

Meisamy, S., P. J. Bolan, E. H. Baker, M. G. Pollema, C. T. Le, F. Kelcz, M. C. Lechner, B. A. Luikens, R. A. Carlson, K. R. Brandt, K. K. Amrami, M. T. Nelson, L. I. Everson, T. H. Emory, T. M. Tuttle, D. Yee, and M. Garwood. 2005. Adding in vivo quantitative 1H MR spectroscopy to improve diagnostic accuracy of breast MR imaging: Preliminary results of observer performance study at 4.0 T. *Radiology* 236(2):465–475.

Melton, L. J., 3rd, S. H. Kan, M. A. Frye, H. W. Wahner, W. M. O'Fallon, and B. L. Riggs. 1989. Epidemiology of vertebral fractures in women. *American Journal of Epidemiology* 129(5):1000–1011.

Melton, L. J., 3rd, E. A. Chrischilles, C. Cooper, A. W. Lane, and B. L. Riggs. 1992. Perspective. How many women have osteoporosis? *Journal of Bone and Mineral Research* 7(9):1005–1010.

Menacker, F., and B. E. Hamilton. 2010. Recent trends in cesarean delivery in the United States. *NCHS Data Brief* (35):1–8.

Mendez, M. F. 2006. The accurate diagnosis of early-onset dementia. *International Journal of Psychiatry in Medicine* 36(4):401–412.

Menke, R., and H. Flynn. 2009. Relationships between stigma, depression, and treatment in white and African American primary care patients. *Journal of Nervous Mental Disorder* 197(6): 407–411.

Meredith, L. S., M. Orlando, N. Humphrey, P. Camp, and C. D. Sherbourne. 2001. Are better ratings of the patient-provider relationship associated with higher quality care for depression? *Medical Care* 39(4):349–360.

Metcalfe, K. A. 2009. Oophorectomy for breast cancer prevention in women with *BRCA1* or *BRCA2* mutations. *Women's Health* 5(1):63–68.

Middeldorp, S. 2005. Oral contraceptives and the risk of venous thromboembolism. *Gender Medicine* 2 (Suppl. A):S3–S9.

Mieres, J. H., L. J. Shaw, A. Arai, M. J. Budoff, S. D. Flamm, W. G. Hundley, T. H. Marwick, L. Mosca, A. R. Patel, M. A. Quinones, R. F. Redberg, K. A. Taubert, A. J. Taylor, G. S. Thomas, and N. K. Wenger. 2005. Role of noninvasive testing in the clinical evaluation of women with suspected coronary artery disease: Consensus statement from the Cardiac Imaging Committee, Council on Clinical Cardiology, and the Cardiovascular Imaging and Intervention Committee, Council on Cardiovascular Radiology and Intervention, American Heart Association. *Circulation* 111(5):682–696.

Migliorelli, R., A. Teson, L. Sabe, M. Petracchi, R. Leiguarda, and S. E. Starkstein. 1995. Prevalence and correlates of dysthymia and major depression among patients with Alzheimers disease. *American Journal of Psychiatry* 152(1):37–44.

Mikhail, G. W. 2005. Coronary heart disease in women. *British Medical Journal* 331(7515): 467–468.

Miller, A. B., T. To, C. J. Baines, and C. Wall. 2000. Canadian National Breast Screening Study-2: 13-year results of a randomized trial in women aged 50–59 years. *Journal of the National Cancer Institute* 92(18):1490–1499.

———. 2002. The Canadian National Breast Screening Study-1: Breast cancer mortality after 11 to 16 years of follow-up: A randomized screening trial of mammography in women age 40 to 49 years. *Annals of Internal Medicine* 137(5 Pt. 1):305–312.

Miller, A. H., S. Ancoli-Israel, J. E. Bower, L. Capuron, and M. R. Irwin. 2008. Neuroendocrine-immune mechanisms of behavioral comorbidities in patients with cancer. *Journal Clinical Oncology* 26(6):971–982.

Miller, B. A., E. J. Feuer, and B. F. Hankey. 1991. The increasing incidence of breast cancer since 1982: Relevance of early detection. *Cancer Causes and Control* 2(2):67–74.

Miller, K., M. Wang, J. Gralow, M. Dickler, M. Cobleigh, E. A. Perez, T. Shenkier, D. Cella, and N. E. Davidson. 2007. Paclitaxel plus bevacizumab versus paclitaxel alone for metastatic breast cancer. *New England Journal of Medicine* 357(26):2666–2676.

Milner, K. A., M. Funk, S. Richards, R. M. Wilmes, V. Vaccarino, and H. M. Krumholz. 1999. Gender differences in symptom presentation associated with coronary heart disease. *American Journal of Cardiology* 84(4):396–399.

Mink, P. J., A. R. Folsom, T. A. Sellers, and L. H. Kushi. 1996. Physical activity, waist-to-hip ratio, and other risk factors for ovarian cancer: A follow-up study of older women. *Epidemiology* 7(1):38–45.

Minkoff, H. 1997. HIV disease in pregnancy. Introduction. *Obstetrics and Gynecology Clinics of North America* 24(4):XI-XVII.

Minkoff, H., and L. M. Mofenson. 1994. The role of obstetric interventions in the prevention of pediatric human immunodeficiency virus infection. *American Journal of Obstetrics and Gynecology* 171(5):1167–1175.

Minkoff, H., R. Hershow, D. H. Watts, M. Frederick, I. Cheng, R. Tuomala, J. Pitt, C. D. Zorrilla, H. Hammill, S. K. Adeniyi-Jones, and B. Thompson. 2003. The relationship of pregnancy to human immunodeficiency virus disease progression. *American Journal of Obstetrics and Gynecology* 189(2):552–559.

Miranda, J., J. Siddique, T. R. Belin, and L. P. Kohn-Wood. 2005. Depression prevalence in disadvantaged young black women—African and Caribbean immigrants compared to US-born African Americans. *Social Psychiatry Psychiatric Epidemiology* 40(4):253–258.

Modjtahedi, B. S., S. P. Modjtahedi, and H. I. Maibach. 2006. Gender: A possible determinant in dosing of dermatologic drugs—An overview. *Cutaneous and Ocular Toxicology* 25(3):195–210.

Moerman, E. J., K. Teng, D. A. Lipschitz, and B. Lecka-Czernik. 2004. Aging activates adipogenic and suppresses osteogenic programs in mesenchymal marrow stroma/stem cells: The role of PPAR-gamma2 transcription factor and TGF-beta/BMP signaling pathways. *Aging Cell* 3(6):379–389.

Mollerup, S., D. Ryberg, A. Hewer, D. H. Phillips, and A. Haugen. 1999. Sex differences in lung cyp1a1 expression and DNA adduct levels among lung cancer patients. *Cancer Research* 59(14):3317–3320.

Mollerup, S., K. Jorgensen, G. Berge, and A. Haugen. 2002. Expression of estrogen receptors alpha and beta in human lung tissue and cell lines. *Lung Cancer* 37(2):153–159.

Monninkhof, E. M., S. G. Elias, F. A. Vlems, I. van der Tweel, A. J. Schuit, D. W. Voskuil, F. E. van Leeuwen, and TFPAC. 2007. Physical activity and breast cancer: A systematic review. *Epidemiology* 18(1):137–157.

Montgrain, P. R., R. Quintana, Y. Rascon, D. W. Burton, L. J. Deftos, A. Casillas, and R. H. Hastings. 2007. Parathyroid hormone-related protein varies with sex and androgen status in nonsmall cell lung cancer. *Cancer* 110(6):1313–1320.

Moore, A. L., O. Kirk, A. M. Johnson, C. Katlama, A. Blaxhult, M. Dietrich, R. Colebunders, A. Chiesi, J. D. Lungren, and A. N. Phillips. 2003. Virologic, immunologic, and clinical response to highly active antiretroviral therapy: The gender issue revisited. *Journal of Acquired Immune Deficiency Syndromes* 32(4):452–461.

Moore, D. H. 2006. Cervical cancer. *Obstetrics and Gynecology* 107(5):1152–1161.

Moore, D. H., J. A. Blessing, R. P. McQuellon, H. T. Thaler, D. Cella, J. Benda, D. S. Miller, G. Olt, S. King, J. F. Boggess, and T. F. Rocereto. 2004. Phase III study of cisplatin with or without paclitaxel in stage IVB, recurrent, or persistent squamous cell carcinoma of the cervix: A gynecologic oncology group study. *Journal Clinical Oncology* 22(15):3113–3119.

Moore, R. D., I. Fortgang, J. Keruly, and R. E. Chaisson. 1996. Adverse events from drug therapy for human immunodeficiency virus disease. *American Journal of Medicine* 101(1):34–40.

Moore, R. D., J. C. Keruly, and R. E. Chaisson. 2001. Incidence of pancreatitis in HIV-infected patients receiving nucleoside reverse transcriptase inhibitor drugs. *AIDS* 15(5):617–620.

Mora, S., R. J. Glynn, J. Hsia, J. G. MacFadyen, J. Genest, and P. M. Ridker. 2010. Statins for the primary prevention of cardiovascular events in women with elevated high-sensitivity C-reactive protein or dyslipidemia: Results from the justification for the use of statins in prevention: An intervention trial evaluating rosuvastatin (JUPITER) and meta-analysis of women from primary prevention trials. *Circulation* 121(9):1069–1077.

Morris, M., P. J. Eifel, J. Lu, P. W. Grigsby, C. Levenback, R. E. Stevens, M. Rotman, D. M. Gershenson, and D. G. Mutch. 1999. Pelvic radiation with concurrent chemotherapy compared with pelvic and para-aortic radiation for high-risk cervical cancer. *New England Journal of Medicine* 340(15):1137–1143.

Mosca, L., L. J. Appel, E. J. Benjamin, K. Berra, N. Chandra-Strobos, R. P. Fabunmi, D. Grady, C. K. Haan, S. N. Hayes, D. R. Judelson, N. L. Keenan, P. McBride, S. Oparil, P. Ouyang, M. C. Oz, M. E. Mendelsohn, R. C. Pasternak, V. W. Pinn, R. M. Robertson, K. Schenck-Gustafsson, C. A. Sila, S. C. Smith, Jr., G. Sopko, A. L. Taylor, B. W. Walsh, N. K. Wenger, and C. L. Williams. 2004. Evidence-based guidelines for cardiovascular disease prevention in women. *Circulation* 109(5):672–693.

Mosca, L., A. H. Linfante, E. J. Benjamin, K. Berra, S. N. Hayes, B. W. Walsh, R. P. Fabunmi, J. Kwan, T. Mills, and S. L. Simpson. 2005. National study of physician awareness and adherence to cardiovascular disease prevention guidelines. *Circulation* 111(4):499–510.

Mosca, L., H. Mochari, A. Christian, K. Berra, K. Taubert, T. Mills, K. A. Burdick, and S. L. Simpson. 2006. National study of women's awareness, preventive action, and barriers to cardiovascular health. *Circulation* 113(4):525–534.

Mosca, L., C. L. Banka, E. J. Benjamin, K. Berra, C. Bushnell, R. J. Dolor, T. G. Ganiats, A. S. Gomes, H. L. Gornik, C. Gracia, M. Gulati, C. K. Haan, D. R. Judelson, N. Keenan, E. Kelepouris, E. D. Michos, L. K. Newby, S. Oparil, P. Ouyang, M. C. Oz, D. Petitti, V. W. Pinn, R. F. Redberg, R. Scott, K. Sherif, S. C. Smith, Jr., G. Sopko, R. H. Steinhorn, N. J. Stone, K. A. Taubert, B. A. Todd, E. Urbina, N. K. Wenger, Expert Panel/Writing Group; American Heart Association; American Academy of Family Physicians; American College of Obstetricians and Gynecologists; American College of Cardiology Foundation; Society of Thoracic Surgeons; American Medical Women's Association; Centers for Disease Control and Prevention; Office of Research on Women's Health; Association of Black Cardiologists; American College of Physicians; World Heart Federation; National Heart, Lung, and Blood Institute; American College of Nurse Practitioners. 2007. Evidence-based guidelines for cardiovascular disease prevention in women: 2007 update. *Circulation* 115(11):1481–1501. [erratum appears in circulation. 2007 Apr 17;115(15):E407].

Mosca, L., H. Mochari-Greenberger, R. J. Dolor, L. K. Newby, and K. J. Robb. 2010. Twelve-year follow-up of American women's awareness of cardiovascular disease risk and barriers to heart health. *Circulation* 3(2):120–127.

Mosselman, S., J. Polman, and R. Dijkema. 1996. ER beta: Identification and characterization of a novel human estrogen receptor. *FEBS Letters* 392(1):49–53.

Muñoz, N. 2000. Human papillomavirus and cancer: The epidemiological evidence. *Journal of Clinical Virology* 19(1-2):1–5.

Muñoz, N., F. X. Bosch, S. de Sanjose, R. Herrero, X. Castellsague, K. V. Shah, P. J. F. Snijders, C. J. L. M. Meijer, and the International Agency for Research on Cancer Multicenter Cervical Cancer Study Group. 2003. Epidemiologic classification of human papillomavirus types associated with cervical cancer. *New England Journal of Medicine* 348(6):518–527.

Muntz, E., and W. Logan. 1979. Focal spot size and scatter suppression in magnification mammography. *American Journal of Roentgeneology* 133(3):453–459.

Murray, C. J. L., and A. D. Lopez. 1997. Alternative projections of mortality and disability by cause 1990–2020: Global burden of disease study. *Lancet* 349(9064):1498–1504.

Murray, J. A., S. B. Moore, C. T. Van Dyke, B. D. Lahr, R. A. Dierkhising, A. R. Zinsmeister, L. J. Melton, 3rd, C. M. Kroning, M. El-Yousseff, and A. J. Czaja. 2007. HLA DQ gene dosage and risk and severity of celiac disease. *Clinical Gastroenterology and Hepatology* 5(12):1406–1412.

Nazroo, J. Y., A. C. Edwards, and G. W. Brown. 1997. Gender differences in the onset of depression following a shared life event: A study of couples. *Psychological Medicine* 27(1):9–19.

NCI (National Cancer Institute). 2008. *SEER Cancer Statistics Review, 1975–2005.* http://seer.cancer. gov/csr/1975_2005/results_merged/sect_05_cervix_uteri.pdf (accessed August 20, 2009).

———. 2009a. *Adjuvant and Neoadjuvant Therapy for Breast Cancer.* http://www.cancer.gov/ cancertopics/factsheet/therapy/adjuvant-breast (accessed April 8, 2010).

———. 2009b. *SEER Stat Fact Sheets: Cancer of the Corpus and Uterus.* www. seer. cancer. gov/ statfacts/html/corp. html (accessed August 20, 2009).

———. 2010a. *Fast Stats: Age-Adjusted U. S. Mortality Rates by Cancer Site All Ages, All Races, Female, 1975–2007.* http://seer.cancer.gov/faststats/selections.php?#Output (accessed August 12, 2010).

———. 2010b. *SEER Cancer Statistics Review, 1975–2007.* http://seer.cancer.gov/csr/1975_2007/ sections.html (accessed May 28, 2010).

———. 2010c. *SEER Cancer Statistics Review, 1975–2007.* http://seer.cancer.gov/statfacts/html/ cervix.html#incidence-mortality (accessed August 20, 2010).

———. 2010d. *SEER Stat Fact Sheets: Ovary.* Bethesda, MD: National Cancer Institute.

———. 2010e. *SEER Stat Fact Sheets: Corpus and Uterus.* http://seer.cancer.gov/statfacts/html/corp. html (accessed August 10, 2010).

———. 2010f. *SEER Fact Sheets: Cancer of the Lung and Bronchus.* http://seer.cancer.gov/statfacts/ html/lungb.html (accessed August 3, 2010).

Negro, A., B. K. Brar, and K. F. Lee. 2004. Essential roles of HER2/ERBB2 in cardiac development and function. *Recent Progress in Hormone Research* 59:1–12.

Nelson, H. D., K. Tyne, A. Naik, C. Bougatsos, B. K. Chan, and L. Humphrey. 2009a. Screening for breast cancer: An update for the US Preventive Services Task Force. *Annals of Internal Medicine* 151(10):727–737.

Nelson, H. D., R. Fu, J. C. Griffin, P. Nygren, M. E. Smith, and L. Humphrey. 2009b. Systematic review: Comparative effectiveness of medications to reduce risk for primary breast cancer. *Annals of Internal Medicine* 151(10):703–715.

Nelson, H. H., D. C. Christiani, E. J. Mark, J. K. Wiencke, J. C. Wain, and K. T. Kelsey. 1999. Implications and prognostic value of K-ras mutation for early-stage lung cancer in women. *Journal of the National Cancer Institute* 91(23):2032–2038.

Netting, E. E., and F. G. Williams. 1996. Case manager-physician collaboration: Implications for professional identity, roles, and relationships. *Health and Social Work* 21(3):216–216.

Nicastri, E., C. Angeletti, L. Palmisano, L. Sarmati, A. Chiesi, A. Geraci, M. Andreoni, and S. Vella. 2005. Gender differences in clinical progression of HIV-1-infected individuals during long-term highly active antiretroviral therapy. *AIDS* 19(6):577–583.

Niklason, L. T., B. T. Christian, L. E. Niklason, D. B. Kopans, D. E. Castleberry, B. H. Opsahl-Ong, C. E. Landberg, P. J. Slanetz, A. A. Giardino, R. Moore, D. Albagli, M. C. DeJule, P. F. Fitzgerald, D. F. Fobare, B. W. Giambattista, R. F. Kwasnick, J. Liu, S. J. Lubowski, G. E. Possin, J. F. Richotte, C. Y. Wei, and R. F. Wirth. 1997. Digital tomosynthesis in breast imaging. *Radiology* 205(2):399–406.

NIMH (National Institute of Mental Health). 2009. *Women and Depression: Discovering Hope.* http://www.nimh.nih.gov/health/publications/women-and-depression-discovering-hope/complete-index.shtml (accessed April 19, 2010).

NOF (National Osteoporosis Foundation). 2002. *America's Bone Health: The State of Osteoporosis and Low Bone Mass.* http://www.nof.org/advocacy/prevalence/ (accessed June 3, 2010).

Nolen-Hoeksema, S. 2004. The response styles theory. In *Depressive Rumination: Nature, Theroy, and Treatment,* edited by C. Papageorgiou and A. Wells. New York: Wiley. Pp. 107–124.

Nolen-Hoeksema, S., J. Larson, and C. Grayson. 1999. Explaining the gender difference in depressive symptoms. *Journal of Personality and Social Psychology* 77(5):1061–1072.

Norman, S. A., S. L. Potashnik, M. L. Galantino, A. M. De Michele, L. House, and A. R. Localio. 2007. Modifiable risk factors for breast cancer recurrence: What can we tell survivors? *Journal of Women's Health* 16(2):177–190.

Nusbaum, R., and C. Isaacs. 2007. Management updates for women with a *BRCA1* or *BRCA2* mutation. *Molecular Diagnosis and Therapy* 11(3):133–144.

Nygaard, I., M. D. Barber, K. L. Burgio, K. Kenton, S. Meikle, J. Schaffer, C. Spino, W. E. Whitehead, J. Wu, and D. J. Brody. 2008. Prevalence of symptomatic pelvic floor disorders in US women. *Journal of the American Medical Association* 300(11):1311–1316.

Nystrom, L., I. Andersson, N. Bjurstam, J. Frisell, B. Nordenskjold, and L. E. Rutqvist. 2002. Long-term effects of mammography screening: Updated overview of the Swedish randomised trials. *Lancet* 359(9310):909–919.

O'Donoghue, M., W. E. Boden, E. Braunwald, C. P. Cannon, T. C. Clayton, R. J. de Winter, K. A. Fox, B. Lagerqvist, P. A. McCullough, S. A. Murphy, R. Spacek, E. Swahn, L. Wallentin, F. Windhausen, and M. S. Sabatine. 2008. Early invasive vs conservative treatment strategies in women and men with unstable angina and non-ST-segment elevation myocardial infarction: A meta-analysis. *Journal of the American Medical Association* 300(1):71–80.

O'Keefe-McCarthy, S. 2008. Women's experiences of cardiac pain: A review of the literature. *Canadian Journal of Cardiovascular Nursing* 18(3):18–25.

Office of Environmental Health Hazard Assessment. 2005. *Proposed Identification of Environmental Tobacco Smoke as a Toxic Air Contaminant.* http://www.oehha.org/air/environmental_tobacco/2005etsfinal.html (accessed August 12, 2010).

Office of National Drug Control Policy. 2006. *Results from the 2006 National Survey on Drug Use and Health: National Findings.* Edited by the US Department of Health and Human Services, Substance Abuse and Mental Health Services Administration Office of Applied Studies.

Office of the Surgeon General. 2006. *Surgeon General's Report—The Health Consequences of Involuntary Exposure to Tobacco Smoke.* Atlanta, GA: US Department of Health and Human Services, Centers for Disease Control and Prevention, Coordinating Center for Health Promotion, National Center for Chronic Disease Prevention and Health Promotion, Office on Smoking and Health.

Okolo, S. 2008. Incidence, aetiology and epidemiology of uterine fibroids. *Best Practice and Research. Clinical Obstetrics and Gynaecology* 22(4):571–588.

Olopade, O. I., T. A. Grushko, R. Nanda, and D. Huo. 2008. Advances in breast cancer: Pathways to personalized medicine. *Clinical Cancer Research* 14(24):7988–7999.

Olsen, O., and P. C. Gotzsche. 2001. Cochrane review on screening for breast cancer with mammography. *Lancet* 358(9290):1340–1342.

Olson, J. A., Jr., L. M. McCall, P. Beitsch, P. W. Whitworth, D. S. Reintgen, P. W. Blumencranz, A. M. Leitch, S. Saha, K. K. Hunt, and A. E. Giuliano. 2008. Impact of immediate versus delayed axillary node dissection on surgical outcomes in breast cancer patients with positive sentinel nodes: Results from American College of Surgeons oncology group trials Z0010 and Z0011. *Journal of Clinical Oncology* 26(21):3530–3535.

Olsson, S. E., S. K. Kjaer, K. Sigurdsson, O. E. Iversen, M. Hernandez-Avila, C. M. Wheeler, G. Perez, D. R. Brown, L. A. Koutsky, E. H. Tay, P. Garcia, K. A. Ault, S. M. Garland, S. Leodolter, G. W. Tang, D. G. Ferris, J. Paavonen, M. Lehtinen, M. Steben, F. X. Bosch, J. Dillner, E. A. Joura, S. Majewski, N. Munoz, E. R. Myers, L. L. Villa, F. J. Taddeo, C. Roberts, A. Tadesse, J. Bryan, R. Maansson, S. Vuocolo, T. M. Hesley, A. Saah, E. Barr, and R. M. Haupt. 2009. Evaluation of quadrivalent HPV 6/11/16/18 vaccine efficacy against cervical and anogenital disease in subjects with serological evidence of prior vaccine type HPV infection. *Human Vaccines* 5(10):696–704.

Osann, K. E., H. Anton-Culver, T. Kurosaki, and T. Taylor. 1993. Sex differences in lung-cancer risk associated with cigarette smoking. *International Journal of Cancer* 54(1):44–48.

Osborne, C. K. 1998. Tamoxifen in the treatment of breast cancer. *New England Journal of Medicine* 339(22):1609–1618.

OTA (US Congress Office of Technology Assessment). 1994. *Hip Fracture Outcomes in People Age 50 and Over—Background Paper.* OTA-BP-H-120. Washington, DC: US Government Printing Office.

Ouellette, D., G. Desbiens, C. Emond, and G. Beauchamp. 1998. Lung cancer in women compared with men: Stage, treatment, and survival. *Annals of Thoracic Surgery* 66(4):1140–1143; discussion 1143–1144.

Padian, N. S., S. C. Shiboski, and N. P. Jewell. 1991. Female-to-male transmission of human-immunodeficiency-virus. *Journal of the American Medical Association* 266(12):1664–1667.

Padian, N. S., A. van der Straten, G. Ramjee, T. Chipato, G. de Bruyn, K. Blanchard, S. Shiboski, E. T. Montgomery, H. Fancher, H. Cheng, M. Rosenblum, M. van der Laan, N. Jewell, and J. McIntyre. 2007. Diaphragm and lubricant gel for prevention of HIV acquisition in southern African women: A randomised controlled trial. *Lancet* 370(9583):251–261.

Palella, F. J., K. M. Delaney, A. C. Moorman, M. O. Loveless, J. Fuhrer, G. A. Satten, D. J. Aschman, S. D. Holmberg. 1998. Declining morbidity and mortality among patients with advanced human immunodeficiency virus infection. *New England Journal of Medicine* 338(13):853–860.

Palm, N. W., and R. Medzhitov. 2009. Pattern recognition receptors and control of adaptive immunity. *Immunological Reviews* 227:221–233.

Palumbo, P., B. Holland, T. Dobbs, C. P. Pau, C. C. Luo, E. J. Abrams, S. Nesheim, P. Vink, R. Respess, and M. Bulterys. 2001. Antiretroviral resistance mutations among pregnant human immunodeficiency virus type 1-infected women and their newborns in the United States: Vertical transmission and clades. *Journal of Infectious Diseases* 184(9):1120–1126.

Papakostas, G. I., M. E. Thase, M. Fava, J. C. Nelson, and R. C. Shelton. 2007. Are antidepressant drugs that combine serotonergic and noradrenergic mechanisms of action more effective than the selective serotonin reuptake inhibitors in treating major depressive disorder? A meta-analysis of studies of newer agents. *Biological Psychiatry* 62(11):1217–1227.

Pappas, G., S. Queen, W. Hadden, and G. Fisher. 1993. The increasing disparity in mortality between socioeconomic groups in the United States, 1960 and 1986. *New England Journal of Medicine* 329(2):103–109.

Pariante, C. M., and A. H. Miller. 2001. Glucocorticoid receptors in major depression: Relevance to pathophysiology and treatment. *Biological Psychiatry* 49(5):391–404.

Partridge, A. H., and E. P. Winer. 2009. On mammography—more agreement than disagreement. *New England Journal of Medicine* 361(26):2499–2501.

Patel, A. V., C. Rodriguez, A. L. Pavluck, M. J. Thun, and E. E. Calle. 2006a. Recreational physical activity and sedentary behavior in relation to ovarian cancer risk in a large cohort of U. S. women. *American Journal of Epidemiology* 163(8):709–716.

Patel, K. K., B. Butler, and K. B. Wells. 2006b. What is necessary to transform the quality of mental health care. *Health Affairs* 25(3):681–693.

Patterson, K. B., S. E. Cohn, J. Uyanik, M. Hughes, M. Smurzynski, and J. J. Eron. 2009. Treatment responses in antiretroviral treatment-naive premenopausal and postmenopausal HIV-infected-women: An analysis from AIDS Clinical Trials Group Studies. *Clinical Infectious Diseases* 49(3):473–476.

Pav, M., H. Kovaru, A. Fiserova, E. Havrdova, and V. Lisa. 2008. Neurobiological aspects of depressive disorder and antidepressant treatment: Role of glia. *Physiological Research* 57(2):151–164.

Pearman, T. 2008. Psychosocial factors in lung cancer: Quality of life, economic impact, and survivorship implications. *Journal of Psychosocial Oncology* 26(1):69–80.

Pernerstorfer-Schoen, H., B. Jilma, A. Perschler, S. Wichlas, K. Schindler, A. Schindl, A. Rieger, O. F. Wagner, and P. Quehenberger. 2001. Sex differences in HAART-associated dyslipidaemia. *AIDS* 15(6):725–734.

Pernis, A. B. 2007. Estrogen and CD4(+) T cells. *Current Opinion in Rheumatology* 19(5):414–420.

Perron, B. E., B. Alexander-Eitzman, D. Watkins, R. J. Taylor, R. Baser, H. W. Neighbors, and J. S. Jackson. 2009. Ethnic differences in delays to treatment for substance use disorders: African Americans, black Caribbeans and non-Hispanic whites. *Journal of Psychoactive Drugs* 41(4):369–377.

Peters, W. A., III, P. Y. Liu, R. J. Barrett, II, R. J. Stock, B. J. Monk, J. S. Berek, L. Souhami, P. Grigsby, W. Gordon, Jr., and D. S. Alberts. 2000. Concurrent chemotherapy and pelvic radiation therapy compared with pelvic radiation therapy alone as adjuvant therapy after radical surgery in high-risk early-stage cancer of the cervix. *Journal Clinical Oncology* 18(8):1606–1613.

Petter, A., K. Heim, M. Guger, A. Ciresa-Ko Nig, N. Christensen, M. Sarcletti, U. Wieland, H. Pfister, R. Zangerle, and R. Hopfl. 2000. Specific serum IgG, IgM and IgA antibodies to human papillomavirus types 6, 11, 16, 18 and 31 virus-like particles in human immunodeficiency virus-seropositive women. *Journal of General Virology* 81(3):701–708.

Pietschmann, P., M. Rauner, W. Sipos, and K. Kerschan-Schindl. 2009. Osteoporosis: An age-related and gender-specific disease—A mini-review. *Gerontology* 55(1):3–12.

Pines, A. 2009. Lifestyle and diet in postmenopausal women. *Climacteric* 12(Suppl. 1):62–65.

Pisano, E. D., and M. J. Yaffe. 2005. Digital mammography. *Radiology* 234(2):353–362.

Pisano, E. D., C. Gatsonis, E. Hendrick, M. Yaffe, J. K. Baum, S. Acharyya, E. F. Conant, L. L. Fajardo, L. Bassett, C. D'Orsi, R. Jong, M. Rebner, and the Digital Mammographic Imaging Screening Trial Investigators Group. 2005. Diagnostic performance of digital versus film mammography for breast-cancer screening. *New England Journal of Medicine* 353(17):1773–1783.

Planchard, D., Y. Loriot, A. Goubar, F. Commo, and J-C. Soria. 2009. Differential expression of biomarkers in men and women. *Seminars in Oncology* 36(6):553–565.

Plassman, B. L., K. M. Langa, G. G. Fisher, S. G. Heeringa, D. R. Weir, M. B. Ofstedal, J. R. Burke, M. D. Hurd, G. G. Potter, W. L. Rodgers, D. C. Steffens, R. J. Willis, and R. B. Wallace. 2007. Prevalence of dementia in the United States: The aging, demographics, and memory study. *Neuroepidemiology* 29(1-2):125–132.

Plummer, F. A., J. N. Simonsen, D. W. Cameron, J. O. Ndinya-Achola, J. K. Kreiss, M. N. Gakinya, P. Waiyaki, M. Cheang, P. Piot, A. R. Ronald, and E. N. Ngugi. 1991. Cofactors in male-female sexual transmission of human immunodeficiency virus type 1. *Journal of Infectious Diseases* 163(2):233–239.

Poplack, S. P., T. D. Tosteson, C. A. Kogel, and H. M. Nagy. 2007. Digital breast tomosynthesis: Initial experience in 98 women with abnormal digital screening mammography. *American Journal of Roentgeneology* 189(3):616–623.

Prentice, R. L., C. A. Thomson, B. Caan, F. A. Hubbell, G. L. Anderson, S. A. Beresford, M. Pettinger, D. S. Lane, L. Lessin, S. Yasmeen, B. Singh, J. Khandekar, J. M. Shikany, S. Satterfield, and R. T. Chlebowski. 2007. Low-fat dietary pattern and cancer incidence in the Women's Health Initiative dietary modification randomized controlled trial. *Journal of the National Cancer Institute* 99(20):1534–1543.

Press, M. F., M. C. Pike, V. R. Chazin, G. Hung, J. A. Udove, M. Markowicz, J. Danyluk, W. Godolphin, M. Sliwkowski, R. Akita, M. C. Paterson, and D. J. Slamon. 1993. HER-2/NEU expression in node-negative breast cancer: Direct tissue quantitation by computerized image analysis and association of overexpression with increased risk of recurrent disease. *Cancer Research* 53(20):4960–4970.

Press, M. F., R. S. Finn, D. Cameron, A. Di Leo, C. E. Geyer, I. E. Villalobos, A. Santiago, R. Guzman, A. Gasparyan, Y. Ma, K. Danenberg, A. M. Martin, L. Williams, C. Oliva, S. Stein, R. Gagnon, M. Arbushites, and M. T. Koehler. 2008. HER-2 gene amplification, HER-2 and epidermal growth factor receptor MRNA and protein expression, and lapatinib efficacy in women with metastatic breast cancer. *Clinical Cancer Research* 14(23):7861–7870.

Price, J. L., and P. D. Butler. 1970. The reduction of radiation and exposure time in mammography. *British Journal of Radiology* 43(508):251–255.

Quan, M. L., and D. McCready. 2009. The evolution of lymph node assessment in breast cancer. *Journal of Surgical Oncology* 99(4):194–198.

Quattrocchi, E., and H. Kourlas. 2004. Teriparatide: A review. *Clinical Therapeutics* 26(6): 841–854.

Quintana, F. J., and I. R. Cohen. 2001. Autoantibody patterns in diabetes-prone NOD mice and in standard C57BL/6 mice. *Journal of Autoimmunity* 17(3):191–197.

Quyyumi, A. A. 2006. Women and ischemic heart disease: Pathophysiologic implications from the Women's Ischemia Syndrome Evaluation (WISE) study and future research steps. *Journal of the American College of Cardiology* 47(3 Suppl.1):S66–S71.

Ramjee, G., N. S. Morar, M. Alary, L. Mukenge-Tshibaka, B. Vuylsteke, V. Ettiegne-Traore, V. Chandeying, S. A. Karim, and L. Van Damme. 2000. Challenges in the conduct of vaginal microbicide effectiveness trials in the developing world. *AIDS* 14(16):2553–2557.

Ravdin, P., K. Cronin, N. Howlader, C. Berg, R. Chlebowski, E. Feuer, B. Edwards, and D. Berry. 2007. The decrease in breast-cancer incidence in 2003 in the United States. *New England Journal of Medicine* 356:1670–1674.

Read, J. S. 2000. Cesarean section delivery to prevent vertical transmission of human immunodeficiency virus type 1 associated risks and other considerations. *Annals of the New York Academy of Sciences* 918:115–121.

Rebbeck, T. R., N. D. Kauff, and S. M. Domchek. 2009. Meta-analysis of risk reduction estimates associated with risk-reducing salpingo-oophorectomy in *BRCA1* or *BRCA2* mutation carriers. *Journal of the National Cancer Institute* 101(2):80–87.

Reinhardt, P. P., B. Reinhardt, J. L. Lathey, and S. A. Spector. 1995. Human cord blood mononuclear cells are preferentially infected by non-syncytium-inducing, macrophage-tropic human immunodeficiency virus type 1 isolates. *Journal of Clinical Microbiology* 33(2):292–297.

Revicki, D. A., J. Siddique, L. Frank, J. Y. Chung, B. L. Green, J. Krupnick, M. Prasad, and J. Miranda. 2005. Cost-effectiveness of evidence-based pharmacotherapy or cognitive behavior therapy compared with community referral for major depression in predominantly low-income minority women. *Archives of General Psychiatry* 62(8):868–875.

Rich-Edwards, J. W., J. E. Manson, C. H. Hennekens, and J. E. Buring. 1995. The primary prevention of coronary heart disease in women. *New England Journal of Medicine* 332(26):1758–1766.

Ridker, P. M., J. E. Buring, N. R. Cook, and N. Rifai. 2003. C-reactive protein, the metabolic syndrome, and risk of incident cardiovascular events: An 8-year follow-up of 14 719 initially healthy American women. *Circulation* 107(3):391–397.

Ridker, P. M., N. R. Cook, I. M. Lee, D. Gordon, J. M. Gaziano, J. E. Manson, C. H. Hennekens, and J. E. Buring. 2005. A randomized trial of low-dose aspirin in the primary prevention of cardiovascular disease in women. *New England Journal of Medicine* 352(13):1293–1304.

Ridker, P. M., J. G. MacFadyen, F. A. Fonseca, J. Genest, A. M. Gotto, J. J. Kastelein, W. Koenig, P. Libby, A. J. Lorenzatti, B. G. Nordestgaard, J. Shepherd, J. T. Willerson, and R. J. Glynn. 2009. Number needed to treat with rosuvastatin to prevent first cardiovascular events and death among men and women with low low-density lipoprotein cholesterol and elevated high-sensitivity C-reactive protein: Justification for the use of statins in prevention: An intervention trial evaluating rosuvastatin (JUPITER). *Circulation. Cardiovascular Quality and Outcomes* 2(6):616–623.

Risch, H. A., G. R. Howe, M. Jain, J. D. Burch, E. J. Holowaty, and A. B. Miller. 1993. Are female smokers at higher risk for lung cancer than male smokers?: A case–control analysis by histologic type. *American Journal of Epidemiology* 138(5):281–293.

Roett, M. A., and P. Evans. 2009. Ovarian cancer: An overview. *American Family Physician* 80(6): 609–616.

Ronckers, C. M., C. A. Erdmann, and C. E. Land. 2005. Radiation and breast cancer: A review of current evidence. *Breast Cancer Research* 7(1):21–32.

Ronco, G., N. Segnan, P. Giorgi-Rossi, M. Zappa, G. P. Casadei, F. Carozzi, P. D. Palma, A. Del Mistro, S. Folicaldi, A. Gillio-Tos, G. Nardo, C. Naldoni, P. Schincaglia, M. Zorzi, M. Confortini, and J. Cuzick. 2006. Human papillomavirus testing and liquid-based cytology: Results at recruitment from the new technologies for cervical cancer randomized controlled trial. *Journal of the National Cancer Institute* 98(11):765–774.

Rooney, P. H., C. Telfer, M. C. McFadyen, W. T. Melvin, and G. I. Murray. 2004. The role of cytochrome P450 in cytotoxic bioactivation: Future therapeutic directions. *Current Cancer Drug Targets* 4:257–265.

Rose, P. G., B. N. Bundy, E. B. Watkins, J. T. Thigpen, G. Deppe, M. A. Maiman, D. L. Clarke-Pearson, and S. Insalaco. 1999. Concurrent cisplatin-based radiotherapy and chemotherapy for locally advanced cervical cancer. *New England Journal of Medicine* 340(15):1144–1153.

Rosenberg, S., L. Goodman, F. Osher, M. Swartz, S. Essock, M. Butterfield, N. Constantine, G. Wolford, and M. Salyers. 2001. Prevalence of HIV, hepatitis B, and hepatitis C in people with severe mental illness. *Journal of Public Health* 91:31–37.

Rosenfeld, A. G. 2006. State of the heart: Building science to improve women's cardiovascular health. *American Journal of Critical Care* 15(6):556–566.

Rougier-Chapman, D., S. Key, and J. Ryan. 2001. Uterine artery embolization for the treatment of symptomatic fibroid disease. *Applied Radiology* (September):11–17.

Rowell, S., B. Newman, J. Boyd, and M. C. King. 1994. Inherited predisposition to breast and ovarian cancer. *American Journal of Human Genetics* 55(5):861–865.

Rubinstein, W. S. 2004. Hereditary breast cancer in Jews. *Familial Cancer* 3(3-4):249–257.

Rubtsov, A. V., K. Rubtsova, J. W. Kappler, and P. Marrack. 2010. Genetic and hormonal factors in female-biased autoimmunity. *Autoimmunity Reviews* 9(7):494–498.

Rush, A. J., M. Fava, S. R. Wisniewski, P. W. Lavori, M. H. Trivedi, H. A. Sackeim, M. E. Thase, A. A. Nierenberg, F. M. Quitkin, T. M. Kashner, D. J. Kupfer, J. F. Rosenbaum, J. Alpert, J. W. Stewart, P. J. McGrath, M. M. Biggs, K. Shores-Wilson, B. D. Lebowitz, L. Ritz, and G. Niederehe. 2004. Sequenced treatment alternatives to relieve depression (STAR*D): Rationale and design. *Controlled Clinical Trials* 25(1):119–142.

Sambrook, P., and C. Cooper. 2006. Osteoporosis. *Lancet* 367:2010–2018.

SAMHSA (Substance Abuse and Mental Health Services Administration). 2005. *Cocaine Use: 2002 and 2003. The NSDUH Report* http://www.oas.samhsa.gov/2k5/cocaine/cocaine.htm (accessed August 12, 2010).

———. 2008. *Treatment Episode Data Set (TEDS) Highlights—2006: National Admissions to Substance Abuse Treatment Services, Drug and Alcohol Services Information System Series.* Rockville, MD: Office of Applied Studies.

Sanne, I., H. Mommeja-Marin, J. Hinkle, J. A. Bartlett, M. M. Lederman, G. Maartens, C. Wakeford, A. Shaw, J. Quinn, R. G. Gish, and F. Rousseau. 2005. Severe hepatotoxicity associated with nevirapine use in HIV-infected subjects. *Journal of Infectious Diseases* 191(6):825–829.

Sardanelli, F., F. Podo, G. D'Agnolo, A. Verdecchia, M. Santaquilani, R. Musumeci, G. Trecate, S. Manoukian, S. Morassut, C. de Giacomi, M. Federico, L. Cortesi, S. Corcione, S. Cirillo, V. Marra, A. Cilotti, C. Di Maggio, A. Fausto, L. Preda, C. Zuiani, A. Contegiacomo, A. Orlacchio, M. Calabrese, L. Bonomo, E. Di Cesare, M. Tonutti, P. Panizza, and A. Del Maschio. 2007. Multicenter comparative multimodality surveillance of women at genetic-familial high risk for breast cancer (HIBCRIT study): Interim results. *Radiology* 242(3):698–715.

Sarkar, K., and F. W. Miller. 2004. Possible roles and determinants of microchimerism in autoimmune and other disorders. *Autoimmunity Reviews* 3(6):454–463.

Saslow, D., C. Boetes, W. Burke, S. Harms, M. O. Leach, C. D. Lehman, E. Morris, E. Pisano, M. Schnall, S. Sener, R. A. Smith, E. Warner, M. Yaffe, K. S. Andrews, and C. A. Russell. 2007. American Cancer Society guidelines for breast screening with MRI as an adjunct to mammography. *CA: A Cancer Journal for Clinicians* 57(2):75–89.

Sattler, F. R., D. Qian, S. Louie, D. Johnson, W. Briggs, V. DeQuattro, and M. P. Dube. 2001. Elevated blood pressure in subjects with lipodystrophy. *AIDS* 15(15):2001–2010.

Scarpellini, F., M. Sbracia, S. Lecchini, and L. Scarpellini. 2002. Anti-angiogenesis treatment with thalidomide in endometriosis: A pilot study. *Fertility and Sterility* 78(Suppl. 1):S87.

Schapira, D. V., R. A. Clark, P. A. Wolff, A. R. Jarrett, N. B. Kumar, and N. M. Aziz. 1994. Visceral obesity and breast cancer risk. *Cancer* 74(2):632–639.

Scheidt-Nave, C., E. Barrett-Connor, D. L. Wingard, B. A. Cohn, and S. L. Edelstein. 1991. Sex differences in fasting glycemia as a risk factor for ischemic heart disease death. *American Journal of Epidemiology* 133(6):565–576.

Schiffman, M., and P. E. Castle. 2005. The promise of global cervical-cancer prevention. *New England Journal of Medicine* 353(20):2101–2104.

Schlecht, N. F., S. Kulaga, J. Robitaille, S. Ferreira, M. Santos, R. A. Miyamura, E. Duarte-Franco, T. E. Rohan, A. Ferenczy, L. L. Villa, and E. L. Franco. 2001. Persistent human papillomavirus infection as a predictor of cervical intraepithelial neoplasia. *Journal of the American Medical Association* 286(24):3106–3114.

Schmidt, P. J. 2005. Mood, depression, and reproductive hormones in the menopausal transition. *American Journal of Medicine* 118 (Suppl. 12B):54–58.

Schrag, D., K. M. Kuntz, J. E. Garber, and J. C. Weeks. 2000. Life expectancy gains from cancer prevention strategies for women with breast cancer and BRCA1 or BRCA2 mutations. *Journal of the American Medical Association* 283(5):617–624.

Schrenk, P., R. Rieger, A. Shamiyeh, and W. Wayand. 2000. Morbidity following sentinel lymph node biopsy versus axillary lymph node dissection for patients with breast carcinoma. *Cancer* 88(3):608–614.

Schubert, E. L., M. K. Lee, H. C. Mefford, R. H. Argonza, J. E. Morrow, J. Hull, J. L. Dann, and M. C. King. 1997. *BRCA2* in American families with four or more cases of breast or ovarian cancer: Recurrent and novel mutations, variable expression, penetrance, and the possibility of families whose cancer is not attributable to *BRCA1* or *BRCA2*. *American Journal of Human Genetics* 60(5):1031–1040.

Schulman, K. A., J. A. Berlin, W. Harless, J. F. Kerner, S. Sistrunk, B. J. Gersh, R. Dube, C. K. Taleghani, J. E. Burke, S. Williams, J. M. Eisenberg, and J. J. Escarce. 1999. The effect of race and sex on physicians' recommendations for cardiac catheterization. *New England Journal of Medicine* 340(8):618–626.

Schulz, M., P. H. Lahmann, E. Riboli, and H. Boeing. 2004. Dietary determinants of epithelial ovarian cancer: A review of the epidemiologic literature. *Nutrition and Cancer* 50(2):120–140.

Seigneurin, A., M. Colonna, L. Remontet, P. Delafosse, and R. Ecochard. 2008. Artefact-free trends in breast cancer incidence over two decades in a whole French Département. *Breast Journal* 17(6):580–586.

Shapiro, S. 1988. *Periodic Screening for Breast Cancer: The Health Insurance Plan Project and Its Sequelae, 1963–1986.* Baltimore, MD: Johns Hopkins University Press.

Shapiro, S., W. Venet, and P. Strax. 1988. Current results of the breast cancer screening randomized trial: The Health Insurance Plan (HIP) of Greater New York Study. In *Screening for Breast Cancer*, edited by N. E. Day and A. B. Miller. Lewiston, NY: Hans Huber Publishers. Pp. 3–15.

Sharftsein, S. 1999. Healthcare policy and opportunities for psychotherapy and psychoanalysis. In *The Challenage to Psychoanalysis and Psychotherapy: Soluations for the Future*, edited by S. de Schill and S. Lebovich. Philidelphia, PA: Jessica Kingsley Publishers.

Sharpe, N. 2002. Clinical trials and the real world: Selection bias and generalisability of trial results. *Cardiovascular Drugs and Therapy* 16(1):75–77.

Shavers, V. L., and M. L. Brown. 2002. Racial and ethnic disparities in the receipt of cancer treatment. *Journal of the National Cancer Institute* 94(5):334–357.

Shaw, L. J., R. Bugiardini, and C. N. Merz. 2009. Women and ischemic heart disease: Evolving knowledge. *Journal of the American College of Cardiology* 54(17):1561–1575.

Shepherd, J., S. M. Cobbe, I. Ford, C. G. Isles, A. R. Lorimer, P. W. MacFarlane, J. H. McKillop, and C. J. Packard. 1995. Prevention of coronary heart disease with pravastatin in men with hypercholesterolemia. West of Scotland Coronary Prevention Study Group. *New England Journal of Medicine* 333(20):1301–1307.

Sherman, M. E., M. H. Schiffman, A. T. Lorincz, R. Herrero, M. L. Hutchinson, C. Bratti, D. Zahniser, J. Morales, A. Hildesheim, K. Helgesen, D. Kelly, M. Alfaro, F. Mena, I. Balmaceda, L. Mango, and M. Greenberg. 1997. Cervical specimens collected in liquid buffer are suitable for both cytologic screening and ancillary human papillomavirus testing. *Cancer* 81(2):89–97.

Sherman, M. E., M. Mendoza, K. R. Lee, R. Ashfaq, G. G. Birdsong, M. E. Corkill, K. M. McIntosh, S. L. Inhorn, D. J. Zahniser, G. Baber, C. Barber, and M. H. Stoler. 1998. Performance of liquid-based, thin-layer cervical cytology: Correlation with reference diagnoses and human papillomavirus testing. *Modern Pathology* 11(9):837–843.

Sherman, M. E., S. S. Wang, J. Carreon, and S. S. Devesa. 2005. Mortality trends for cervical squamous and adenocarcinoma in the United States. Relation to incidence and survival. *Cancer* 103(6):1258–1264.

Sherwin, B. B. 2003. Estrogen and cognitive functioning in women. *Endocrine Reviews* 24(2):133–151.

Shriver, S. P., H. A. Bourdeau, C. T. Gubish, D. L. Tirpak, A. L. Davis, J. D. Luketich, and J. M. Siegfried. 2000. Sex-specific expression of gastrin-releasing peptide receptor: Relationship to smoking history and risk of lung cancer. *Journal of the National Cancer Institute* 92(1):24–33.

Shtern, F. 1992. Digital mammography and related technologies: A perspective from the National Cancer Institute. *Radiology* 183(3):629–630.

Shumaker, S. A., C. Legault, L. Kuller, S. R. Rapp, L. Thal, D. S. Lane, H. Fillit, M. L. Stefanick, S. L. Hendrix, C. E. Lewis, K. Masaki, and L. H. Coker. 2004. Conjugated equine estrogens and incidence of probable dementia and mild cognitive impairment in postmenopausal women: Women's Health Initiative Memory Study. *Journal of the American Medical Association* 291(24):2947–2958.

Sichel, D., and J. W. Drischoll. 1999. *Women's Moods, Women's Minds: What Every Woman Must Know About Hormones, the Brain and Emotional Health*. New York: Harper Collins Publishers, Inc.

Siebers, A. G., P. J. Klinkhamer, J. M. Grefte, L. F. Massuger, J. E. Vedder, A. Beijers-Broos, J. Bulten, and M. Arbyn. 2009. Comparison of liquid-based cytology with conventional cytology for detection of cervical cancer precursors: A randomized controlled trial. *Journal of the American Medical Association* 302(16):1757–1764.

Silva, W. A., and M. M. Karram. 2005. Scientific basis for use of grafts during vaginal reconstructive procedures. *Current Opinions in Obstetrics and Gynecology* 17(5):519–529.

Simard, J. F., and K. H. Costenbader. 2007. What can epidemiology tell us about systemic lupus erythematosus? *International Journal of Clinical Practice* 61(7):1170–1180.

Simon, G. E., M. VonKorff, C. Rutter, and E. Wagner. 2000. Randomised trial of monitoring, feedback, and management of care by telephone to improve treatment of depression in primary care. *British Medical Journal* 320(7234):550–554.

Simon, G. E., E. J. Ludman, S. Tutty, B. Operskalski, and M. VonKorff. 2004. Telephone psychotherapy and telephone care management for primary care patients starting antidepressant treatment: A randomized controlled trial. *Journal of the American Medical Association* 292(8):935–942.

Simon, G. R., M. Extermann, A. Chiappori, C. C. Williams, M. Begum, R. Kapoor, E. B. Haura, R. Ismail-Khan, M. J. Schell, S. J. Antonia, and G. Bepler. 2008. Phase 2 trial of docetaxel and gefitinib in the first-line treatment of patients with advanced nonsmall-cell lung cancer (NSCLC) who are 70 years of age or older. *Cancer* 112(9):2021–2029.

Sirey, J. A., M. L. Bruce, G. S. Alexopoulos, D. A. Perlick, P. Raue, S. J. Friedman, and B. S. Meyers. 2001. Perceived stigma as a predictor of treatment discontinuation in young and older outpatients with depression. *American Journal of Psychiatry* 158(3):479–481.

Siris, E. S., P. D. Miller, E. Barrett-Connor, K. G. Faulkner, L. E. Wehren, T. A. Abbott, M. L. Berger, A. C. Santora, and L. M. Sherwood. 2001. Identification and fracture outcomes of undiagnosed low bone mineral density in postmenopausal women: Results from the National Osteoporosis Risk Assessment. *Journal of the American Medical Association* 286(22):2815–2822.

Siris, E. S., Y. T. Chen, T. A. Abbott, E. Barrett-Connor, P. D. Miller, L. E. Wehren, and M. L. Berger. 2004. Bone mineral density thresholds for pharmacological intervention to prevent fractures. *Archives of Internal Medicine* 164(10):1108–1112.

Skaane, P., S. Hofvind, and A. Skjennald. 2007. Randomized trial of screen-film versus full-field digital mammography with soft-copy reading in population-based screening program: Follow-up and final results of Oslo II Study. *Radiology* 244(3):708–717.

Slamon, D., and M. Pegram. 2001. Rationale for trastuzumab (herceptin) in adjuvant breast cancer trials. *Seminars in Oncology* 28(Suppl. 3):13–19.

Slamon, D. J., G. M. Clark, S. G. Wong, W. J. Levin, A. Ullrich, and W. L. McGuire. 1987. Human breast cancer: Correlation of relapse and survival with amplification of the HER-2/NEU oncogene. *Science* 235(4785):177–182.

Slamon, D. J., W. Godolphin, L. A. Jones, J. A. Holt, S. G. Wong, D. E. Keith, W. J. Levin, S. G. Stuart, J. Udove, A. Ullrich, and M. F. Press. 1989. Studies of the HER-2/NEU proto-oncogene in human breast and ovarian cancer. *Science* 244(4905):707–712.

Slattery, D. A., A. L. Hudson, and D. J. Nutt. 2004. Invited review: The evolution of antidepressant mechanisms. *Fundamental and Clinical Pharmacology* 18(1):1–21.

Smith, D. K., D. L. Warren, D. Vlahov, P. Schuman, M. D. Stein, B. L. Greenberg, and S. D. Holmberg. 1997. Design and baseline participant characteristics of the Human Immunodeficiency Virus Epidemiology Research (HER) Study: A prospective cohort study of human immunodeficiency virus infection in US women. *American Journal of Epidemiology* 146(6):459–469.

Smith, R. A., S. W. Duffy, R. Gabe, L. Tabar, A. M. Yen, and T. H. Chen. 2004. The randomized trials of breast cancer screening: What have we learned? *Radiologic Clinics of North America* 42(5):793–806.

Smith, R. A., V. Cokkinides, and O. W. Brawley. 2009. Cancer screening in the United States, 2009: A review of current American Cancer Society guidelines and issues in cancer screening. *CA: A Cancer Journal for Clinicians* 59(1):27–41.

Smith-McCune, K. K., S. Shiboski, M. Z. Chirenje, T. Magure, J. Tuveson, Y. Ma, M. Da Costa, A. B. Moscicki, J. M. Palefsky, R. Makunike-Mutasa, T. Chipato, A. van der Straten, and G. F. Sawaya. 2010. Type-specific cervico-vaginal human papillomavirus infection increases risk of HIV acquisition independent of other sexually transmitted infections. *PLoS One* 5(4):e10094.

Sobieszczyk, M. E., D. R. Hoover, K. Anastos, K. Mulligan, T. Tan, Q. Shi, W. Gao, C. Hyman, M. H. Cohen, S. R. Cole, M. W. Plankey, A. M. Levine, and J. Justman. 2008. Prevalence and predictors of metabolic syndrome among HIV-infected and HIV-uninfected women in the Women's Interagency HIV Study. *Journal of Acquired Immune Deficiency Syndromes* 48(3):272–280.

Solomon, D. H., M. A. Brookhart, T. K. Gandhi, A. Karson, S. Gharib, E. J. Orav, S. Shaykevich, A. Licari, D. Cabral, and D. W. Bates. 2004. Adherence with osteoporosis practice guidelines: A multilevel analysis of patient, physician, and practice setting characteristics. *American Journal of Medicine* 117(12):919–924.

Solomon, D. H., J. S. Finkelstein, P. S. Wang, and J. Avorn. 2005. Statin lipid-lowering drugs and bone mineral density. *Pharmacoepidemiology and Drug Safety* 14(4):219–226.

Sparano, J. A., L. J. Goldstein, B. H. Childs, S. Shak, D. Brassard, S. Badve, F. L. Baehner, R. Bugarini, S. Rowley, E. Perez, L. N. Shulman, S. Martino, N. E. Davidson, G. W. Sledge, and R. Gray. 2009. Relationship between topoisomerase 2A RNA expression and recurrence after adjuvant chemotherapy for breast cancer. *Clinical Cancer Research* 15(24):7693–7700.

Spitz, M. R., Q. Wei, Q. Dong, C. I. Amos, and X. Wu. 2003. Genetic susceptibility to lung cancer: The role of DNA damage and repair. *Cancer Epidemiology, Biomarkers and Prevention* 12(8):689–698.

Ssali, F., W. Stohr, P. Munderi, A. Reid, A. S. Walker, D. M. Gibb, P. Mugyenyi, C. Kityo, H. Grosskurth, J. Hakim, H. Byakwaga, E. Katabira, J. H. Darbyshire, and C. F. Gilks. 2006. Prevalence, incidence and predictors of severe anaemia with zidovudine-containing regimens in African adults with HIV infection within the DART Trial. *Antiviral Therapy* 11(6):741–749.

Stabile, L. P., A. L. Davis, C. T. Gubish, T. M. Hopkins, J. D. Luketich, N. Christie, S. Finkelstein, and J. M. Siegfried. 2002. Human non-small cell lung tumors and cells derived from normal lung express both estrogen receptor alpha and beta and show biological responses to estrogen. *Cancer Research* 62(7):2141–2150.

Stadtmauer, E. A., A. O'Neill, L. J. Goldstein, P. A. Crilley, K. F. Mangan, J. N. Ingle, I. Brodsky, S. Martino, H. M. Lazarus, J. K. Erban, C. Sickles, and J. H. Glick. 2000. Conventional-dose chemotherapy compared with high-dose chemotherapy plus autologous hematopoietic stem-cell transplantation for metastatic breast cancer. Philadelphia bone marrow transplant group. *New England Journal of Medicine* 342(15):1069–1076.

Stefanick, M. L. 2006. Risk-benefit profiles of raloxifene for women. *New England Journal of Medicine* 355(2):190–192.

Steinhubl, S. R., W. A. Tan, J. M. Foody, and E. J. Topol. 1999. Incidence and clinical course of thrombotic thrombocytopenic purpura due to ticlopidine following coronary stenting. *Journal of the American Medical Association* 281(9):806–810.

Stewart, D., M. Gossop, J. Marsden, T. Kidd, and S. Treacy. 2003. Similarities in outcomes for men and women after drug misuse treatment: Results from the National Treatment Outcome Research Study (NTORS). *Drug and Alcohol Review* 22(1):35–41.

Stone, G. W., C. L. Grines, D. A. Cox, E. Garcia, J. E. Tcheng, J. J. Griffin, G. Guagliumi, T. Stuckey, M. Turco, J. D. Carroll, B. D. Rutherford, and A. J. Lansky. 2002. Comparison of angioplasty with stenting, with or without abciximab, in acute myocardial infarction. *New England Journal of Medicine* 346(13):957–966.

Stoskopf, C., Y. Kim, and S. Glover. 2001. Dual diagnosis: HIV and mental illness, a population-based study. *Community Mental Health Journal* 37(6):469–479.

Sturmer, M., H. W. Doerr, and L. Gurtler. 2009. Human immunodeficiency virus: 25 years of diagnostic and therapeutic strategies and their impact on hepatitis B and C virus. *Medical Microbiology Immunology* 198(3):147–155.

Sundar, S. S., R. J. Gornall, and S. T. Kehoe. 2005. Advances in the management of cervical cancer. *Menopause International* 11(3):91–95.

Suzich, J. A., S. J. Ghim, F. J. Palmer-Hill, W. I. White, J. K. Tamura, J. A. Bell, J. A. Newsome, A. B. Jenson, and R. Schlegel. 1995. Systemic immunization with papillomavirus L1 protein completely prevents the development of viral mucosal papillomas. *Proceedings of the National Academy of Sciences of the United States of America* 92(25):11553–11557.

Suzuki, R., N. Orsini, L. Mignone, S. Saji, and A. Wolk. 2008. Alcohol intake and risk of breast cancer defined by estrogen and progesterone receptor status—A meta-analysis of epidemiological studies. *International Journal of Cancer* 122(8):1832–1841.

Swica, Y. 2007. The transdermal patch and the vaginal ring: Two novel methods of combined hormonal contraception. *Obstetrics and Gynecology Clinics of North America* 34(1): viii, 31–42.

Szodoray, P., B. Nakken, J. Gaal, R. Jonsson, A. Szegedi, E. Zold, G. Szegedi, J. G. Brun, R. Gesztelyi, M. Zeher, and E. Bodolay. 2008. The complex role of vitamin D in autoimmune diseases. *Scandinavian Journal of Immunology* 68(3):261–269.

Tabar, L., G. Fagerberg, H. H. Chen, S. W. Duffy, C. R. Smart, A. Gad, and R. A. Smith. 1995. Efficacy of breast cancer screening by age. New results from the swedish two-county trial. *Cancer* 75(10):2507–2517.

Takeuchi, D. T., M. Alegria, J. S. Jackson, and D. R. Williams. 2007. Immigration and mental health: Diverse findings in Asian, black, and Latino populations. *American Journal of Public Health* 97(1):11–12.

Tamres, L. K., D. Janicki, and V. S. Helgeson. 2002. Sex differences in coping behavior: A meta-analytic review and an examination of relative coping. *Personality and Social Psychology Review* 6(1):2–30.

Tang, B. M., G. D. Eslick, C. Nowson, C. Smith, and A. Bensoussan. 2007. Use of calcium or calcium in combination with vitamin D supplementation to prevent fractures and bone loss in people aged 50 years and older: A meta-analysis. *Lancet* 370(9588):657–666.

Tanis, K. Q., and R. S. Duman. 2007. Intracellular signaling pathways pave roads to recovery for mood disorders. *Annals of Medicine* 39(7):531–544.

Tao, X., W. Hu, P. T. Ramirez, and J. J. Kavanagh. 2008. Chemotherapy for recurrent and metastatic cervical cancer. *Gynecologic Oncology* 110(3 Suppl. 2):S67–S71.

Tay, S-K., and K-J. Tay. 2004. Passive cigarette smoking is a risk factor in cervical neoplasia. *Gynecologic Oncology* 93(1):116–120.

Taylor, A. J., L. C. Gary, T. Arora, D. J. Becker, J. R. Curtis, M. L. Kilgore, M. A. Morrisey, K. G. Saag, R. Matthews, H. Yun, W. Smith, and E. Delzell. 2010. Clinical and demographic factors associated with fractures among older Americans. *Osteoporosis International* Jun 18. [Epub ahead of print].

Taylor, V. M., Y. Yasui, N. Burke, T. Nguyen, E. Acorda, H. Thai, P. Qu, and J. C. Jackson. 2004. Pap testing adherence among Vietnamese American women. *Cancer Epidemiology, Biomarkers and Prevention* 13(4):613–619.

Tetrault, J. M., R. A. Desai, W. C. Becker, D. A. Fiellin, J. Concato, and L. E. Sullivan. 2008. Gender and non-medical use of prescription opioids: Results from a national US survey. *Addiction* 103(2):258–268.

Thomas, L., L. A. Doyle, and M. J. Edelman. 2005. Lung cancer in women: Emerging differences in epidemiology, biology, and therapy. *Chest* 128(1):370–381.

Thun, M. J., S. J. Henley, and E. E. Calle. 2002. Tobacco use and cancer: An epidemiologic perspective for geneticists. *Oncogene* 21(48 Review Issue 6):7307–7325.

Thun, M. J., L. M. Hannan, L. L. Adams-Campbell, P. Boffetta, J. E. Buring, D. Feskanich, W. D. Flanders, H. J. Sun, K. Katanoda, L. N. Kolonel, I. M. Lee, T. Marugame, J. R. Palmer, E. Riboli, T. Sobue, E. Avila-Tang, L. R. Wilkens, and J. M. Samet. 2008. Lung cancer occurrence in never-smokers: An analysis of 13 cohorts and 22 cancer registry studies. *PLoS Medicine* 5(9):1357–1371.

Tien, P. C., S. R. Cole, C. M. Williams, R. Li, J. E. Justman, M. H. Cohen, M. Young, N. Rubin, M. Augenbraun, and C. Grunfeld. 2003. Incidence of lipoatrophy and lipohypertrophy in the Women's Interagency HIV Study. *Journal of Acquired Immune Deficiency Syndromes* 34(5):461–466.

Tien, P. C., Y. Barron, J. E. Justman, C. Hyman, M. H. Cohen, M. Young, A. Kovacs, and S. R. Cole. 2007. Antiretroviral therapies associated with lipoatrophy in HIV-infected women. *AIDS Patient Care and STDs* 21(5):297–305.

Tillman, G. F., S. G. Orel, M. D. Schnall, D. J. Schultz, J. E. Tan, and L. J. Solin. 2002. Effect of breast magnetic resonance imaging on the clinical management of women with early-stage breast carcinoma. *Journal Clinical Oncology* 20(16):3413–3423.

Tolaymat, L. L., and A. M. Kaunitz. 2007. Long-acting contraceptives in adolescents. *Current Opinion in Obstetrics and Gynecology* 19(5):453–460.

Tosteson, A. N., N. K. Stout, D. G. Fryback, S. Acharyya, B. A. Herman, L. G. Hannah, and E. D. Pisano. 2008. Cost-effectiveness of digital mammography breast cancer screening. *Annals of Internal Medicine* 148(1):1–10.

Towfighi, A., J. L. Saver, R. Engelhardt, and B. Ovbiagele. 2007. A midlife stroke surge among women in the United States. *Neurology* 69(20):1898–1904.

Towfighi, A., L. Zheng, and B. Ovbiagele. 2009. Sex-specific trends in midlife coronary heart disease risk and prevalence. *Archives of Internal Medicine* 169(19):1762–1766.

Trimble, C. L., J. M. Genkinger, A. E. Burke, S. C. Hoffman, K. J. Helzlsouer, M. Diener-West, G. W. Comstock, and A. J. Alberg. 2005. Active and passive cigarette smoking and the risk of cervical neoplasia. *Obstetrics and Gynecology* 105(1):174–181.

Trussell, J., and L. L. Wynn. 2008. Reducing unintended pregnancy in the United States. *Contraception* 77(1):1–5.

Tsao, A. S., D. Liu, J. J. Lee, M. Spitz, and W. K. Hong. 2006. Smoking affects treatment outcome in patients with advanced nonsmall cell lung cancer. *Cancer* 106(11):2428–2436.

Tumbarello, M., R. Rabagliati, K. De Gaetano Donati, S. Bertagnolio, E. Tamburrini, E. Tacconelli, and R. Cauda. 2003. Older HIV-positive patients in the era of highly active antiretroviral therapy: Changing of a scenario. *AIDS* 17(1):128–131.

Tyrer, J., S. W. Duffy, and J. Cuzick. 2004. A breast cancer prediction model incorporating familial and personal risk factors. *Statistics in Medicine* 23(7):1111–1130.

Uetrecht, J. 2009. Immune-mediated adverse drug reactions. *Chemical Research in Toxicology* 22(1): 24–34.

Uhlenhuth, E. H., and E. S. Paykel. 1973. Symptom intensity and life events. *Archives of General Psychiatry* 28(4):473–477.

Unutzer, J., W. Katon, C. M. Callahan, J. W. Williams, Jr., E. Hunkeler, L. Harpole, M. Hoffing, R. D. Della Penna, P. H. Noel, E. H. B. Lin, P. A. Arean, M. T. Hegel, L. Tang, T. R. Belin, S. Oishi, and C. Langston. 2002. Collaborative care management of late-life depression in the primary care setting: A randomized controlled trial. *Journal of the American Medical Association* 288(22):2836–2845.

US Preventive Services Task Force. 2002. Screening for breast cancer: Recommendations and rationale. *Annals of Internal Medicine* 137(5 Pt. 1):344–346.

———. 2009. Screening for breast cancer: US Preventive Services Task Force recommendation statement. *Annals of Internal Medicine* 151(10):716–726.

Vaccarino, V., L. Parsons, N. R. Every, H. V. Barron, and H. M. Krumholz. 1999. Sex-based differences in early mortality after myocardial infarction. National registry of myocardial infarction 2 participants. *New England Journal of Medicine* 341(4):217–225.

Vaccarino, V., S. S. Rathore, N. K. Wenger, P. D. Frederick, J. L. Abramson, H. V. Barron, A. Manhapra, S. Mallik, and H. M. Krumholz. 2005. Sex and racial differences in the management of acute myocardial infarction, 1994 through 2002. *New England Journal of Medicine* 353(7):671–682.

Vainio, H., and F. Bianchini. 2002a. IARC handbooks of cancer prevention. In *Weight Control and Physical Activity.* Vol. 6. Lyon, France: International Agency for Research on Cancer Press.

———. 2002b. *Breast Cancer Screening, IARC Handbooks of Cancer Prevention, Vol. 7.* Lyon, France: International Agency for Research on Cancer Press.

Vallbohmer, D., J. Brabender, D. Y. Yang, K. Danenberg, P. M. Schneider, R. Metzger, A. H. Holscher, and P. V. Danenberg. 2006. Sex differences in the predictive power of the molecular prognostic factor HER2/NEU in patients with non-small-cell lung cancer. *Clinical Lung Cancer* 7(5):332–337.

van Benthem, B. H., P. Vernazza, R. A. Coutinho, and M. Prins. 2002. The impact of pregnancy and menopause on CD4 lymphocyte counts in HIV-infected women. *AIDS* 16(6):919–924.

van't Veer, L. J., S. Paik, and D. F. Hayes. 2005. Gene expression profiling of breast cancer: A new tumor marker. *Journal Clinical Oncology* 23(8):1631–1635.

Vandamme, A. M. 2008. Cellulose sulfate for prevention of HIV infection. *New England Journal of Medicine* 359(19):2066–2067.

Vannucci, S. J., L. B. Willing, S. Goto, N. J. Alkayed, R. M. Brucklacher, T. L. Wood, J. Towfighi, P. D. Hurn, and I. A. Simpson. 2001. Experimental stroke in the female diabetic, DB/DB, mouse. *Journal of Cerebral Blood Flow and Metabolism* 21(1):52–60.

Varghese, B., J. E. Maher, T. A. Petermen, B. M. Branson, and R. W. Steketee. 2002. Reducing the risk of sexual HIV transmission: Quantifying the per-act risk for HIV on the basis of choice of partner, sex act, and condom use. *Sexually Transmitted Diseases* 29(1):38–43.

Vassilakos, P., F. de Marval, M. Munoz, G. Broquet, and A. Campana. 1998. Human papillomavirus (HPV) DNA assay as an adjunct to liquid-based pap test in the diagnostic triage of women with an abnormal pap smear. *International Journal of Gynaecology and Obstetrics* 61(1):45–50.

Vega, W. A., B. Kolody, S. Aguilar-Gaxiola, E. Alderete, R. Catalano, and J. Caraveo-Anduaga. 1998. Lifetime prevalence of DSM-III-R psychiatric disorders among urban and rural Mexican Americans in California. *Archives of General Psychiatry* 55(9):771–778.

Vera, M., C. Perez-Pedrogo, S. E. Huertas, M. L. Reyes-Rabanillo, D. Juarbe, A. Huertas, M. L. Reyes-Rodriguez, and W. Chaplin. 2010. Collaborative care for depressed patients with chronic medical conditions: A randomized trial in Puerto Rico. *Psychiatric Services* 61(2):144–150.

Veronesi, U., P. Maisonneuve, N. Rotmensz, B. Bonanni, P. Boyle, G. Viale, A. Costa, V. Sacchini, R. Travaglini, G. D'Aiuto, P. Oliviero, F. Lovison, G. Gucciardo, M. R. del Turco, M. G. Muraca, M. A. Pizzichetta, S. Conforti, and A. Decensi. 2007. Tamoxifen for the prevention of breast cancer: Late results of the Italian randomized tamoxifen prevention trial among women with hysterectomy. *Journal of the National Cancer Institute* 99(9):727–737.

Viard, J. P., A. Mocroft, A. Chiesi, O. Kirk, B. Roge, G. Panos, N. Vetter, J. N. Bruun, M. Johnson, and J. D. Lundgren. 2001. Influence of age on CD4 cell recovery in human immunodeficiency virus-infected patients receiving highly active antiretroviral therapy: Evidence from the Euro-SIDA study. *Journal of Infectious Diseases* 183(8):1290–1294.

Vigna-Taglianti, F., S. Vadrucci, F. Faggiano, G. Burkhart, R. Siliquini, and M. R. Galanti. 2009. Is universal prevention against youths' substance misuse really universal? Gender-specific effects in the EU-Dap school-based prevention trial. *Journal of Epidemiology and Community Health* 63(9):722–728.

Vinnicombe, S., S. M. Pinto Pereira, V. A. McCormack, S. Shiel, N. Perry, and I. M. dos Santos Silva. 2009. Full-field digital versus screen-film mammography: Comparison within the UK breast screening program and systematic review of published data. *Radiology* 251(2):347–358.

Visbal, A. L., B. A. Williams, F. C. Nichols, 3rd, R. S. Marks, J. R. Jett, M. C. Aubry, E. S. Edell, J. A. Wampfler, J. R. Molina, and P. Yang. 2004. Gender differences in non-small-cell lung cancer survival: An analysis of 4,618 patients diagnosed between 1997 and 2002. *Annals of Thoracic Surgery* 78(1):209–215.

Vogel, V. G., J. P. Costantino, D. L. Wickerham, W. M. Cronin, R. S. Cecchini, J. N. Atkins, T. B. Bevers, L. Fehrenbacher, E. R. Pajon, Jr., J. L. Wade, III, A. Robidoux, R. G. Margolese, J. James, S. M. Lippman, C. D. Runowicz, P. A. Ganz, S. E. Reis, W. McCaskill-Stevens, L. G. Ford, V. C. Jordan, N. Wolmark, and the National Surgical Adjuvant Breast and Bowel Project (NSABP). 2006. Effects of tamoxifen vs raloxifene on the risk of developing invasive breast cancer and other disease outcomes: The NSABP study of tamoxifen and raloxifene (STAR) P-2 trial. *Journal of the American Medical Association* 295(23):2727–2741.

Walboomers, J. M., M. V. Jacobs, M. M. Manos, F. X. Bosch, J. A. Kummer, K. V. Shah, P. J. Snijders, J. Peto, C. J. Meijer, and N. Muñoz. 1999. Human papillomavirus is a necessary cause of invasive cervical cancer worldwide. *Journal of Pathology* 189(1):12–19.

Walkup, J., S. Crystal, and U. Sambamoorthi. 1999. Schizophrenia and major affective disorder among Medicaid recipients with HIV/AIDS in New Jersey. *American Journal of Public Health* 89(7):1101–1103.

Wallenius, M., J. F. Skomsvoll, W. Koldingsnes, E. Rodevand, K. Mikkelsen, C. Kaufmann, and T. K. Kvien. 2009. Comparison of work disability and health-related quality of life between males and females with rheumatoid arthritis below the age of 45 years. *Scandinavian Journal of Rheumatology* 38(3):178–183.

Ward, R. K., and M. A. Zamorski. 2002. Benefits and risks of psychiatric medications during pregnancy. *American Family Physician* 66(4):629–636.

Warner, E., D. B. Plewes, K. A. Hill, P. A. Causer, J. T. Zubovits, R. A. Jong, M. R. Cutrara, G. DeBoer, M. J. Yaffe, S. J. Messner, W. S. Meschino, C. A. Piron, and S. A. Narod. 2004. Surveillance of *BRCA1* and *BRCA2* mutation carriers with magnetic resonance imaging, ultrasound, mammography, and clinical breast examination. *Journal of the American Medical Association* 292(11):1317–1325.

Warner-Schmidt, J. L., and R. S. Duman. 2008. VEGF as a potential target for therapeutic intervention in depression. *Current Opinion in Pharmacology* 8(1):14–19.

Warren, M. 2000. The expanding role of the female condom. *AIDS Analysis Africa* 10(5):8–10.

Wasserheit, J. N. 1992. Epidemiological synergy. Interrelationships between human immunodeficiency virus infection and other sexually transmitted diseases. *Sexually Transmitted Disease* 19(2):61–77.

Wassertheil-Smoller, S., S. Hendrix, M. Limacher, G. Heiss, C. Kooperberg, A. Baird, T. Kotchen, J. D. Curb, H. Black, J. E. Rossouw, A. Aragaki, M. Safford, E. Stein, S. Laowattana, and W. J. Mysiw. 2003. Effect of estrogen plus progestin on stroke in postmenopausal women: The Women's Health Initiative: A randomized trial. *Journal of the American Medical Association* 289(20):2673–2684.

Watts, N. B., and D. L. Diab. 2010. Long-term use of bisphosphonates in osteoporosis. *Journal of Clinical Endocrinology and Metabolism* 95(4):1555–1565.

Way, C. M. 2007. Safety of newer antidepressants in pregnancy. *Pharmacotherapy* 27(4):546–552.

Wei, Q., L. Cheng, C. I. Amos, L. E. Wang, Z. Guo, W. K. Hong, and M. R. Spitz. 2000. Repair of tobacco carcinogen-induced DNA adducts and lung cancer risk: A molecular epidemiologic study. *Journal of the National Cancer Institute* 92(21):1764–1772.

Weiss, E. L., J. G. Longhurst, and C. M. Mazure. 1999. Childhood sexual abuse as a risk factor for depression in women: Psychosocial and neurobiologica correlates. *American Journal of Psychiatry* 156:816–828.

Weiss, R. B. 1999. The randomized trials of dose-intensive therapy for breast cancer: What do they mean for patient care and where do we go from here? *Oncologist* 4(6):450–458.

Weissman, A. M., B. T. Levy, A. J. Hartz, S. Bentler, M. Donohue, V. L. Ellingrod, and K. L. Wisner. 2004. Pooled analysis of antidepressant levels in lactating mothers, breast milk, and nursing infants. *American Journal of Psychiatry* 161(6):1066–1078.

Welch, H. G., and J. Mogielnicki. 2002. Presumed benefit: Lessons from the American experience with marrow transplantation for breast cancer. *British Medical Journal* 324(7345):1088–1092.

Werner-Wasik, M., C. Scott, M. L. Graham, C. Smith, R. W. Byhardt, M. Roach, 3rd, and E. J. Andras. 1999. Interfraction interval does not affect survival of patients with non-small cell lung cancer treated with chemotherapy and/or hyperfractionated radiotherapy: A multivariate analysis of 1076 RTOG patients. *International Journal of Radiation Oncology, Biology, Physics* 44(2):327–331.

Wheatley-Price, P., C. Ma, L. F. Ashcroft, M. Nankivell, R. J. Stephens, S. C. White, P. Lorigan, N. Thatcher, F. H. Blackhall, and F. A. Shepherd. 2009. The strength of female sex as a prognostic factor in small-cell lung cancer: A pooled analysis of chemotherapy trials from the Manchester Lung Group and Medical Research Council Clinical Trials Unit. *Annals of Oncology* 21(2):232–237.

White, E., C. Y. Lee, and A. R. Kristal. 1990. Evaluation of the increase in breast cancer incidence in relation to mammography use. *Journal of the National Cancer Institute* 82(19):1546–1552.

White, I. D. 2008. The assessment and management of sexual difficulties after treatment of cervical and endometrial malignancies. *Clinical Oncology* 20(6):488–496.

White, L. N., and M. R. Spitz. 1993. Cancer risk and early detection assessment. *Seminars in Oncology Nursing* 9(3):188–197.

WHO (World Health Organization). 2010. *WHO Fracture Risk Assessment Tool.* http://www.sheffield.ac.uk/FRAX/ (accessed April 5, 2010).

Wilkins, C. H., and S. J. Birge. 2005. Prevention of osteoporotic fractures in the elderly. *American Journal of Medicine* 118(11):1190–1195.

Williams, D. R., H. M. Gonzalez, H. Neighbors, R. Nesse, J. M. Abelson, J. Sweetman, and J. S. Jackson. 2007. Prevalence and distribution of major depressive disorder in African Americans, Caribbean blacks, and non-Hispanic whites: Results from the National Survey of American Life. *Archives of General Psychiatry* 64(3):305–315.

Winer, E. P., C. Hudis, H. J. Burstein, A. C. Wolff, K. I. Pritchard, J. N. Ingle, R. T. Chlebowski, R. Gelber, S. B. Edge, J. Gralow, M. A. Cobleigh, E. P. Mamounas, L. J. Goldstein, T. J. Whelan, T. J. Powles, J. Bryant, C. Perkins, J. Perotti, S. Braun, A. S. Langer, G. P. Browman, and M. R. Somerfield. 2005. American Society of Clinical Oncology technology assessment on the use of aromatase inhibitors as adjuvant therapy for postmenopausal women with hormone receptor-positive breast cancer: Status report 2004. *Journal Clinical Oncology* 23(3):619–629.

Winer, R. L., J. P. Hughes, Q. Feng, S. O'Reilly, N. B. Kiviat, K. K. Holmes, and L. A. Koutsky. 2006. Condom use and the risk of genital human papillomavirus infection in young women. *New England Journal of Medicine* 354(25):2645–2654.

Wingo, P. A., J. King, J. Swan, S. S. Coughlin, J. S. Kaur, J. A. Erb-Alvarez, J. Jackson-Thompson, and T. G. Arambula Solomon. 2008. Breast cancer incidence among American Indian and Alaska native women: US, 1999–2004. *Cancer* 113(5 Suppl.):1191–1202.

Wisner, K. L., K. Peindl, and B. H. Hanusa. 1993. Relationship of psychiatric illness to childbearing status: A hospital-based epidemiologic study. *Journal of Affective Disorders* 28(1):39–50.

Wolff, A. C., M. E. Hammond, J. N. Schwartz, K. L. Hagerty, D. C. Allred, R. J. Cote, M. Dowsett, P. L. Fitzgibbons, W. M. Hanna, A. Langer, L. M. McShane, S. Paik, M. D. Pegram, E. A. Perez, M. F. Press, A. Rhodes, C. Sturgeon, S. E. Taube, R. Tubbs, G. H. Vance, M. van de Vijver, T. M. Wheeler, and D. F. Hayes. 2007. American Society of Clinical Oncology/College of American Pathologists guideline recommendations for human epidermal growth factor receptor 2 testing in breast cancer. *Journal Clinical Oncology* 25(1):118–145.

Wong, G. C., R. P. Giugliano, and E. M. Antman. 2003. Use of low-molecular-weight heparins in the management of acute coronary artery syndromes and percutaneous coronary intervention. *Journal of the American Medical Association* 289(3):331–342.

Wong, K. H., K. C. Chan, and S. S. Lee. 2001. Sex differences in nevirapine rash. *Clinical Infectious Diseases* 33(12):2096–2098.

Woodman, C. B. J., S. I. Collins, and L. S. Young. 2007. The natural history of cervical HPV infection: Unresolved issues. *Nature Reviews: Cancer* 7(1):11–22.

Wright, T. C. 2007. Cervical cancer screening in the 21st century: Is it time to retire the pap smear? *Clinical Obstetrics and Gynecology* 50(2):313–323.

Wright, T. C., Jr., L. S. Massad, C. J. Dunton, M. Spitzer, E. J. Wilkinson, and D. Solomon. 2007. 2006 consensus guidelines for the management of women with abnormal cervical cancer screening tests. *American Journal of Obstetrics and Gynecology* 197(4):346–355.

Writing Group for the Women's Health Initiative Investigators. 2002. Risks and benefits of estrogen plus progestin in healthy postmenopausal women: Principal results from the Women's Health Initiative Randomized Controlled Trial. *Journal of the American Medical Association* 288(3):321–333.

Xu, J., K. D. Kochanek, S. L. Muphy, and B. Tejada-Vera. 2010. *National Vital Statistics Report. Deaths: Final Data for 2007.* HHS (Department of Health and Human Services).

Yamamoto, H., I. Sekine, K. Yamada, H. Nokihara, N. Yamamoto, H. Kunitoh, Y. Ohe, and T. Tamura. 2008. Gender differences in treatment outcomes among patients with non-small cell lung cancer given a combination of carboplatin and paclitaxel. *Oncology* 75(3-4):169–174.

Yan, G., Y. Fu, and D. Faustman. 1997. Reduced expression of TAP1 and LMP2 antigen-processing genes in the nonobese diabetic (NOD) mouse due to a mutation in their shared bidirectional promoter. *Journal of Immunology* 159(6):3068–3080.

Yang, W. T., S. Carkaci, L. Chen, C-J. Lai, A. Sahin, G. J. Whitman, and C. C. Shaw. 2007. Dedicated cone-beam breast CT: Feasibility study with surgical mastectomy specimens. *American Journal of Roentgeneology* 189(6):1312–1315.

Young, E. A., S. G. Kornstein, S. M. Marcus, A. T. Harvey, D. Warden, S. R. Wisniewski, G. K. Balasubramani, M. Fava, M. H. Trivedi, and A. John Rush. 2009. Sex differences in response to citalopram: A STAR*D report. *Journal of Psychiatric Research* 43(5):503–511.

Xu J. Q., K. D. Kochanek, S. L. Murphy, B. Tejada-Vera. 2010. Deaths: Final data for 2007. *National Vital Statistics Reports* 58(19). Hyattsville, MD: National Center for Health Statistics. 2010.

Yusuf, S., S. R. Mehta, F. Zhao, B. J. Gersh, P. J. Commerford, M. Blumenthal, A. Budaj, T. Wittlinger, and K. A. A. Fox. 2003. Early and late effects of clopidogrel in patients with acute coronary syndromes. *Circulation* 107(7):966–972.

Zaino, R. J., J. Kauderer, C. L. Trimble, S. G. Silverberg, J. P. Curtin, P. C. Lim, and D. G. Gallup. 2006. Reproducibility of the diagnosis of atypical endometrial hyperplasia: A Gynecologic Oncology Group Study. *Cancer* 106(4):804–811.

Zakaria, S., and A. C. Degnim. 2007. Prophylactic mastectomy. *Surgical Clinics of North America* 87(2):317–331.

Zang, E. A., and E. L. Wynder. 1996. Differences in lung cancer risk between men and women: Examination of the evidence. *Journal of the National Cancer Institute* 88(3-4):183–192.

Zeferino, L. C., and S. F. Derchain. 2006. Cervical cancer in the developing world. *Best Practice and Research, Clinical Obstetrics and Gynaecology* 20(3):339–354.

Zell, J., W. Tsang, T. Taylor, R. Mehta, and H. Anton-Culver. 2009. Prognostic impact of human epidermal growth factor-like receptor 2 and hormone receptor status in inflammatory breast cancer (IBC): Analysis of 2,014 IBC patient cases from the California cancer registry. *Breast Cancer Research* 11(1):R9.

Zhou, J., X. Y. Sun, D. J. Stenzel, and I. H. Frazer. 1991. Expression of vaccinia recombinant HPV 16 L1 and L2 ORF proteins in epithelial cells is sufficient for assembly of HPV virion-like particles. *Virology* 185(1):251–257.

zur Hausen, H. 2009. Papillomaviruses in the causation of human cancers—A brief historical account. *Virology* 384(2):260–265.

4

Methodologic Issues in Women's Health Research

In reviewing and evaluating research on women's health, the committee considered not only conditions[1] and health determinants but also the types of research conducted. This chapter addresses methodologic issues with respect to women's health, looking at study design, subject sampling, outcome measures, and analysis. The Women's Health Initiative (WHI) is then discussed as an example of what has been learned about methods of women's health research from the studies already conducted. The information in this chapter helps the committee address question 4 from Box 1-4, whether the most appropriate research methods are being used to study women's health.

STUDY DESIGN

Research can be conducted on molecules, cells, and animals (basic research); on individuals or populations (clinical or observational studies); and on health systems (health-services and health-policy research). Each type of study has strengths and weaknesses, and progress generally requires congruence of evidence from multiple studies of different designs. For example, progress in breast and cervical cancer came through basic and experimental clinical research and other epidemiologic studies that provided support for similar conclusions (see Chapters 2 and 3).

Two major types of clinical studies are observational studies and clinical trials. An observational study is a study in which investigators do not manipulate the use of or deliver an intervention (that is, they do not assign subjects to treatment

---

[1] For brevity, the committee uses the term *conditions* to mean diseases, disorders, and conditions.

and control groups) but only observe and measure outcomes in subjects who are (or are not, in the case of a comparison group) exposed to an intervention (for example, a smoking ban that decreases secondhand smoke exposure) (Rosenbaum, 2002). Such studies have less control of potential confounders than do experimental studies, such as randomized controlled trials, and are more prone to selection bias and to bias in the choice of comparison populations. Observational studies provide information for identifying associations and are especially useful for generating hypotheses for further testing; they are less useful for determining causality. The Nurses' Health Study (NHS) and the Study of Women's Health Across the Nation (SWAN) are examples of large observational studies. The NHS was originally intended to investigate the potential long-term consequences of oral contraceptives and later adapted to investigate factors that influence women's health, especially in preventing cancer (NHS, 2008). SWAN was designed to collect information on the natural history of menopause (SWAN, 2010).

A randomized clinical trial is a prospective experiment in which investigators assign an eligible sample of people randomly to one or more treatment groups and a control group and follow subjects' outcomes. Randomized clinical trials are usually considered the best for testing the efficacy of a treatment or intervention (Rosenbaum, 2002). The Women's Health Study (WHS) was a randomized clinical trial in which the interventions were aspirin and vitamin E (WHS, 2009). The WHI consisted of both an observational study and three blinded, randomized clinical trial components that had hormone therapy, calcium and vitamin D, or dietary and exercise modification as the interventions (WHI, 2010). The randomized clinical trial in the WHI identified a risk of heart disease to be associated with combination estrogen hormone therapy, which was previously thought to be cardioprotective, and it confirmed the risk of breast cancer, venous thromboembolism, and stroke. Confidence in those results facilitated a decision to halt the study and led to a rapid change in prescribing practices (WHI, 2010).

Randomized clinical trials, however, have limitations of their own. Because of the expense and number of subjects needed to assess a given drug or other treatment, it is not possible to change key variables. The ability to extrapolate the results to a larger population might also be limited (Rosenbaum, 2002). In addition, ethical and practical considerations of the studies, including the ethics of placebo controls, need to be taken into account.

SUBJECT SAMPLING

If study results are to be extrapolated to the general population, the research sample needs to reflect the general population. Ensuring that research can be applied to the general population requires more than simply incorporating members of a subpopulation as part of the overall sample; it requires adequate numbers to ensure the statistical power to evaluate effects in that subpopulation. It is important to note that using gender or sex as a control variable is not the same as examining the effects of gender or sex on a given outcome. Thus, the issue is not simply including women in trials but including sufficient numbers to test effects on both women and men. To be fully informative, findings need to be reported separately by sex or gender. If a subpopulation, such as women in this case, is excluded or underrepresented in the sample, it is difficult to know whether the results will apply to the subpopulation or whether it would have responded differently. For example, that lack of data can delay translation of research findings on effective treatments to the excluded or underrepresented subpopulation or can lead to adverse outcomes because of inappropriate application to one population of treatments developed on another.

It might seem obvious that poor clinical outcomes can occur if it is presumed that there are no sex or gender differences when they do exist, but false inferences and bad outcomes can also result from a presumption of sex or gender differences when such differences do not exist (Baumeister, 1988). For example, the first randomized clinical trial of estrogen therapy, the Coronary Drug Project, was done in men. That study was discontinued prematurely because of a lack of evidence of a positive effect and a trend toward increased cardiovascular mortality in the treated group (The Coronary Drug Project Research Group, 1973). The doses in the trial were much higher than those given to women, so the results were thought not to be relevant to women, and estrogen therapy continued to be prescribed to women to reduce cardiovascular risks. More than 20 years after the study, postmenopausal hormones were still among the top-selling drugs in the United States—an estimated 15 million women were taking them (Hersh et al., 2004). Conversely, statins (that is, 3-hydroxy-3-methylglutaryl coenzyme A reductase inhibitors) were first shown to be effective in lowering cholesterol in a Scottish trial in men (Shepherd et al., 1995). Of 5 randomized controlled trials published in 1994–1998, the Scottish trial was in men only, and the other 4 included 14–19% women. That small number of women in statin trials limited conclusions for women and led to questions about the extrapolation of the data to women. LaRosa and colleagues (1999) conducted a meta-analysis of data from those trials and concluded that the risk reduction from statins is similar in men and women.[2] Meta-analyses, however, are not optimal, especially when evaluating the leading cause of mortality in women, and more recently the efficacy and safety of statins, especially for primary prevention, has been questioned and is still being evaluated (Abramson and Wright, 2007; Mascitelli and Pezzetta, 2007; McPherson and Kavaslar, 2007; Ridker, 2010).

Before 1987, women were underrepresented in key randomized controlled trials because of policies that limited or prevented their participation mainly owing to concern about potential exposures of fetuses. Changes in National In-

---

[2]LaRosa and colleagues (1999) searched the Medline database from 1966 to 1998. Therefore, most of the studies found were probably designed and initiated before the enactment of Public Law 103-43.

stitutes of Health (NIH) and Food and Drug Administration (FDA) regulations and policies, starting in 1987, addressed that underrepresentation and aimed to increase the enrollment of women and analysis of data on women in clinical trials (GAO, 1992, 2000; Merkatz and Junod, 1994). Progress has been made since then in increasing enrollment of women. Women made up 51.7% and 60.0% of participants in NIH extramural and intramural clinical research in 1995 and 2008, respectively (HHS, 2009). The highest percentage, 64.2%, was seen in 2002; that corresponds to when large women-only studies related to breast cancer, menopause, and cardiovascular diseases (the WHS, the WHI, and SWAN) were conducted (HHS, 2009). The sex distribution in all the minority-group participants in 2008 was similar to that in the nonminority population; women made up 59.15% of minority-group participants (HHS, 2009).[3]

Data from clinical trials that looked at specific end points have provided additional insight into the participation of women and minorities. A recent analysis of FDA clinical trials found that although the number of trials enrolling women and the proportion of participants who are female participating in phase I trials have increased since 2001, women are still underrepresented (Pinnow et al., 2009). Stewart and colleagues (2007) found higher enrollments of women than of men in their study of cooperative group surgical oncology trials, primarily because of the large number of breast-cancer trials. Members of racial and ethnic minorities and older persons were less likely to be enrolled in the trials than were whites and younger subjects.

Human immunodeficiency virus (HIV) research historically has had low representation of women. Of the women who were eligible to participate in the largest cohort study of HIV-infected women in the United States (the Women's Interagency HIV Study), about half would have been ineligible, on the basis of exclusion criteria, to participate in 20 of the AIDS Clinical Trials Group studies, which are among the largest HIV clinical-trial groups in the United States (Gandhi et al., 2005). Those results are consistent with an earlier meta-analysis published in abstract form that found that in 49 randomized controlled trials of antiretrovirals in 1990–2000, women averaged only 12.25% of the participants (Pardo et al., 2002).

In studies of cardiovascular disease, clinical-trial subjects have not been representative of the general population (Lloyd-Jones et al., 2001; Pedone and Lapane, 2003); one study discussed the predominance of men in cardiovascular trials (Sharpe, 2002). In 19 randomized controlled trials open to both men and

---

[3]Although these findings should be interpreted with caution because the Office of Management and Budget (OMB) changed minority classifications between 1995 and 2007 (HHS, 2009), data indicate that minority enrollment was 36.7% in 1995. It peaked in 2006 at 43.1% and dropped to 28.6% in 2008 (HHS, 2009). The aggregated extramural and intramural data from 2008 (using the 1977 OMB standards in a combined race–ethnicity format) show that "Black or African American" had the highest proportion of participation (15.8% of enrollees), followed by "Asian/Pacific Islander" (2.6%) and "Hispanic not White" (4.6%).

women that examined myocardial infarction, stroke, or death, the mean percentage of female subjects was only 27%.[4] Only 13 of those studies presented sex-based analyses (Kim and Menon, 2009). A review of the literature by the Agency for Healthcare Research and Quality indicated that studies of coronary heart disease rarely included women in adequate numbers for analysis of the data by sex (Grady et al., 2003).

Part of the reason for the low participation of women is that many cardiovascular-disease clinical trials had inclusion criteria that were more appropriate for men than for women (Grady et al., 2003). Such inclusion criteria as early age of onset of myocardial infarction and chest pain as a presenting symptom will favor enrollment of men because women are on the average older at disease onset, are less likely than men to report chest pain during a heart attack, and are more likely to report other symptoms (Bairey Merz et al., 2006; Canto et al., 2007).

Even when women are included in clinical trials, having too few of them can be a barrier to obtaining statistically significant results related to women. Freedman and colleagues (1995) suggested conducting large clinical trials for conditions in which there is a priori evidence of sex differences. The NIH guidelines require inclusion of women and minorities in phase III clinical trials unless there is substantial evidence that sex differences do not exist (Bennett and the Board on Health Sciences Policy of the Institute of Medicine, 1993; Freedman et al., 1995). That implies that earlier research—including cells, animals, and phase I and II clinical trials—must have addressed potential sex differences sufficiently to support a choice not to include women in phase III clinical trials in numbers adequate for assessing sex differences. Underrepresentation of women in earlier phases could lead to interventions or treatments that are less effective or more toxic in women. For example, dose regimens are determined in phase I clinical trials, and conducting such studies mostly in men would result in drug doses based on male anatomy (Chen et al., 2000). Data indicate that women continue to be underrepresented in trials. For example, Jagsi (2009) found that women comprised only 38.8% of participants in non–sex-specific prospective clinical studies.

Because women might not be included in studies in adequate numbers to obtain a valid statistical analysis, another potential method of obtaining useful data on women is to perform meta-analysis of aggregated published data. That, however, requires that multiple studies be sufficiently similar in design (for example, having similar inclusion criteria and dosing regimens) and in clinical outcomes to be aggregated and also that the studies provide data on women separately (Berlin and Ellenberg, 2009). However, most clinical trials do not publish results on key subgroups of interest. Even when results on subgroups are published, the data

---

[4]The studies were funded by the National Heart, Lung, and Blood Institute and published in 1997–2006. Sex-specific studies were excluded.

are typically presented in different ways among studies and difficult to combine in a meta-analysis (Berlin and Ellenberg, 2009).

Combining data on individual subjects from randomized trials is another approach for enhancing statistical power that increases the number of subjects available for analysis in clinical subgroups. Pooling of data on individual subjects overcomes the limitations of meta-analysis and allows use of more sensitive statistical methods, including analysis of survival times, multivariable models, and tests for treatment-by-covariate interactions (Samsa et al., 2005). It also enables the assessment of the combined effect of treatment for multiple end points—combining benefits and risks to capture net "value" (Antithrombotic Trialists Collaboration, 2009). However, the technique poses logistical challenges and requires collaboration among trial groups and support from funding agencies (Bravata et al., 2007).

A Bayesian approach could also be used to determine whether sex or gender differences exist, and that information could form the basis of further research. The Bayesian approach is an iterative one that adds more subjects from a subgroup on the basis of probabilities estimated from previous or preliminary results (Berry, 2006). In Bayesian analysis, the effect in a small number of women could be compared with the effect in a larger sample of men (or vice versa). If the distribution of results for several outcomes is the same between the sexes or genders, the study can proceed and continue to include a small number of women and to conduct periodic analyses to determine whether sex or gender differences are evident. If the distributions are different, the next phase of the clinical trial would incorporate larger numbers of women to assess the differences. This method could be applied to individual and pooled trials.

An alternative to executing clinical trials with women and men and analyzing sex- or gender-specific data is to conduct women-only studies, particularly in cases in which there are gaps in knowledge about women. That has been done in a few men-only studies that demonstrated the benefit of a drug. For example, the original Physicians Health Study was a randomized controlled trial in men that found that daily aspirin led to a significant reduction in myocardial infarction but not in cardiovascular death (Hennekens and Buring, 1989; Hennekens and Eberlein, 1985). It was not known whether the results would be the same in women. Later the women-only WHS had slightly different results: daily aspirin lowered the risk of stroke but did not affect the risk of myocardial infarction or cardiovascular death (Ridker et al., 2005). Sex differences were then examined in a study that pooled individual-level data from 6 primary-prevention randomized trials and 16 secondary-prevention randomized trials (looking for prevention after a coronary event), including both the sex-specific trials discussed above. No sex differences in the effect of aspirin on overall serious cardiovascular events were seen, and the risk of cardiovascular events was reduced in both men and women. However, there were slight sex differences in aspirin's value in primary prevention (depending on the statistical analysis): less primary prevention of major coronary events and more primary prevention of strokes were seen in women than in men. No sex differences were seen in secondary prevention of either end point—aspirin was protective in both sexes (Antithrombotic Trialists Collaboration, 2009). Overall, the authors concluded that aspirin is beneficial for protecting against secondary events in both women and men but that protection against primary events needs to be weighed against the risks posed by daily aspirin for both sexes.

OUTCOME MEASURES

Female-Appropriate End Points

Sex and gender differences need to be considered not only for inclusion and exclusion criteria but also when determining the end points to be studied. If study end points are based on male pathophysiology, clinical outcomes relevant to women will be missed. For example, women are more likely to have unstable angina (DeCara, 2003), unrecognized myocardial infarction (Sheifer et al., 2001), and stroke as cardiovascular outcomes than men (Lloyd-Jones et al., 2009; Towfighi et al., 2007). If a clinical trial looking at a cardiovascular-disease treatment assesses fatal and nonfatal myocardial infarction as its outcome but does not assess such events as unstable angina that are more common in women, it will underestimate the prevalence of cardiovascular disease in women and be biased against finding a treatment effect in women.

Quality of Life as an End Point

Incidence and 5-year survival rates are often the end points evaluated in clinical trials, including studies of women's health; fewer studies assess morbidity or health-related quality-of-life (HRQoL) end points. The focus of research on mortality is also reflected in the relative lack of attention paid to conditions associated more closely with morbidity than with mortality, such as autoimmune disease, thyroid disease, and nonmalignant gynecologic disorders. Many of those chronic disabling disorders and depressive and anxiety disorders affect women more than men (Rieker and Bird, 2005), and women, when surveyed, generally report worse health than men even though men have shorter life expectancy and lower age of onset of such diseases as cardiovascular disease (Rieker and Bird, 2005). In addition, women rank quality-of-life end points high when considering what aspects of health matter to them, and this points to the need to assess HRQoL end points in women (Fryback et al., 2007).

One challenge in including HRQoL end points in studies is the need for consistent and accurate metrics for them. In particular for women's health, including metrics that measure what matters to women is important. Metrics for HRQoL end points have been developed as interest in assessing them in observational studies, clinical trials, and health-services research has increased. Measures of HRQoL end points can reflect specific symptoms, constellations of symptoms associated with specific conditions, or the combined effects on overall well-being that reflect symptoms that affect HRQoL (that is, quantify a global measure of quality of life) (Gold et al., 2002). HRQoL metrics, such as the *SF-36*, which is a short-form health survey with 36 questions, quantify quality of life in terms of domains (for example, physical, psychologic, economic, spiritual, and social) and allow comparisons among conditions, but some may lack sensitivity to sex- and gender-specific issues (such as menopause and premenstrual-syndrome symptoms), and some are affected by sex and gender (Fleishman and Lawrence, 2003). Research is beginning to identify and improve understanding of those differences to capture quality-of-life end points for women better (Fryback et al., 2007). Improved measures of HRQoL in women will help not only in assessing women's health but in communicating risks and benefits associated with treatment and intervention options to women and to facilitate informed decision making for female patients—an important aspect of translating research into practice, which is discussed further in Chapter 5.

ANALYSIS

Including adequate numbers of women in clinical trials is necessary but not sufficient to ensure that results are applicable to women. Despite improved inclusion of women in trials funded by NIH and reviewed by FDA, there has been a lag in the routine analysis and reporting of data by sex (GAO, 2000, 2001). Often there is no mention of separate male and female analysis in publications, and it is not possible to know whether an analysis by sex was not conducted or was conducted but not reported, especially inasmuch as negative findings are often not reported. Many trials are designed to test an intervention, not to test whether the intervention is safe and effective in both men and women.

Another consideration is that the volume of health-research data is expanding, and new initiatives are underway to capture those data. The initiatives include developing a health-information-technology infrastructure and large databases, including the i2b2, the Cancer Biomedical Informatics Grid, improvement in the Medicare and Medicaid claims databases, and use of distributed data networks for an FDA sentinel system to detect adverse drug events (Bach et al., 2002; Kakazu et al., 2004; Murphy et al., 2006; Platt et al., 2009). If those technologies are to achieve their full potential in improving women's health, the ability to capture and analyze sex- and gender-specific data needs to be considered during the design of such systems (Brittle and Bird, 2007; McKinley et al., 2002; Weisman, 2000). Additionally, data relevant to women's health needs to be captured better in health-services research (for example, by using metrics of care quality specific to women) so that there can be more accurate measures of the translation of research findings into health-care services and delivery (Chou et al., 2007a,b; Correa-de-Araujo, 2004; NCQA, 2010).

METHODOLOGIC LESSONS FROM THE WOMEN'S HEALTH INITIATIVE

Much has been learned from the WHI about how to design women's health research (see Appendix C for details of this study). The WHI, which is the largest clinical study done exclusively on women, was designed as a study of primary prevention of diseases of aging (coronary heart disease, breast and colorectal cancer, and hip and other fractures), but it also assessed other end points (stroke, venous and pulmonary emboli, ovarian and endometrial cancer, gall bladder disease, cognition, and death). A global index was developed as a summary measure of the effect of treatment for potentially life-threatening events (Resnick et al., 2006, 2009). The WHI consisted of an observational study that was designed to identify predictors of disease in women and a clinical trial that consisted of three randomized components (Anderson et al., 2003):

1. trials that evaluated the effects of the postmenopausal hormone therapy, conjugated equine estrogen (Premarin™) on heart disease, fractures, and breast and colorectal cancer in 10,739 postmenopausal women who did not have uteruses, or conjugated equine estrogen plus medroxyprogesterone (Prempro™) in 16,608 postmenopausal women who had uteruses;
2. a trial that assessed whether a calcium and vitamin D supplement reduces the risk of colorectal cancer and the frequency of hip and other fractures in over 36,000 postmenopausal women; and
3. a trial that assessed the effects of a diet low in fat and high in fruits, vegetables, and grains on breast cancer, colorectal cancer, and heart disease in almost 49,000 postmenopausal women.

The hormone-therapy component of the WHI was initiated to assess the risks and benefits associated with menopausal hormone therapy (estrogen or estrogen plus progestin) and to help to settle controversies about the efficacy of those therapies in preventing cardiovascular disease (HHS, 2010). Basic research had suggested a cardioprotective effect of estrogen in animals (Gerhard-Herman et al., 2000); data from individual studies and pooled data from observational studies, such as the NHS, found a significantly lower risk of coronary heart disease in postmenopausal women who were on estrogen alone (Barrett-Connor and Grady, 1998; Grady et al., 1992; Grodstein et al., 1996, 2000; Stampfer and Colditz, 1991); and data from a randomized controlled trial (the Postmenopausal Estrogen/Progestin Interventions [PEPI]) that examined intermediate end points (lipid profiles) as proxies for coronary heart disease found a somewhat beneficial effect of PEPI (reducing low-density–lipoprotein cholesterol and increasing high-density–lipoprotein cholesterol by 10–15%) (Espeland et al., 1998). The NHS specifically showed decreased rates of coronary heart disease and of death from cardiovascular disease, but no effect on the rate of stroke, with estrogen therapy (Stampfer et al., 1991). At the time, hormone therapy was routinely prescribed from menopause on, and many thought it likely that the WHI would be halted prematurely because the beneficial effects of such therapy on cardiovascular disease would be demonstrated early in the study (IOM, 1993).

At the same time, however, other randomized controlled trials—such as the Heart and Estrogen/Progestin Replacement Study (HERS), which examined heart attacks and death from coronary heart disease (Herrington et al., 2000), and the Estrogen Replacement and Atherosclerosis (ERA) study, which examined lipid concentrations, angiographic end points, and cardiovascular events—did not show that estrogen plus progestin prevented further heart attacks or death from coronary heart disease in postmenopausal women who had heart disease and, in the case of HERS, actually resulted in a higher rate of coronary heart disease soon after initiation of treatment (Grady et al., 2000; Herrington et al., 2000; Hulley et al., 1998). Earlier, the Framingham Study, the only prospective observational study designed specifically to measure coronary–heart-disease end points, did not show beneficial effects of estrogen on mortality from all causes or from cardiovascular disease (Wilson et al., 1985). The Framingham Study differed from other observational studies in its inclusion of angina and systematic ascertainment of silent myocardial infarction through routine electrocardiography. Those examples highlight the importance of including study end points that reflect both female and male physiology. It is noteworthy that the observational studies showed effects similar to those in the WHI of both hormone treatments for disease outcomes other than cardiovascular disease (that is, breast, colorectal, and endometrial cancer; stroke; and venous thromboembolism) (WHI, 2010).

Because the WHI was a large, randomized controlled trial that looked at multiple end points, it provided more definitive results than the previous conflicting findings. That design helped to detect an increased risk of stroke and a lack of effect (increase or decrease) on heart disease in the estrogen-only portion of the WHI, and it enabled scientific confidence in those results (Anderson et al., 2004). That led to the halting of the studies for safety reasons (HHS, 2004).

The conflicting results on coronary heart disease in the NHS and the WHI led to exploration of new statistical methods to adjust for potential confounders in the use of nonrandomized observational data. One method, the use of propensity scores, was able to replicate the WHI's findings on coronary heart disease better when applied to the observational data (Hernán et al., 2008; Tannen et al., 2007).

The WHI illustrates the utility of developing a composite score to assess benefits and risks together and among diseases. The WHI's "global index" gave equal weight to the effects of hormone therapy on specific monitored outcomes—

coronary heart disease, stroke, pulmonary embolism, breast and colorectal cancer, hip fractures, and death. It was helpful in understanding the net effect of hormone therapy on those clinical outcomes. One limitation of the index, however, is in making decisions about treatment for menopause symptoms. The index does not include the effect of hormone therapy on menopausal symptoms, because the hormone-therapy component of the WHI was designed to evaluate effects on diseases of aging, not on menopause symptoms. The index also did not include dementia, urinary incontinence, and other end points that might affect treatment decisions. To be most useful for treatment decisions, a global measure of net effect should include all clinically relevant end points, especially those of greatest importance to women. The end points need to be weighted (either equally or differently) in an index; this can be done by using analytic decision models in which end points can be weighted implicitly according to their likelihood of occurrence, effect on mortality, and effect on HRQoL. The WHI recruited a large number of older, postmenopausal women and was relatively successful in meeting not only its overall recruitment goals but also its recruitment goals for minority women (Hays et al., 2003), and lessons can be learned from its recruitment strategies (Limacher, 2003). In addition, the lack of information on the social roles of the women in the WHI (for example, marital history) limits the ability to assess barriers to behavioral change, especially for the dietary arm.

The WHI also pointed to the importance of considering the timing and duration of treatment in observational studies. Some researchers pointed to the treatment of older postmenopausal women and questioned the generalizability of the findings to women who take hormone therapy at earlier stages for menopausal symptoms (Harman et al., 2004). A reanalysis of the data from the NHS demonstrated the importance of accounting for age, timing and duration of treatment, and the onset of adverse events in observational studies, with the reanalysis yielding results for the NHS closer to WHI than originally reported (Hernán et al., 2008). That reanalysis generated some controversy (Stampfer, 2008), but does point to the importance of timing issues in studies and the potential for novel analytical techniques to shed light on study differences (Hernán and Robins, 2008; Hernán et al., 2008; Hoover, 2008; Prentice, 2008; Wilcox and Wacholder, 2008; Willet et al., 2008).

SUMMARY

There are several lessons to be learned regarding methodologic and statistical approaches to women's health research. Etiology and risk factors can be investigated with well-designed and well-executed observational studies that measure and adjust for known confounders, ensure appropriate ascertainment of end points (especially coronary heart disease, whose ascertainment is more challenging), and use appropriate statistical techniques to analyze data. Caution needs to be exercised in extrapolating from studies that use biomarkers rather than clinical outcomes. In using biomarkers for clinical outcomes, it is crucial that the measures selected be relevant to women, especially in clinical studies that involve both women and men. For example, the results of observational studies that reported on the effect of hormone therapy on lipids were interpreted as proxy evidence of their effect on coronary–heart-disease end points, but this was not confirmed or supported in randomized controlled trials that examined these end points.

Single-sex studies like the WHI can provide valuable information and fill in research gaps—especially in, for example, coronary heart disease—in clinical trials where women have been underrepresented. Most clinical trials, however, now include both women and men, and it will be critical to develop new methods and approaches to analysis of data by subgroup. After many years, the analysis of data by sex is still inadequate, and it is unclear whether adequate numbers of women are being enrolled in clinical trials to allow adequate analysis (GAO, 2000, 2001).

The limitations of randomized controlled trials, such as expense and the number of subjects needed, are reflected in questions that arose regarding the randomized controlled trials of the WHI. One question was related to the choice of hormone therapy—conjugated equine estrogen with progestin (Prempro™) and without progestin (Premarin™). Conjugated equine estrogen is a complex compound, and it is not known whether these results would apply to estradiol alone. It is also not known whether other routes of administration—dermal or intranasal—would have produced different results or whether different types of progestin would have different effects on coronary heart disease.

CONCLUSIONS

- Women need to be considered in the design, inclusion and exclusion criteria, recruitment, outcome measures, and analysis of research. Adequate numbers of women need to be enrolled in studies to allow statistically significant sex-based analyses, study outcomes need to include symptoms and effects seen in women, analyses need to be conducted to determine sex or gender differences, and the results of the analyses need to be published. A number of design and analytic techniques can be explored to improve sex-specific analyses while limiting the increase in sample size.
- Much research focuses on improving disease survival; insufficient attention has been paid to improving disease-related morbidity (for example, autoimmune diseases that affect a large number of women and the health effects that follow breast-cancer treatment and recovery) and especially to wellness and quality of life as health outcomes.

RECOMMENDATIONS

- In the absence of a compelling reason not to, it should be assumed that there are sex differences in conditions (that is, sex matters), so research studies should be designed to include women in sufficient numbers to allow the resulting data to be analyzed.
  - Basic research should include analysis of effects in females. Information from this basic research can guide the focus of sex and gender differences in clinical studies.
  - Sex and gender differences in the manifestation of disease should be considered in the design of research to incorporate the spectrum of outcomes that are relevant to women. Government and other funding agencies should ensure adequate participation of women and reporting of sex-stratified analyses in health research. One possible mechanism would be to expand the role of data-safety monitoring boards to monitor participation, efficacy, and adverse outcomes by sex.
  - Given the practical limitations in the size of research studies, research designs and statistical techniques that facilitate analysis of data on subgroups—without substantially increasing the overall size of a study population—should be explored. Conferences or meetings with a specific goal of developing consensus guidelines or recommendations on such study methods (for example, the use of Bayesian statistics and the pooling of data across study groups) should be convened by NIH and other federal agencies and relevant professional organizations.
  - To gain knowledge from existing studies that individually do not have sufficient numbers of female subjects for separate analysis, the director of the Department of Health and Human Services Office of the National Coordinator for Health Information Technology should support development and application of mechanisms for pooling patient and subject data to answer research questions that are not definitively answered by single studies.
  - For approval of medical products (drugs, devices, and biologics) coming to market, FDA should enforce compliance with the requirement for sex-stratified analyses of efficacy and safety and should take these analyses into account in regulatory decisions.
  - When it is possible, analysis of clinical research should be stratified by sex and should include power calculations to prevent type II errors in interpretation that might lead to withholding of therapy from women.
  - The International Committee of Medical Journal Editors and editors of relevant journals not represented on that committee should adopt as a guideline that all papers that report the outcomes of clinical trials report outcomes in men and women separately except for trials involving sex-specific conditions (such as endometrial cancer and prostatic cancer). NIH should sponsor a meeting to facilitate establishment of such guidelines.

○ The federal government should ensure that a data infrastructure is designed to capture data in forms that facilitate its analysis by sex and gender.

• Research should be conducted on women's quality of life, including the development of better measures to compare effects not only of health conditions but of interventions and treatments on quality of life. The end points or outcomes examined in studies should include quality-of-life outcomes (for example, functional status, mobility, and pain) in addition to mortality.

REFERENCES

Abramson, J., and J. M. Wright. 2007. Are lipid-lowering guidelines evidence-based? *Lancet* 369(9557):168–169.

Anderson, G., J. Manson, R. Wallace, B. Lund, D. Hall, S. Davis, S. Shumaker, C. Y. Wang, E. Stein, and R. L. Prentice. 2003. Implementation of the women's health initiative study design. *Annals of Epidemiology* 13(9 Suppl.):S5–S17.

Anderson, G., M. Limacher, A. Assaf, T. Bassford, S. Beresford, H. Black, D. Bonds, R. Brunner, R. Brzyski, B. Caan, R. Chlebowski, D. Curb, M. Gass, J. Hays, G. Heiss, S. Hendrix, B. Howard, J. Hsia, A. Hubbell, R. Jackson, K. Johnson, H. Judd, J. Kotchen, L. Kuller, A. LaCroix, D. Lane, R. Langer, N. Lasser, C. Lewis, J. Manson, K. Margolis, J. Ockene, M. O'Sullivan, L. Phillips, R. Prentice, C. Ritenbaugh, J. Robbins, J. Rossouw, G. Sarto, M. Stefanick, L. Van Horn, J. Wactawski-Wende, R. Wallace, and S. Wassertheil-Smoller. 2004. Effects of conjugated equine estrogen in postmenopausal women with hysterectomy: The women's health initiative randomized controlled trial. *Journal of the American Medical Association* 291(14):1701–1712.

Antithrombotic Trialists Collaboration. 2009. Aspirin in the primary and secondary prevention of vascular disease: Collaborative meta-analysis of individual participant data from randomised trials. *Lancet* 373(9678):1849–1860.

Bach, P. B., E. Guadagnoli, D. Schrag, N. Schussler, and J. L. Warren. 2002. Patient demographic and socioeconomic characteristics in the SEER-Medicare database applications and limitations. *Medical Care* 40(8 Suppl.):IV19–IV25.

Bairey Merz, C. N., L. J. Shaw, S. E. Reis, V. Bittner, S. F. Kelsey, M. Olson, B. D. Johnson, C. J. Pepine, S. Mankad, B. L. Sharaf, W. J. Rogers, G. M. Pohost, A. Lerman, A. A. Quyyumi, and G. Sopko. 2006. Insights from the NHLBI-sponsored Women's Ischemia Syndrome Evaluation (WISE) study: Part II: Gender differences in presentation, diagnosis, and outcome with regard to gender-based pathophysiology of atherosclerosis and macrovascular and microvascular coronary disease. *Journal of the American College of Cardiology* 47(3 Suppl.):S21–S29.

Barrett-Connor, E., and D. Grady. 1998. Hormone replacement therapy, heart disease, and other considerations. *Annual Review of Public Health* 19:55–72.

Baumeister, R. F. 1988. Should we stop studying sex differences altogether? [editorial]. *American Psychologist* 43:1092–1095.

Bennett, J. C., and the Board on Health Sciences Policy of the Institute of Medicine. 1993. Inclusion of women in clinical trials—policies for population subgroups. *New England Journal of Medicine* 329(4):288–292.

Berlin, J. A., and S. S. Ellenberg. 2009. Inclusion of women in clinical trials. *BMC Medicine* 7:56.

Berry, D. A. 2006. Bayesian clinical trials. *Nature Reviews Drug Discovery* 5(1):27–36.

Bravata, D. M., A. L. Gienger, K. M. McDonald, V. Sundaram, M. V. Perez, R. Varghese, J. R. Kapoor, R. Ardehali, D. K. Owens, and M. A. Hlatky. 2007. Systematic review: The comparative effectiveness of percutaneous coronary interventions and coronary artery bypass graft surgery. *Annals of Internal Medicine* 147(10):703–716.

Brittle, C., and C. E. Bird. 2007. *Literature Review on Effective Sex- and Gender-Based Systems/Models of Care.* Arlington, VA: Uncommon Insights.

Canto, J. G., R. J. Goldberg, M. M. Hand, R. O. Bonow, G. Sopko, C. J. Pepine, and T. Long. 2007. Symptom presentation of women with acute coronary syndromes: Myth vs reality. *Archives of Internal Medicine* 167(22):2405–2413.

Chen, M. L., S. C. Lee, M. J. Ng, D. J. Schuirmann, L. J. Lesko, and R. L. Williams. 2000. Pharmacokinetic analysis of bioequivalence trials: Implications for sex-related issues in clinical pharmacology and biopharmaceutics. *Clinical Pharmacology and Therapeutics* 68(5):510–521.

Chou, A. F., S. H. Scholle, C. S. Weisman, A. S. Bierman, R. Correa-de-Araujo, and L. Mosca. 2007a. Gender disparities in the quality of cardiovascular disease care in private managed care plans. *Women's Health Issues* 17(3):120–130.

Chou, A. F., L. Wong, C. S. Weisman, S. Chan, A. S. Bierman, R. Correa-de-Araujo, and S. H. Scholle. 2007b. Gender disparities in cardiovascular disease care among commercial and medicare managed care plans. *Women's Health Issues* 17(3):139–149.

The Coronary Drug Project Research Group. 1973. The Coronary Drug Project: Findings leading to discontinuation of the 2.5-mg/day estrogen group. *Journal of the American Medical Association* 226(6):652–657.

Correa-de-Araujo, R. 2004. A wake-up call to advance women's health. *Women's Health Issues* 14(2):31–34.

DeCara, J. M. 2003. Noninvasive cardiac testing in women. *Journal of the American Medical Women's Association* 58(4):254–263.

Espeland, M. A., S. M. Marcovina, V. Miller, P. D. Wood, C. Wasilauskas, R. Sherwin, H. Schrott, and T. L. Bush. 1998. Effect of postmenopausal hormone therapy on lipoprotein(a) concentration. PEPI investigators. Postmenopausal estrogen/progestin interventions. *Circulation* 97(10): 979–986.

Fleishman, J. A., and W. F. Lawrence. 2003. Demographic variation in SF-12 scores: True differences or differential item functioning? *Medical Care* 41(7 Suppl.):III75–III86.

Freedman, L. S., R. Simon, M. A. Foulkes, L. Friedman, N. L. Geller, D. J. Gordon, and R. Mowery. 1995. Inclusion of women and minorities in clinical trials and the NIH revitalization act of 1993—the perspective of NIH clinical trialists. *Controlled Clinical Trials* 16(5):277–285; discussion 286–289, 293–309.

Fryback, D. G., N. C. Dunham, M. Palta, J. Hanmer, J. Buechner, D. Cherepanov, S. A. Herrington, R. D. Hays, R. M. Kaplan, T. G. Ganiats, D. Feeny, and P. Kind. 2007. US norms for six generic health-related quality-of-life indexes from the National Health Measurement Study. *Medical Care* 45(12):1162–1170.

Gandhi, M., N. Ameli, P. Bacchetti, G. B. Sharp, A. L. French, M. Young, S. J. Gange, K. Anastos, S. Holman, A. Levine, and R. M. Greenblatt. 2005. Eligibility criteria for HIV clinical trials and generalizability of results: The gap between published reports and study protocols. *AIDS* 19(16):1885–1896.

GAO (General Acounting Office). 1992. *Women's Health: FDA Needs to Ensure More Study of Gender Differences in Prescription Drug Testing: Report to Congressional Requesters.* Washington, DC: GAO.

———. 2000. *Women's Health: NIH Has Increased Its Efforts to Include Women in Research: Report to Congressional Requesters.* Washington, DC: GAO.

———. 2001. *Women's Health: Women Sufficiently Represented in New Drug Testing, but FDA Oversight Needs Improvement.* Washington, DC: GAO.

Gerhard-Herman, M., N. Hamburg, and P. Ganz. 2000. Hormone replacement therapy and cardiovascular risk. *Current Cardiology Reports* 2(4):288–292.

Gold, M. R., D. Stevenson, and D. G. Fryback. 2002. HALYS and QALYS and DALYS, oh my: Similarities and differences in summary measures of population health. *Annual Review of Public Health* 23(1):115–134.

Grady, D., S. M. Rubin, D. B. Petitti, C. S. Fox, D. Black, B. Ettinger, V. L. Ernster, and S. R. Cummings. 1992. Hormone therapy to prevent disease and prolong life in postmenopausal women. *Annals of Internal Medicine* 117(12):1016–1037.

Grady, D., N. K. Wenger, D. Herrington, S. Khan, C. Furberg, D. Hunninghake, E. Vittinghoff, and S. Hulley. 2000. Postmenopausal hormone therapy increases risk for venous thromboembolic disease. The Heart and Estrogen/Progestin Replacement Study. *Annals of Internal Medicine* 132(9):689–696.

Grady, D., L. Chaput, and M. Kristof. 2003. Results of systematic review of research on diagnosis and treatment of coronary heart disease in women. In *Evidence Report/Technology Assessment*. No. 80. (Prepared by the University of California, San Francisco—Stanford Evidence-based Practice Center under Contract No 290-97-0013.) AHRQ Publication No. 03-0035. Rockville, MD: Agency for Healthcare Research and Quality.

Grodstein, F., M. J. Stampfer, J. E. Manson, G. A. Colditz, W. C. Willett, B. Rosner, F. E. Speizer, and C. H. Hennekens. 1996. Postmenopausal estrogen and progestin use and the risk of cardiovascular disease. *New England Journal of Medicine* 335(7):453-461.

Grodstein, F., J. E. Manson, G. A. Colditz, W. C. Willett, F. E. Speizer, and M. J. Stampfer. 2000. A prospective, observational study of postmenopausal hormone therapy and primary prevention of cardiovascular disease. *Annals of Internal Medicine* 133(12):933–941.

Harman, S. M., E. A. Brinton, T. Clarkson, C. B. Heward, H. S. Hecht, R. H. Karas, D. R. Judelson, and F. Naftolin. 2004. Is the WHI relevant to HRT started in the perimenopause? *Endocrine* 24(3):195–202.

Hays, J., J. R. Hunt, F. A. Hubbell, G. L. Anderson, M. Limacher, C. Allen, and J. E. Rossouw. 2003. The Women's Health Initiative recruitment methods and results. *Annals of Epidemiology* 13(9 Suppl.):S18–S77.

Hennekens, C. H., and J. E. Buring. 1989. Methodologic considerations in the design and conduct of randomized trials: The US Physicians' Health Study. *Controlled Clinical Trials* 10(4 Suppl.):142S–150S.

Hennekens, C. H., and K. Eberlein. 1985. A randomized trial of aspirin and beta-carotene among US Physicians. *Preventive Medicine* 14(2):165–168.

Hernán, M. A., and J. M. Robins. 2008. Authors' response, part I: Observational studies analyzed like randomized experiments: Best of both worlds. *Epidemiology* 19(6):789–792.

Hernán, M. A., A. Alonso, R. Logan, F. Grodstein, K. B. Michels, W. C. Willett, J. E. Manson, and J. M. Robins. 2008. Observational studies analyzed like randomized experiments: An application to postmenopausal hormone therapy and coronary heart disease. *Epidemiology* 19(6):766–779.

Herrington, D. M., D. M. Reboussin, K. B. Brosnihan, P. C. Sharp, S. A. Shumaker, T. E. Snyder, C. D. Furberg, G. J. Kowalchuk, T. D. Stuckey, W. J. Rogers, D. H. Givens, and D. Waters. 2000. Effects of estrogen replacement on the progression of coronary-artery atherosclerosis. *New England Journal of Medicine* 343(8):522–529.

Hersh, A. L., M. L. Stefanick, and R. S. Stafford. 2004. National use of postmenopausal hormone therapy: Annual trends and response to recent evidence. *Journal of the American Medical Association* 291(1):47–53.

HHS (US Department of Health and Human Services). 2004. *NHLBI Advisory for Physicians on the WHI Trial of Conjugated Equine Estrogens Versus Placebo.* http://www.nhlbi.nih.gov/whi/e-a_advisory.htm (accessed April 12, 2010).

———. 2009. *Monitoring Adherence to the NIH Policy on the Inclusion of Women and Minorities as Subjects in Clinical Research.*

———. 2010. *Women's Health Initiative.* http://orwh.od.nih.gov/inclusion/FinalAnnualReport2007.pdf (accessed May 6, 2010).

Hoover, R. N. 2008. The sound and the fury: Was it all worth it? *Epidemiology* 19(6):780–782; discussion 789–793.

Hulley, S., D. Grady, T. Bush, C. Furberg, D. Herrington, B. Riggs, and E. Vittinghoff. 1998. Randomized trial of estrogen plus progestin for secondary prevention of coronary heart disease in postmenopausal women. Heart and Estrogen/progestin Replacement Study (HERS) Research Group. *Journal of the American Medical Association* 280(7):605–613.

IOM (Institute of Medicine). 1993. *An Assessment of the NIH Women's Health Initiative.* Washington, DC: National Academy Press.

Jagsi, R., A. R. Motomura, S. Amarnath, A. Jankovic, N. Sheets, and P. A. Ubel. 2009. Underrepresentation of women in high-impact published clinical cancer research. *Cancer* 115(14): 3293–3301.

Kakazu, K. K., L. W. Cheung, and W. Lynne. 2004. The cancer biomedical informatics grid (caBIG): Pioneering an expansive network of information and tools for collaborative cancer research. *Hawaii Medical Journal* 63(9):273–275.

Kim, E. S., and V. Menon. 2009. Status of women in cardiovascular clinical trials. *Arteriosclerosis, Thrombosis, and Vascular Biology* 29(3):279–283.

LaRosa, J. C., J. He, and S. Vupputuri. 1999. Effect of statins on risk of coronary disease: A meta-analysis of randomized controlled trials. *Journal of the American Medical Association* 282(24):2340–2346.

Limacher, M. C. 2003. Recruitment and retention: Lessons learned from the Women's Health Initiative. In *Science Meets Reality: Recruitment and Retention of Women in Clinical Studies, and the Critical Role of Relevance. A Report of the Task Force Sponsored by the NIH Office of Women's Health,* edited by HHS. Washington, DC.

Lloyd-Jones, D., R. Adams, M. Carnethon, G. De Simone, T. B. Ferguson, K. Flegal, E. Ford, K. Furie, A. Go, K. Greenlund, N. Haase, S. Hailpern, M. Ho, V. Howard, B. Kissela, S. Kittner, D. Lackland, L. Lisabeth, A. Marelli, M. McDermott, J. Meigs, D. Mozaffarian, G. Nichol, C. O'Donnell, V. Roger, W. Rosamond, R. Sacco, P. Sorlie, R. Stafford, J. Steinberger, T. Thom, S. Wasserthiel-Smoller, N. Wong, J. Wylie-Rosett, and Y. Hong. 2009. Heart disease and stroke statistics—2009 update: A report from the American Heart Association Statistics Committee and Stroke Statistics Subcommittee. *Circulation* 119(3):480–486.

Lloyd-Jones, D. M., C. J. O'Donnell, R. B. D'Agostino, J. Massaro, H. Silbershatz, and P. W. F. Wilson. 2001. Applicability of cholesterol-lowering primary prevention trials to a general population: The Framingham Heart Study. *Archives of Internal Medicine* 161(7):949–954.

Mascitelli, L., and F. Pezzetta. 2007. Statins for primary prevention of coronary artery disease. *Lancet* 369(9567):1078–1079; author reply 1079.

McKinley, E. D., J. W. Thompson, J. Briefer-French, L. S. Wilcox, C. S. Weisman, and W. C. Andrews. 2002. Performance indicators in women's health: Incorporating women's health in the health plan employer data and information set (HEDIS). *Women's Health Issues* 12(1):46–58.

McPherson, R., and N. Kavaslar. 2007. Statins for primary prevention of coronary artery disease. *Lancet* 369(9567):1078; author reply 1079.

Merkatz, R. B., and S. W. Junod. 1994. Historical background of changes in FDA policy on the study and evaluation of drugs in women. *Academic Medicine* 69(9):703–707.

Murphy, S. N., M. E. Mendis, D. A. Berkowitz, I. Kohane, and H. C. Chueh. 2006. Integration of clinical and genetic data in the i2b2 architecture. *AMIA Annual Symposium Proceedings*:1040.

NCQA (National Committee for Quality Assurance). 2010. *HEDIS 2010 Measures.* http://www.ncqa.org/tabid/59/Default.aspx (accessed March 23, 2010).

NHS (Nurse's Health Study). 2008. *History of the Nurse's Health Study.* http://www.channing.harvard.edu/nhs/index.php/history/ (accessed March 9, 2010).

Pardo, M., M. Ruiz, A. Gimeno, L. Navarro, A. Garcia, M. Tarazona, and M. Aznar. 2002. *Gender Bias in Clinical Trials of AIDS Drugs.* Paper read at International Conference on AIDS, July 7–12, 2002; Barcelona, Spain.

Pedone, C., and K. Lapane. 2003. Generalizability of guidelines and physicians' adherence. Case study on the Sixth Joint National Committee's Guidelines on Hypertension. *BMC Public Health* 3(1):24.

Pinnow, E., P. Sharma, A. Parekh, N. Gevorkian, and K. Uhl. 2009. Increasing participation of women in early phase clinical trials approved by the FDA. *Women's Health Issues* 19(2):89–93.

Platt, R., M. Wilson, K. A. Chan, J. S. Benner, J. Marchibroda, and M. McClellan. 2009. The new sentinel network—improving the evidence of medical-product safety. *New England Journal of Medicine* 361(7):645–647.

Prentice, R. L. 2008. Data analysis methods and the reliability of analytic epidemiologic research. *Epidemiology* 19(6):785–788; discussion 789–793.

Resnick, S. M., P. M. Maki, S. R. Rapp, M. A. Espeland, R. Brunner, L. H. Coker, I. A. Granek, P. Hogan, J. K. Ockene, and S. A. Shumaker. 2006. Effects of combination estrogen plus progestin hormone treatment on cognition and affect. *Journal of Clinical Endocrinology and Metabolism* 91(5):1802–1810.

Resnick, S. M., M. A. Espeland, Y. An, P. M. Maki, L. H. Coker, R. Jackson, M. L. Stefanick, R. Wallace, and S. R. Rapp. 2009. Effects of conjugated equine estrogens on cognition and affect in postmenopausal women with prior hysterectomy. *Journal of Clinical Endocrinology and Metabolism* 94(11):4152–4161.

Ridker, P. M. 2010. Statin therapy for low-LDL, high-hsCRP patients: From JUPITER to CORONA. *Clinical Chemistry* 56(4):505–507.

Ridker, P. M., N. R. Cook, I. M. Lee, D. Gordon, J. M. Gaziano, J. E. Manson, C. H. Hennekens, and J. E. Buring. 2005. A randomized trial of low-dose aspirin in the primary prevention of cardiovascular disease in women. *New England Journal of Medicine* 352(13):1293–1304.

Rieker, P. P., and C. E. Bird. 2005. Rethinking gender differences in health: Why we need to integrate social and biological perspectives. *Journals of Gerontology. Series B, Psychological Sciences and Series B, Psychological Sciences and Social Sciences* 60(Special Issue 2):S40–S47.

Rosenbaum, P. R. 2002. *Observational Studies.* 2nd ed. New York: Springer-Verlag.

Samsa, G., G. Hu, and M. Root. 2005. Combining information from multiple data sources to create multivariable risk models: Illustration and preliminary assessment of a new method. *Journal of Biomedicine and Biotechnology* 2005(2):113–123.

Sharpe, N. 2002. Clinical trials and the real world: Selection bias and generalisability of trial results. *Cardiovascular Drugs and Therapy* 16(1):75–77.

Sheifer, S. E., T. A. Manolio, and B. J. Gersh. 2001. Unrecognized myocardial infarction. *Annals of Internal Medicine* 135(9):801–811.

Shepherd, J., S. M. Cobbe, I. Ford, C. G. Isles, A. R. Lorimer, P. W. MacFarlane, J. H. McKillop, and C. J. Packard. 1995. Prevention of coronary heart disease with pravastatin in men with hypercholesterolemia. West of Scotland Coronary Prevention Study Group. *New England Journal of Medicine* 333(20):1301–1307.

Stampfer, M. J. 2008. ITT for observational data: Worst of both worlds? *Epidemiology* 19(6):783–784; discussion 789–793.

Stampfer, M. J., and G. A. Colditz. 1991. Estrogen replacement therapy and coronary heart disease: A quantitative assessment of the epidemiologic evidence. *Preventive Medicine* 20(1):47–63.

Stampfer, M. J., G. A. Colditz, W. C. Willett, J. E. Manson, B. Rosner, F. E. Speizer, and C. H. Hennekens. 1991. Postmenopausal estrogen therapy and cardiovascular disease. Ten-year follow-up from the Nurses' Health Study. *New England Journal of Medicine* 325(11):756–762.

Stewart, J. H., A. G. Bertoni, J. L. Staten, E. A. Levine, and C. P. Gross. 2007. Participation in surgical oncology clinical trials: Gender-, race/ethnicity-, and age-based disparities. *Annals of Surgical Oncology* 14(12):3328–3334.

SWAN (Study of Women's Health Across the Nation). 2010. *Swan History.* http://www.swanstudy.org/history.asp (accessed April 9, 2010).

Tannen, R. L., M. G. Weiner, D. Xie, and K. Barnhart. 2007. Estrogen affects post-menopausal women differently than estrogen plus progestin replacement therapy. *Human Reproduction* 22(6):1769–1777.

Towfighi, A., J. L. Saver, R. Engelhardt, and B. Ovbiagele. 2007. A midlife stroke surge among women in the United States. *Neurology* 69(20):1898–1904.

Weisman, C. S. 2000. Advocating for gender-specific health care: A historical perspective. *Journal of Gender-Specific Medicine* 3(3):22–24.

WHI (Women's Health Initiative). 2010. *About Women's Health Initiative.* http://whi.org/about/ (accessed April 8, 2010).

WHS (Women's Health Study). 2009. *Women's Health Study (WHS): A Randomized Trial of Low-dose Aspirin and Vitamin E in the Primary Prevention of Cardiovascular Disease and Cancer.* http://clinicaltrials.gov/ct/show/NCT00000479 (accessed April 9, 2010).

Wilcox, A., and S. Wacholder. 2008. Observational data and clinical trials: Narrowing the gap? *Epidemiology* 19(6):765.

Willet, W. C., J. E. Manson, and F. Grodstein. 2008. Author's response, part II. *Epidemiology* 19(6):793.

Wilson, P. W., R. J. Garrison, and W. P. Castelli. 1985. Postmenopausal estrogen use, cigarette smoking, and cardiovascular morbidity in women over 50. The Framingham Study. *New England Journal of Medicine* 313(17):1038–1043.

5

Transforming Discovery to Impact: Translation and Communication of Findings of Women's Health Research

The previous chapters document substantial progress in research on women's health. This chapter examines first the factors that shape translation of research findings on women's health into use by health-care providers and public-health practitioners and, second, how those factors shape communication of research findings to women. The chapter closes with case studies of the Women's Health Initiative (WHI), breast and cervical cancer and cardiovascular disease (CVD) to illustrate successes of—or obstacles to—translation into improvements in women's health and communication of research findings to women. The information in this chapter addresses questions 5 and 6 in Box 1-4, which deal with whether research findings are being translated in a way that affects practice and whether they are being communicated effectively to women.

Many of the barriers to the translation and communication of research findings are similar between women's and men's health. Those barriers have been reviewed in other Institute of Medicine (IOM) reports (2001a,b, 2002a, 2006a,b), and their analysis is beyond the scope of this report. In this chapter, the committee highlights the issues that it considered especially relevant to women's health.

TRANSLATION OF FINDINGS INTO PRACTICE

The steps in translation, communication, and application of research findings into practice and policies that lead to health improvements are complex. Each step involves different and sometimes competing factions—patients, providers, payers, purchasers, and manufacturers—and multiple processes. There are questions regarding who should transmit research information (investigators, government, industry, or the press), what the message should be (complex information or basic elements), how the message should be framed (regarding an individual or a population), how the information should be transmitted (in scientific publications or by professional organizations, medical practitioners, or the mass media), who the target audience of the message is (health-care providers, women, or both), who uses the information, and, ultimately, what the individual woman, does with the information (Bero et al., 1998; Berwick, 2003; IOM, 2001a; Kreuter and Wray, 2003; Rogers, 1995).

The steps in translating research discoveries into practice are outlined in Figure 5-1. The initial step generally occurs with the publication of results in peer-reviewed scientific journals. For some topics, the news media may immediately report the findings, as in the coverage of the WHI. If research findings will affect clinical practice, professional societies may develop clinical-practice guidelines. At each step, constraints associated with current practices limit the translation of findings into improved services. In cases where there are uncertainties or contradictory research findings, guidelines from different organizations can differ or updated guidelines might reflect recent data and contradict previous guidelines, leading to confusion. For example, if research findings are not analyzed or presented separately for women and men, this might decrease their utility in addressing women's needs, including the development of women-specific

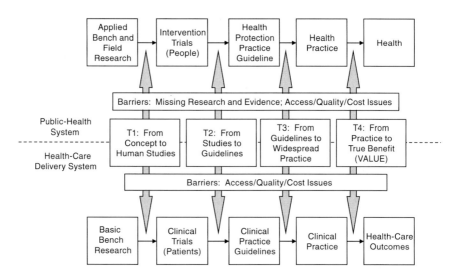

FIGURE 5-1 The process for translating research into practice. The top half of figure shows the path for a public-health system. The bottom half shows the path for health-care delivery systems.
SOURCE: Modified from a presentation by Dr. Julie Gerberding to the House Committee on Appropriations, Subcommittee on Labor, Health and Human Services, Education and Related Agencies, March 5, 2008.

guidelines. Although there are exceptions, such as the women-specific guidelines for CVD issued by the American Heart Association (AHA) (Mosca et al., 2004a), most practice guidelines are not sex specific.

Government agencies and professional organizations play an important role in the translation of research findings into policy and practice. For example, in light of findings from the Breast Cancer Prevention Trial showing that tamoxifen reduced the incidence of invasive breast cancer in women at high risk for the disease (Cuzick et al., 2003; Fisher et al., 1998; Lewis, 2007; Mamounas et al., 2005; Powles et al., 1998; Veronesi et al., 1998, 2007), the Food and Drug Administration (FDA) required modification of the language on the label for tamoxifen (FDA, 1998). Government agencies and professional organizations have also developed campaigns to disseminate research findings to both health-care providers and women. For example, the National Heart Lung and Blood Institute, the Department of Health and Human Services (HHS) Office on Women's Health (OWH), and AHA collaborated to develop the Heart Truth campaign to increase women's awareness of their risks of heart disease (HHS, 2010). The campaign has contributed to an increase in awareness compared with that in 1997 (Christian et al., 2007; Mosca et al., 2010).

Barriers Associated with the Nature of Science

Clinically useful findings are almost never generated by a single study but require a multitude of studies of types—basic, clinical, and applied—and require the overall evidence to lay the foundation for a given clinical action. Along the way, different studies may produce dissimilar results. Beyond the uncertainty due to inconsistent findings, uncertainties about the applicability of findings and about inadequate data on the effects of treatments in women can occur when data are not analyzed and reported by sex. Failure to report sex-specific findings has resulted in delays in standard-of-care treatment for women, such as the use of stents, beta blockers, and aspirin for myocardial infarction (Berger et al., 2009; Chauhan et al., 2005; Lansky et al., 2005; Rich-Edwards et al., 1995).

Paradoxically, there are also examples of rapid adoption of unproven interventions, such as transplantation of autologous bone marrow for advanced breast cancer, which was later shown by research not to provide benefit but to increase risk (Farquhar et al., 2003; Rettig et al., 2007). An objective research base with sex-specific information is critical both for the adoption of new approaches and to stop practices that are not beneficial and may actually be harmful.

Barriers Associated with Economic, Social, and Cultural Factors

Economic forces and other nonscientific factors may complicate the interpretation of scientific data and their translation into practice. Conflicts of interest can occur in the conduct of science and the publication of scientific information

(Jagsi et al., 2009; Lexchin and Light, 2006), including findings related to drugs used primarily or exclusively by women. The role of industry in funding research, interpreting results, writing papers, and presenting findings directly to providers and industry's relationships with patient-advocacy organizations can introduce bias (Burton and Rowell, 2003; Herxheimer, 2003; Koch, 2003; Moynihan, 2003; Watkins et al., 2003).

Social and cultural values may also complicate the translation of research into practice. That is most clearly seen in relation to sexual and reproductive health. For example, the adoption of the human papillomavirus (HPV) vaccine, which could prevent the vast majority of cervical cancers, has been slowed, in addition to concerns of parents about safety,[1] because of a number of nonscientific issues. An editorial in the *New England Journal of Medicine* looking at the HPV vaccine highlighted the issues of access to the vaccine, high cost, and concerns focused on purported interference in family life and sexual mores (Charo, 2007). It identified a variety of political efforts to forestall the creation of a mandated vaccination program, which was attacked as an intrusion on parental discretion and an invitation to teenage promiscuity. Other identified barriers to vaccination include misinformation, lack of knowledge, substandard provider–patient communication, parental concerns about the sexual implications of HPV vaccination, and concerns about the manufacturers' influence (Charo, 2007).

The case of the HPV vaccine also demonstrates disparities in the translation of knowledge into health-care services for less-advantaged groups. Specific populations of women—such as those of lower socioeconomic status (SES), those who have low literacy level, illegal immigrants, and those who have language barriers—are likely to be more affected by social barriers or by a lack of knowledge about HPV and the vaccine. For example, the 2007 California Health Interview Survey indicates that 90% of non-Hispanic white women 18–50 years old had heard of HPV, compared with 69% of Latinas (California Health Interview Survey, 2010). Vaccination rates are also lower in Latinas (14.0 %) than in white girls (19.7%) 12–26 years old; the largest discrepancy is in those 19–26 years old: Latinas, 6.7%, and non-Hispanic white women, 14.3% (California Health Interview Survey, 2010). Some studies have examined attitudes toward the HPV vaccine among Latinas, but methodologic shortcomings limit the utility of their results, and the factors that contribute to Latina underuse of the HPV vaccine remain unknown.

Although new knowledge generally benefits the more advantaged to a greater extent, more advantaged women may also be more likely to receive new treatments that have not been thoroughly tested and can have adverse effects that are

---

[1] FDA and Centers for Disease Control and Prevention published postmarketing surveillance data from the Vaccine Adverse Event Reporting System. With the exception of synecope and venous thromboembolic events, no increase in adverse events was seen as compared to other vaccinations (Slade et al., 2009).

discovered only after additional study. Use of hormone therapy is a case in point. Hormone therapy was prescribed more frequently to more affluent, educated women; those women were then at greater risk of developing breast cancer. A recent analysis of the decline in breast-cancer mortality seen after the publication of the WHI findings, which studies have attributed to the decreased use of hormone therapy (Chlebowski et al., 2009; Hausauer et al., 2009; Jemal et al., 2007; Krieger et al., 2010), showed that the greatest decreases in mortality occurred among white women over 50 years old who had estrogen-receptor–positive tumors and lived in counties that had higher mean incomes (Hausauer et al., 2009; Krieger et al., 2010). Smaller decreases were seen in women in other racial or ethnic groups and in poorer areas who were less likely to have been using hormone therapy in the first place (Hausauer et al., 2009; Krieger et al., 2010).

Barriers Associated with Health-Care Providers

The existence and characteristics of substantial problems in our health-care system have been the topic of a multitude of studies and IOM reports (IOM, 2000, 2002b, 2006a, 2009). The problems are not specific to women but constitute a serious barrier to the efficient and effective uptake of information to improve the treatment of women. US adults receive only about half the recommended care, and its quality varies significantly by medical condition. Fragmentation of health care also hinders translation and may be particularly problematic for women. Many women receive their primary care from obstetricians and gynecologists, and others are seen also by other primary-care providers (Bean-Mayberry et al., 2007a). In addition, given the higher rates of comorbidities and late-life illnesses in women than in men (Marcus et al., 2005), women's health issues often encompass a broader array of conditions and comorbidities—such as mental health disorders, bone disorders, CVD, cancers, autoimmune disorders, and violence—in addition to reproductive issues. To have those health needs met, women must see multiple providers, who are often in different places and who do not communicate with one another about the care they are providing. In the current health-care system, it is difficult for women to receive comprehensive evidence-based care in one place.

The HHS OWH funded National Centers of Excellence in Women's Health to address the issue and change the care model for women. The centers were established to provide a comprehensive model of health-care delivery for women and to encourage community outreach, stimulate research in women's health, incorporate research findings into women's health in the clinic and medical-school curriculum, and the provision of leadership positions for women in academic medicine (Goodman et al., 2002). Funding for the centers ceased, however, and without outside support there is a risk that they will not be maintained by academic medical centers (Goodman et al., 2002). Although the Department of Veteran Affairs has established similar centers for women's health (Bean-

Mayberry et al., 2007b), such a model is not widely adopted in other settings. That is especially disappointing in light of the evidence from a survey that women who used the centers of excellence were more satisfied with their health care than comparison populations and that the centers were particularly successful in mammography and breast self-examination and in counseling services related to many of the important determinants of health discussed in Chapter 2, including smoking and violence against women (Goodman et al., 2002).

Barriers in the Health Systems and Health Plans

Health systems and health plans can play an important role in translating evidence-based practices and research advances into clinical practice through the use of public reporting mechanisms and payment incentives. A key example is the Healthcare Effectiveness Data and Information Set (HEDIS), a set of publicly reported health-plan performance measures maintained by the National Committee for Quality Assurance. The measures are routinely collected by managed-care plans through a review of administrative claims data, provider chart abstraction, and member surveys to gauge plan quality, preventive-care services, prenatal care, acute-disease and chronic-disease management, and satisfaction with health plans and doctors (NCQA, 2010). The data are used by some commercial plans and by Medicaid and Medicare managed-care organizations, and plans are evaluated and accredited on the basis of their performance on HEDIS measures. Therefore, there are strong incentives for providers in health plans or networks to meet the standards of care. Although the HEDIS measures have been expanded in recent years to capture conditions that are specific to women more fully, many measures for conditions specific to women are still not included. Furthermore, sex-, race- and ethnicity-specific analysis is rarely conducted on HEDIS measures to investigate possible sex-based differences in care or differential care patterns by race and ethnicity (Bird et al., 2007; McKinley et al., 2002; Weisman, 2000). No comparable, reportable, and uniform data source exists for patients in fee-for-service arrangements, so less is known about the quality of care of women who use those services than about the care of women in managed care (McGlynn et al., 1999).

Reimbursement by government and private insurers influences the provision of services and may determine whether research findings are adopted in clinical practice (Trivedi et al., 2008). For example, although research findings supported the value of breast and cervical cancer screening, many women were not being routinely screened until the Centers for Disease Control and Prevention–funded National Breast and Cervical Cancer Early Detection Program expanded coverage to low-income uninsured women (Henson et al., 1996). In recent years, there has been increased interest in basing reimbursement on practices that have been demonstrated to be effective. Reimbursement decisions might require additional studies of the safety and effectiveness of new treatments, such as comparative-effectiveness studies. Those studies would be more informative if they provided sex-specific analyses of the effectiveness of treatments.

Barriers in Patient Decision Making

Given the fragmentation of care described above, patients often have to coordinate their own care. Those who are seriously ill often have to make a cascade of decisions about their treatment, and even those who are well and who wish to maintain their health and optimize wellness have an array of possibilities. The increased research on women's health has led to more knowledge about women's health, which has translated into heightened awareness of conditions that affect women, the availability of more treatments for some conditions, more information on an expanded number of outcomes of given treatments, the ability to detect potential diseases at earlier stages, and a proliferation of clinical guidelines. Those developments represent progress, but the increase in information and alternatives can overwhelm women who are making decisions.

Most decisions made by patients and providers alike involve weighing options that have uncertain probabilities and anticipating how they will affect overall health and quality of life. Some studies help to clarify the probabilities or value of outcomes, but more often than not new research expands available options that have uncertain outcomes (O'Connor et al., 1999). Studies of decision making have shown that, counter intuitively, some people making choices who are given more options make poorer choices on the average and are less satisfied with their decisions than those who are given fewer options (Schwartz et al., 2002). Expanding options (whether for screening, diagnosis, or treatment) is generally advantageous, especially if these offer different mixes of costs and benefits. However, increasing the number of alternatives also increases uncertainty in decision making and can pose profound challenges for patients and providers. For example, the use of more sensitive tests for cervical cancer lowers the threshold for detecting cervical cancer, decreases specificity, and increases uncertainty about the likelihood of future disease and the benefits of intervention. In other words, a more sensitive test will detect abnormalities in the cervix that are less likely to develop into cervical cancer than are more advanced lesions. A positive test provides a woman and her physician with less information about the risk posed by the lesion than if the lesion had been detected at a more advanced stage (Sundar et al., 2005). The problems posed by uncertainty and multiple options should not preclude developing or offering alternatives or encourage limiting choice. Rather, awareness of the difficulties should foster more research on how best to present complex choices and highlight the need for clear explanations and decision aids for such decisions.

The increased knowledge about multiple end points that might be affected by a treatment decision (that is, if a treatment for one disease might not only decrease the risk of adverse consequences from that disease but also increase the risk of other diseases) introduces additional challenges, including questions as to which end points are most important; how to weigh multiple end points, which might vary in severity, timing, and likelihood; and how to assess composite impact. For example, the WHI reported on dozens of outcomes. There are attempts to report on composite end points (such as the WHI "global index" and a similar index for tamoxifen), but there is no consensus on components of these indexes or their internal weighting (Sundar et al., 2005).

Advances in decision-making science over the last 2 decades provide greater understanding of the barriers to optimal decision making by both providers and patients. Patient preference is playing a larger role in treatment decisions through shared clinical decision making (O'Connor et al., 2007). Decision aids can facilitate communication between patients and providers concerning specific clinical decisions, make information about options and outcomes available, and clarify personal values (O'Connor et al., 1999). Decision aids are particularly helpful when there is no clear right or wrong decision and the evidence supporting different treatment options suggests equipoise. Such aids have proved to be effective, for example, in relation to decisions regarding treatments for breast cancer. In one study, Sepucha and colleagues (2002) randomized breast-cancer patients to an intervention that helped them to prepare for a consultation visit or to usual care. Patients who received consultation planning were more satisfied with their consultation, as were the physicians who treated women in the intervention group. Later studies have shown that those tools not only increase satisfaction but enhance communication and improve decision quality and that such practices can be institutionalized into clinical care, not only in the academic medical setting in which they were developed but in practices that serve rural women (Belkora et al., 2009; Franklin et al., 2009). More sophisticated computerized risk models that can account for many conditions that affect women (such as breast cancer, cervical cancer, and osteoporosis) have been developed and can be used as decision-making tools.

Developments Aimed at Speeding Translation

In women's health, as in all elements of health, there is a large gap between research discoveries and their implementation into practices that result in better outcomes. Increased investment in health research in recent times has resulted in an explosion of discoveries. However, the serendipitous nature of translation and the barriers to the adoption of new discoveries are reflected in the 15–20 years that it typically takes for discoveries to be adopted into clinical practice (Bansal and Barnes, 2008). Several developments are working to speed the process.

One is the emphasis in the National Institutes of Health (NIH) on translational research. Policy makers, administrators, and scientists are increasingly considering how to translate basic-science discoveries at the molecular and animal levels into human-health applications at the clinical and population levels more rapidly. NIH has funded Clinical and Translational Science Awards to medical research institutions to support consortia whose goal is to develop the infrastructure needed to speed translation of research from bench to treatment, from treatment to provider practice, and from provider practice to improved population health (NIH, 2010).

A second development is the emergence of the health-consumer advocacy movement, which has sought a more active role for laypersons in their own health care (Keefe et al., 2006). A number of advocacy groups are devoted to women's health and have pushed for increased research and increased translation of research findings into practice, including groups advocating for research, treatment, and policy changes related to breast cancer and to heart disease in women (Kolker, 2004; Lerner, 2002). For example, the National Breast Cancer Coalition (NBCC) had as one of its main goals "increasing access to screening and treatment for all women." The NBCC has been credited with ensuring congressional funding for the National Breast and Cervical Cancer Early Detection Program and the Breast and Cervical Cancer Prevention and Treatment Act of 2000, which provide funding, respectively, for breast- and cervical-cancer screening and for treatment for women who cannot afford to pay (Lerner, 2002). The NBCC is one of many groups that have contributed to an improvement in women's health, either through the women's health movement in general or through organizations related to specific conditions (Allsop et al., 2004; Keefe et al., 2006; Kolker, 2004).

Third, the movement toward evidence-based practice is creating demand for a more rigorous evaluation of new treatments. Research findings are necessary for evidence-based medicine that can be used to speed the adoption of effective and safe interventions while avoiding interventions that are less effective, ineffective, harmful, or more expensive (IOM, 2008). Pressures for evidence-based medicine arose, in part, from women's experiences with drugs whose adverse health effects and efficacy were supported by inadequate data. Two examples are diethylstilbestrol, which resulted in a rare form of vaginal cancer in the female offspring of women who used it while pregnant (Herbst and Anderson, 1990), and the WHI, which demonstrated that hormone therapy, which without proper trials had been in widespread use to reduce cardiovascular risk in women, was not effective in reducing cardiovascular risk and, in fact, increased the risk of breast cancer in women (Writing Group for the Women's Health Initiative Investigators, 2002).

COMMUNICATION

Women are not passive recipients of care, but active participants in decision making (Braddock et al., 1997). To be effective in that role, however, women need access to clear and accurate information. That need highlights the importance of communicating scientific findings, which can often be complex, in simple, accurate, understandable, and actionable messages. Although a substantial literature provides information on the process of communication itself and on identifying strategies that are effective in the diffusion and adoption of new information and approaches (Rogers, 2003), the findings are not explicitly developed in relation to the communication of research findings to women.

Women's access to research findings and their capacity to use them to improve their health depend on a number of factors, including their SES, race, and ethnicity. Greater uptake of new information by those who have more advantages works to increase disparities when new data are available (Donohue et al., 1975; Viswanath and Finnegan, 1996).

Even when research results are delivered by reliable and objective sources, problems can emerge in communicating them. Some of the problems are derived from the complexity of results, which may generate confusion. An example is the recent statement released by the US Preventive Services Task Force on mammography screening. It reviewed extensive data on the appropriateness of mammography screening for women and on the balance between lives saved through early detection and adverse effects of false-positive results as these varied by age (discussed in case study below) (Nelson et al., 2009). One of the task force's recommendations for women aged 40–49 was that "the decision to start regular, biennial screening mammography before the age of 50 years should be an individual one and take patient context into account, including the patient's values regarding specific benefits and harms" (US Preventive Services Task Force, 2009). The main message received by the public, however, was that women aged 40–49 years should not routinely screen for breast cancer. Another example of the difficulty of disseminating research information, also discussed below, is the WHI, in which messages were communicated rapidly to women in the study but only later to physicians; there was thus a lag in the movement of complete information to clinicians who were receiving questions from and giving advice to female patients before they had it (Bush et al., 2007).

The Internet has added a powerful new dynamic to communicating information (Viswanath and Finnegan, 1996). About four-fifths of American adults use the Internet in their homes, offices, schools, or other locations (Harris Interactive, 2008a), and the population of Internet users increasingly looks like the population of the United States. Initially dominated by men, the population of Internet users is today equally divided between men and women. The Internet has become a common source of health information for people in general and for women in particular. Over 80% of Internet users said that they had looked on line for health information (Harris Interactive, 2008b). The Internet was the third-most frequent (46%) source of information that respondents reported turning to when facing a health problem, behind professionals (83%) and family and friends (51%) (Estabrook et al., 2007). Fewer people turned to print sources of health information (37%), television or radio (16%), government agencies (15%), and libraries (10%) (Estabrook et al., 2007).

Women have consistently engaged in more health-related online activities than men (Tu and Cohen, 2008). A 2006 survey found that 54% of health-information seekers were women, whether they were acting as consumers, caregivers, or "e-patients" (Internet users who seek online health information that is of particular interest to them). The top health topics on which women sought information were specific diseases or medical problems (69%); medical treatments (54%); diet, nutrition, and vitamins (53%); exercise or fitness (46%); and prescription or over-the-counter drugs (39%). Women reported significantly more interest in online information than men about specific diseases, particular treatments, diet, and mental health (Fox, 2006). Another study found that women are more likely than men to look online for support groups to communicate about health conditions (Fallows, 2005).

There is evidence that Internet users, including women, find online health information to be helpful and use it to make decisions about their health. In one survey of e-patients, 31% said that they or someone they knew had been substantially helped by following medical advice or health information found on the Internet, whereas only 3% said that they or someone they knew had been seriously harmed by following advice found online (Fox, 2006). Women who have breast cancer use the Internet to access information about their condition, share experiences, and obtain support (Fogel et al., 2002; Klemm et al., 1998; Sharf, 1997).

As discussed earlier, however, more information is not necessarily better from the health consumer's standpoint. Evidence is emerging that confusion about cancer in general may be having an adverse effect on the American public. In a cross-sectional analysis, Arora and colleagues (2008) found that of the 45% of American adults who had searched for cancer information on the Web, nearly three-fifths expressed concerns about the quality of information, nearly half reported negative experiences when searching for cancer information, and about two-fifths reported frustration in their searching. Compared with those who had a better experience, those experiencing such frustration were more likely to agree that "everything causes cancer," that there are few actions a person can take to prevent cancer, and that it is hard to know what prevention recommendations to follow. Importantly those who had no more than a high-school education were more likely to report having an adverse experience and the other effects mentioned. As the Internet continues to transform how people receive health information and interact with their health-care providers, work is needed to address those concerns and frustrations.

CASE STUDIES IN TRANSLATION AND COMMUNICATION

The Women's Health Initiative

Hormone therapy has been studied, prescribed, debated, hailed, and criticized for more than 70 years (Rymer et al., 2003). From the middle 1960s to 2002, hormone therapy for postmenopausal women (then called hormone-replacement therapy) was commonly prescribed not only for menopause symptoms but because of presumed health benefits, including prevention of chronic disease (Garbe and Suissa, 2004; Rymer et al., 2003). The WHI was designed as a primary prevention study that was, by many, anticipated to demonstrate the preventive effects of hormone therapy for postmenopausal women against CVD. For example, the design of the WHI was reviewed and critiqued by an IOM committee during the early phases of the study (IOM, 1993). One criticism made by the IOM committee was that the informed consent and "stopping rules" for the study were not explicit enough, with the major concern being that "[t]he emergence of new information that may require closing a branch of the [clinical trial] is not unlikely over the next nine years. One branch is at special risk: the near-term effects of hormones on reducing cardiovascular risk factors and event rates may be confirmed early in this project." In July, 2002, when the WHI (see Appendix C for description) stopped its clinical trial of conjugated equine estrogen plus progestin (Prempro™) early (HHS, 2002a), many women's and physicians' opinions and perspectives of hormone therapy changed (Bush et al., 2007). The WHI results demonstrated that rather than reducing the risk of CVD, estrogen plus progestin therapy could increase the risk of CVD and the risk of breast and ovarian cancer (Schonberg et al., 2005). Once it was determined that the treatment could cause harm, the clinical trial was immediately canceled on the advice of a data and safety monitoring board (DSMB) after a mean of 5.2 years of study (HHS, 2002a).[2] The DSMB determined that the increased risk of breast cancer and CVD (stroke and venous thromboembolic disease)—consistent with the results of the previous Heart Estrogen/Progestin Study—outweighed the benefit of lower risk of colorectal cancer and hip and osteoporotic fractures (Prentice and Anderson, 2008). In March of 2004 NIH informed participants of the estrogen-only hormone-therapy trial portion of WHI to stop taking the medication because of what it considered an unacceptable risk of stroke (HHS, 2004).

A search of Pubmed.gov for articles with "Women's Health Initiative" in "All Fields" *OR* "hormone replacement therapy" as a MeSH term, limited to publication dates between July 9, 2002, and July 9, 2003,[3] retrieved over 1,500 publications. Within a month of the announcement, 215 articles on the WHI findings were published in popular media (McIntosh and Blalock, 2005), and a study of local, regional, and national newspapers showed an 8-fold increase in the number of articles about hormone therapy the month after the stopping of the trial compared with periods before the announcement (Haas et al., 2006). A large number of women stopped hormone therapy almost immediately (Barber et al., 2004; Schonberg et al., 2005; Theroux, 2008). Filled prescriptions for hormone therapy dropped by 29%; and new prescriptions in 2003 and 2004 were 73% and

---

[2]The dietary modification study—increases in calcium and vitamin D intake—and the observational study continued to their planned conclusions.

[3]The year after the notice from NIH stopping the clinical trial of conjugated equine estrogen plus progestin (HHS, 2002a).

77% lower, respectively, than in 2001, and they were for different formulations from those in the WHI (Wegienka et al., 2006).

The response from physicians was uneven. A 2004 survey of a multi-disciplinary group of health-care providers determined that 67% of the time respondents overestimated risks when hormone therapy increased risks and overestimated benefits when hormone therapy increased benefits (Williams et al., 2005). A study conducted in 2003 found that nearly half the physicians surveyed did not find the WHI results convincing enough to stop the clinical trial (Power et al., 2008). Physicians who had completed their residency more recently rated evidence from randomized clinical trials as more important, were more inclined to be favorable toward alternative therapies, and were most accepting of the trial results. In contrast, older physicians who had been in practice longer were un-convinced of the need to terminate the trial (Power et al., 2008).

Critiques of the WHI raise criticisms about which results were communicated and how. The stopping of the trial was based on relative risk; relative risk differs from attributable risk, which may not seem significant (Lobo et al., 2006) and which can overstate risk if it reflects "data-mining" (Bluming and Tavris, 2009). Another issue was generalizability. Women in the hormone-therapy study were older and many years past the onset of menopause, so they had other health risks, such as the risk of atherosclerosis, which could have affected study results (Harman et al., 2005; Lobo et al., 2006). Sample selection is an issue in observational studies as well as in clinical trials. In addition to the fact that higher-SES women were more likely to be using hormone therapy, subjects in other hormone-therapy studies may have been affected by "healthy-user bias," in that subjects were healthier, were better educated, had higher incomes, and were inclined to have better compliance than the general population (Harman et al., 2005). Observational studies of healthy users may have led to overestimation of expected benefits of hormone therapy in the WHI, which was a study of a population that was older, more obese, sometimes diabetic, and more often smokers than the women who were using hormone therapy at that time (Harman et al., 2005).

The WHI sample also underrepresented women for whom symptom relief would be a major benefit. Although the primary reason for hormone therapy in menopausal women is to treat for vasomotor symptoms (such as night sweats and hot flashes), the WHI focused on primary prevention of coronary heart disease, cancer, and fractures, and relief of menopausal symptoms was not included as a major end point (Prentice and Anderson, 2008). Women who had severe vasomotor symptoms were excluded from the study, probably to avoid having to randomize some of them to placebo (Lobo et al., 2006).

Women seek health information about hormone therapy from the mass media and health-care professionals. One study indicated that 48% go to health-care providers, 33% to print media, 29% to the Internet, 8% to social networks, and 5% to broadcast media (Breslau et al., 2003). Other reports have said that only 31% go to health-care providers for information on hormone therapy and that the mass media are often primary and trusted sources of new information on hormone therapy (Theroux, 2005). The Internet provides a great deal of information, but it is also a venue for marketing pharmaceutical products, such as hormone therapy.

Some articles in scientific journals and in the popular press have been critical of the WHI and have cast doubt on the validity of its findings. Adding to the confusion about the value of and harm caused by hormone therapy are more recent allegations that pharmaceutical companies that produce hormone-therapy drugs influenced some of the publications that were critical of the study (Singer, 2009). That illustrates how the different goals and interests of science and industry may foster greater controversy and confusion.

The mass media played a large role in the dissemination of the findings of the WHI, which had worldwide ramifications. MacLennan and colleagues (2004) stated on the basis of a survey that most of the 64% of Australian women who stopped taking hormone therapy did so because of published reports. In a survey of Swedish women, "newspaper or magazines" and "television or radio" were the main sources of information for 43.8% and 31.7%, respectively (Hoffmann et al., 2005). In a very small study of 97 US women surveyed, all had heard about the WHI study, and 52% reported changing their use of hormone therapy in response (McIntosh and Blalock, 2005). In a study of women who received a mammogram at a site that is part of the Breast Cancer Surveillance Consortium (327,144 women), "greater average household exposure to newspaper coverage about the results of the [estrogen plus progestion therapy arm of the Women's Health Initiative] (EPT-WHI) was associated with a larger population-based decline in HT use after the publication of the EPT-WHI" (Haas et al., 2007). Among US women who received mammography and were surveyed by Kerlikowske and colleagues (2007), the decline in hormone therapy use was associated with exposure to newspaper coverage of the risks posed by hormone therapy. Taken together, those studies indicate that media coverage of the WHI affected women's decisions regarding continuing that therapy.

After the WHI, women stated confusion and fear in making decisions about hormone therapy. Some women who could have benefited from hormone therapy stopped taking it or refused it for fear of increased risks of other health conditions. Other women who initially ceased hormone therapy began again but often with accompanying worry (French et al., 2006). Women stated that they would like to have their physicians more involved in the decision process (Theroux, 2005). Physicians observed that their patients were confused about hormone therapy and menopausal treatments and that they themselves would like more assistance, perhaps in the form of discussion or decision guides, in counseling patients (Bush et al., 2007; Lobo et al., 2006).

There are important lessons to be learned from the WHI experience. First, the surprising findings from the WHI emphasize the value of generating data through objective research and using them as the basis of decisions in clinical practice. Such treatments as hormone therapy can affect multiple systems; if they are to be used for many years, long-term clinical trials are needed to gain data on their intended use. The data showed that what was then the practice of putting menopausal women on hormone therapy to prevent heart disease did not have this intended effect and in fact was harming them (Chlebowski et al., 2003). Later results confirmed that the health risks posed by long-term use of combination hormone therapy in healthy postmenopausal women persist even a few years after the drugs are stopped and clearly outweigh the benefits. About 3 years after women stopped taking combination hormone therapy, many of the health effects of hormones, such as increased risk of heart disease, were found to be diminished, but the risk of cancer remained elevated (Heiss et al., 2008).

The WHI demonstrated the value of a study design that included a variety of outcomes. Data on multiple end points allow a balancing of disease risks that may be increased, decreased, or unaffected by a given treatment. However, communicating findings that involve balancing benefits in relation to some outcomes and harm in relation to others is challenging. That problem arose in relation to the WHI and in the recent events surrounding guidelines for mammography. In both cases, the large response among women in general is indicative of how engaged women are on topics related to their health.

Cardiovascular Disease

CVD used to be thought of as a male disease, and this meant that less attention was paid to its impact on women. For more than a decade, there have been concerted efforts and calls to action by government agencies and private-sector not-for-profit organizations to reduce the burden of CVD in women through improved awareness, translation of research, and dissemination of information to the public and health-care providers. In 1997, an AHA scientific statement on CVD in women pointed to the growing number of women at risk (Mosca et al., 1997) and suggested that healthy lifestyles for young women should be emphasized, health-care providers should be sensitive to sex differences in CVD, scientists should examine potential sex differences in the pathophysiology of and outcomes related to CVD, research in minority-group women should be expanded, and education should play a pivotal role in communicating and translating scientific developments about women and heart disease. In that year, the AHA launched its national women's heart disease and stroke campaign, highlighting the need for greater awareness of heart disease in women (Mosca et al., 2004b). The Red Dress symbol developed by the National Heart, Lung, and Blood Institute's Heart Truth campaign has become the national icon of the movement toward awareness of heart disease in women (Long et al., 2008).

The first initiative to develop female-specific recommendations to prevent heart disease were published in 1999 and were based on a qualitative review of science, previous guidelines and consensus panel statements, and available gender-specific data (Mosca et al., 1999). The relative lack of data on CVD in women, however, limits the development of better guidelines for clinical care of women (Pepine et al., 2004). A report from the Agency for Healthcare Research and Quality noted the paucity of women enrolled in diagnostic studies and stated that much evidence is based on research done in men (Grady et al., 2003), and an AHA consensus panel concluded that clinical decision making would be greatly improved if sex differences in cardiac-imaging technologies were better understood (Mieres et al., 2005). An expert panel representing a dozen national organizations updated the 1999 guidelines in 2004 and 2007, providing clinical recommendations based on a review and evaluation of gender-specific results of clinical trials (Mosca et al., 2004a, 2007). Hsia and colleagues (2010) applied the 2007 updated AHA guideline categories to the data from the WHI and found that the updated categories predicted coronary events with an accuracy similar to that of the Framingham risk categories.

Although physicians appear to be aware of CVD-prevention guidelines for women, implementation is less than optimal. A survey of randomly selected physicians (primary-care physicians, cardiologists, and gynecologists) found that perception of a woman's risk was the primary determinant of adherence to preventive recommendations (Mosca et al., 2005). Gynecologists, two-thirds of whom reported providing primary care for their female patients, were less aware of national prevention guidelines and had lower self-reported effectiveness in managing risk factors than did the other physicians. Of concern was the finding that fewer than one-fifth of physicians knew that more women than men die of CVD each year and that in specific groups of women who have risk profiles identical with men's, women were more likely to be assigned to a lower risk category than men (Mosca et al., 2005). As this example shows, simply releasing guidelines is not sufficient to change provider knowledge and practice; educational efforts aimed at health-care providers may be needed to improve translation of scientific results into practice.

Women themselves have become more aware of CVD: in 1997, only 30% of women recognized CVD as the leading killer of women, significantly less than the 57% and 54% of women who recognized CVD as the leading killer of women in 2006 and 2009, respectively (Mosca et al., 2010). In turn, greater awareness is linked to a greater likelihood of taking preventive action (Mosca et al., 2006). That association is more pronounced in racial- and ethnic-minority populations, and this suggests that targeted educational campaigns have the potential to reduce disparities in CVD outcomes in women.

Mammography

Mammography has an extensive history of scientific investigation, public and private extramural research funding, clinical care and practice guidelines, government regulations, public exposure in the mass media, confusion, and controversy. It illustrates the interaction of important public and private institutions and organizations, including the role of guidelines and government regulations, that shape the agenda for women's health research and their knowledge, attitudes, and use of findings.

Competing Perspectives and Interests

In relation to any issue, those with different interests and concerns position themselves to build an agenda and shape the "frame" within which people will interpret information to which they are exposed (Hilgartner and Bosk, 1988; McCombs and Shaw, 1977, 1993). They compete in a symbolic "arena" for public attention. The communication media play a major role as gatekeepers to that arena (Gandy, 1982). Media attention, in conjunction with key social and institutional actors (such as news sources), raises, changes, or reinforces the public's perception of the importance of issues (Corbett and Mori, 1999; Viswanath and Finnegan, 2002) and how the public thinks about them (Scheufele and Tewksbury, 2007).

Radiologic technology developed to a point where it was feasible and useful for routine screening for breast cancer in the late 1960s (Gold, 1992; Picard, 1998), and scientific and public controversy surrounding benefits of and risks posed by mammography have existed almost since then. The questions of the early 1970s centered on its promise as a new clinical tool and on the role that it should play for women at different levels of risk. By the middle 1970s, a scientific and clinical consensus was forming around the three-part approach to breast-cancer prevention: breast self-examination (BSE), breast clinical examination (BCE) by a trained health-care provider, and regular mammography for women over 50 years old and for younger women who have a family history of breast cancer (Foster and Costanza, 1984; Gorringe et al., 1978; Green and Taplin, 2003; Justin, 1977). The major clinical trials that would have provided an evidentiary basis of safety, efficacy, benefit, and timing vs risk and outcomes had to yet be developed, but major organizations became engaged in the issues. In 1982 the American Cancer Society (ACS) recommended that women at least 50 years old and younger women who were at risk receive mammograms "every year when feasible" (National Task Force on Breast Cancer Control, 1982). Mammography centers were established nationwide. The economic benefits of the centers to providers and producers introduced an economic variable and new conflicts of interest into women's health care (Blakeslee, 1976). At that time, mammography was not high on the public's or women's agenda, in part because of a taboo about openly discussing cancer in general and breast cancer specifically (Braun, 2003). However, when high-profile women, undoubtedly aided by a re-empowered feminist movement in the United States, spoke out about personal experiences with breast cancer (Braun, 2003; Corbett and Mori, 1999; Subak-Sharpe, 1976), the taboo was substantially diminished, and mass-media stories on breast cancer spiked in 1974 (Corbett and Mori, 1999). That spike in coverage was the largest recorded up to that point and portended increasing media attention to research. Compared with news coverage in the 1960s, news stories increased especially in the category of "screening and diagnosis." Corbett and Mori (1999) found a lagged relationship of about 2 years between media coverage and increased breast-cancer incidence, which suggested an effect on screening behavior. They also observed a potential relationship between increased media coverage and discussion, increased publication of medical research articles, and increased federal funding of breast-cancer research.

Braun (2003) reviewed the history of advocacy by groups seeking to raise public awareness of breast-cancer issues. She described four chronologically overlapping phases, in all of which the mass media played an important role: an early phase, raising public awareness and understanding of the issue ("priming the market"); a second phase, "engaging consumers"; a third phase, "establishing political advocacy"; and finally "taking the advocacy mainstream." In the 1980s women's health-advocacy groups emerged, such as the Susan Komen Race for the Cure, as did the establishment of guidelines that institutionalized the three-part approach to breast-cancer prevention: mammography, BSE, and BCE. By the middle 1990s, private and public advocacy efforts on behalf of research on breast cancer had dramatically increased funding not only through NIH but through the Department of Defense and the US Army.

The increase in emphasis on breast cancer is illustrated in Figure 5-2. Specifically, the graph shows the growth of news coverage of mammography by major US news and wire-service outlets from 1989 through 2008 as reflected in the LexisNexis database. News coverage of mammography roughly doubled from 1989 to 1992 and again from 1992 to 1995. By 1997–1998, the high level of news coverage was continuous, and it was sustained through 2008. That appears to support Braun's (2003) contention that breast-cancer advocacy activity has been strong and steady. Since the late 1990s, breast cancer has become a standard "repertoire" issue on the health agenda in government, science, women's advocacy groups, and the communication media.

Mammography Standards

The successful implementation of the Mammography Quality Standards Act of 1992 (MQSA; Public Law 102-539) and the well-documented improvement in the quality of mammography services available to American women constitute a model for the dissemination and adoption of national standards for other services.

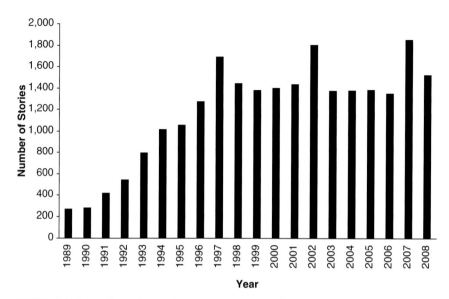

FIGURE 5-2 Number of news items on mammography in major US news and wire-service outlets listed in LexisNexis database, 1989–2008.

The MQSA evolved from a voluntary program created in 1987 by the American College of Radiology to address concerns about variations in mammography quality in the United States (Galkin et al., 1988; Suleiman et al., 1999). Accreditation became tied to evidence that facilities met standards for personnel, equipment, quality-assurance procedures, clinical images, phantom images, and dose. By 1991, one-fourth of the roughly 10,000 mammography units in the country had been accredited by American College of Radiology, and another one-fourth had sought accreditation but failed to meet the standards (McLelland et al., 1991). Following the voluntary program, state and federal legislation required facilities to meet quality standards, with all facilities requiring accreditation under the MQSA by October 1, 1994 (Destouet et al., 2005). Regulations have evolved in response both to new concerns about quality and to the development of new technologies, such as full-field digital mammography (IOM, 2005). There is now substantial research supporting the improvements in quality for patients since the uniform adoption of quality standards under the MQSA. This is an example of how research findings contribute both to the initial development of new screening and treatment services and to the evaluation of their implementation and of the value of mandatory standards in improving the quality of services (Destouet et al., 2005).

The Mass Media and Controversy

There has been continuing scientific study and changing interpretations of research surrounding the use of mammography as a regular screening tool for women's breast health. The process has been complicated by the mass media's interest in "news value," which emphasizes novelty, conflict, and drama. At its best, media coverage generates public attention to and learning about important subjects and builds and sustains an issue on the public agenda. At its worst, it engenders confusion and perhaps fatalism that can lead to inaction (Dunwoody, 1999; Kitzinger and Reilly, 1997; Nelkin, 1995).

For example, in the early 1970s, ACS launched an initiative with NIH to test mammography's detection ability. The partnership established the Breast Cancer Detection Demonstration Project (BCDDP), which engaged some 280,000 women volunteers 35–74 years old in receiving regular mammograms over 5 years (Finkel, 2005). It was not a clinical trial of effectiveness, but a feasibility demonstration involving 29 sites. It was a precursor to the health-care system's potentially widespread investment in expensive technology. As Cunningham (1997) recounted, the project was criticized almost immediately in the media by some scientists and clinicians for its "risk, cost, effectiveness and purpose." The director of the National Cancer Institute raised the question of radiation risks accruing from mammography, especially in women 35–50 years old, in a letter to the physicians at the BCDDP sites, stating his concerns and recommendations (Blakeslee, 1976; Cancer Institute Proposes Limits on Breast X-rays, 1976; Finkel, 2005). Although his recommendations had no official status, media coverage reduced the number of BCDDP volunteers who adhered fully to the demonstration protocol (Cunningham, 1997). This was never formally studied, but it may be that media coverage of the risk of contracting breast cancer from repeated mammography engendered enough uncertainty in the volunteers for many to choose not to continue (Dunwoody, 1999).

A 2001 research letter in the *Lancet* by two Cochrane Collaboration investigators who had conducted a systematic review of mammography sparked considerable controversy that appears to be linked to mass-media coverage (Steele et al., 2005). The investigators had re-examined the clinical trials that formed the basis of mammography guidelines, which were conducted in the 1980s and 1990s (Smith et al., 2004). In summarizing the collective results of those clinical trials, they said that "there is no reliable evidence that screening for breast cancer reduces mortality" (Olsen and Gotzsche, 2001). Steele and colleagues (2005) found that the media appeared to play a large role in the response to the study. Of the newspapers reviewed, only the *Washington Post* reported on the study's finding when it was first published (Steele et al., 2005). However, 2 months later, the *New York Times* reported the findings in a front-page article; after that, there was a spike in coverage of the original findings and responses and statements issued by a number of government agencies. Media coverage of mammography spiked several times over the next year as some investigators reanalyzed the same clinical-trial data and arrived at the opposite conclusion, health and medical organizations took out full-page newspaper advertisements pledging their continued support of mammography, and HHS issued new guidelines continuing to support mammography, which were underscored in a public hearing in the US Senate (HHS, 2002b).

Controversy emerged again in 2009 when an independent scientific panel of the US Preventive Services Task Force issued its findings. The task force had examined the evidence base again from the standpoint of risk of harm from vs benefits of mammography (Mandelblatt et al., 2009). It concluded that women under 50 years old who had no familial or personal history of breast cancer should not be screened routinely, but that "the decision to start regular, biennial screening mammography before the age of 50 years should be an individual one and take patient context into account, including the patient's values regarding specific benefits and harms" (US Preventive Services Task Force, 2009), and that women 50–74 years old should be screened with mammography every 2 years rather than annually. The task force's recommendations were based on its evaluation of conclusions about risk and harm based on how the task force members ranked the quality of available evidence. It suggested—on the basis of the research as it existed, with all its flaws and challenges—that the accepted mammography guidelines interpreted benefits too liberally and harm too conservatively. It used multiple indicators of harm from false-positive results, including psychologic harm from unnecessary anxiety and physical-health risks from additional tests. That is more complicated and harder to understand than a simple balance of lives saved due to one or another treatment and, in many cases, the message that was conveyed was that women under 50 should not routinely be screened for breast cancer.

Media coverage spiked rapidly (Woolf, 2010). One reason for the interest was that professional experts, key institutions, advocacy groups, and the government might have different perspectives, and the report challenged established guidelines developed by those stakeholders. Complicating matters was that its release occurred at the height of the US Senate debate regarding national health-care reform. Opponents of reform efforts seized on the report as evidence that the US government was intent on a policy of "health-care rationing" that would endanger women's health (Woolf, 2010). Individual women testified that if the proposed recommendations had been followed by their health-care providers, they would probably not have survived their breast cancers. Such anecdotes and arguments were easier to convey in brief sound-bites than the more complicated balance of harm vs benefit and the more abstract concept of population-attributable risk. The panel appeared to have been surprised by the intense controversy and did not have an immediate strategy for dealing with the reactions to its report.

The issues illustrated by the controversies surrounding mammography will continue to occur in this and other fields. Science evolves and different groups will have different guidelines and recommendations depending on how they weigh the scientific evidence.

Lessons Learned

The case of mammography illustrates the interaction of the forces and factors of science, politics, economics, and culture that combine with mass-media communication to shape and reshape the research agenda for women's health and the health services that they receive. The process frames the meaning of women's health itself and the interpretation and limits of scientific data. The meaning and interpretation of scientific results is often variable and contentious, especially as findings are translated into clinical recommendations and strategies for improving women's health. The dynamics of the mammography issue offer a case in point about the struggle of conveying in the media the meaning and interpretation of scientific findings given the sometimes conflicting opinions within the scientific community about the findings and how best to effectively convey the messages. Although the portrayal of conflict can increase the salience of an issue so as to gain the public's attention, it can also foster contentiousness among policy makers, scientists, and others. Such conflict runs the risk of discouraging and confusing women potentially to the point of fatalism about the causes and prevention of breast cancer. That impact is greater on those of lower SES, who tend to have poorer health outcomes overall.

CONCLUSIONS

- Barriers delay or preclude the translation of findings of women's health research into practice. Those barriers range from fragmentation of health-care delivery and health-care policies, and reimbursement to the complexity of science and research, challenges in communicating understandable and actionable messages, and consumer confusion and apprehension. Few studies of how to increase the speed or extent of translation of findings related to women's health into clinical practice have been conducted. Clinical-practice guidelines, mandatory standards, reimbursement practices, laws (including public-health laws), and health-professions school curricula and continuing education are some methods of translation that have been used and warrant evaluation for translating research findings on women.
- Women are, in general, a receptive audience for medical messages and information. Many messages, however, are confusing because of conflicting results and uncertainty in data. Improved strategies for communicating research results to the public are needed.

RECOMMENDATIONS

- Research should be conducted on the best ways to translate research findings on women's health into clinical practice and public-health policies rapidly. Research findings should be incorporated at the practitioner level and at the overall public-health systems level through, for example, the use of targeted education programs for practitioners and the development of guidelines. Research on what messages women find confusing and how those messages could be delivered in a more effective manner is needed. As those programs and guidelines are developed and implemented, they should be evaluated to ensure effectiveness.

- HHS should appoint a task force to develop an evidence-based strategy to communicate and market health messages to women that are based on objective research results. In addition to content experts in relevant departments and agencies, the task force should include mass-media and targeted-messaging and marketing experts. The goals of the strategy should include effective communication to the diverse audience of women; increasing awareness of women's health issues and treatments, including prevention and intervention strategies; and decreasing confusion in light of complex and sometimes conflicting health messages. Strategies to explore might include

  ○ requiring a plan for communication and dissemination of findings in government-funded studies to the public, providers, and policy makers, similar to the requirement to have a data and safety monitoring board in those studies;

  ○ establishing a national media advisory panel with experts in women's health, which would be readily available to provide context to reporters, scientists, clinicians, and policy makers at the time of release of important or potentially complex new research reports. (One goal of the panel could be to explain discrepancies and uncertainties in research findings); and

  ○ creation by the HHS OWH of a program dedicated to translation of findings of women's health research into practice.

REFERENCES

Allsop, J., K. Jones, and R. Baggott. 2004. Health consumer groups in the UK: A new social movement? *Sociology of Health & Illness* 26(6):737–756.

Arora, N. K., B. W. Hesse, B. K. Rimer, K. Viswanath, M. L. Clayman, and R. T. Croyle. 2008. Frustrated and confused: The American public rates its cancer-related information-seeking experiences. *Journal of General Internal Medicine* 23(3):223–228.

Bansal, A. T., and M. R. Barnes. 2008. Genomics in drug discovery: The best things come to those who wait. *Current Opinion in Drug Discovery & Development* 11(3):303–310.

Barber, C. A., K. Margolis, R. V. Luepker, and D. K. Arnett. 2004. The impact of the Women's Health Initiative on discontinuation of postmenopausal hormone therapy: The Minnesota Heart Survey (2000–2002). *Journal of Women's Health* 13(9):975–984.

Bean-Mayberry, B., E. M. Yano, N. Bayliss, J. Navratil, C. S. Weisman, and S. H. Scholle. 2007a. Federally funded comprehensive women's health centers: Leading innovation in women's healthcare delivery. *Journal of Women's Health* 16(9):1281–1290.

Bean-Mayberry, B. A., E. M. Yano, C. D. Caffrey, L. Altman, and D. L. Washington. 2007b. Organizational characteristics associated with the availability of women's health clinics for primary care in the veterans health administration. *Military Medicine* 172(8):824–828.

Belkora, J. K., M. K. Loth, S. Volz, and H. S. Rugo. 2009. Implementing decision and communication aids to facilitate patient-centered care in breast cancer: A case study. *Patient Education and Counseling* 77(3):360–368.

Berger, J. S., M. J. Krantz, J. M. Kittelson, and W. R. Hiatt. 2009. Aspirin for the prevention of cardiovascular events in patients with peripheral artery disease: A meta-analysis of randomized trials. *Journal of the American Medical Association* 301(18):1909–1919.

Bero, L. A., R. Grilli, J. M. Grimshaw, E. Harvey, A. D. Oxman, and M. A. Thomson. 1998. Closing the gap between research and practice: An overview of systematic reviews of interventions to promote the implementation of research findings. The Cochrane Effective Practice and Organization of Care Review Group. *British Medical Journal* 317(7156):465–468.

Berwick, D. M. 2003. Disseminating innovations in health care. *Journal of the American Medical Assocation* 289(15):1969–1975.

Bird, C. E., A. M. Fremont, A. S. Bierman, S. Wickstrom, M. Shah, T. Rector, T. Horstman, and J. J. Escarce. 2007. Does quality of care for cardiovascular disease and diabetes differ by gender for enrollees in managed care plans? *Women's Health Issues* 17(3):131–138.

Blakeslee, A. 1976. Women shouldn't fear breast x-rays: Doctor. Associated press wire story. *St. Petersburg Times*, September 5, 15A.

Bluming, A. Z., and C. Tavris. 2009. Hormone replacement therapy: Real concerns and false alarms. *Cancer Journal* 15(2):93–104.

Braddock, C. H., S. D. Fihn, W. Levinson, A. R. Jonsen, and R. A. Pearlman. 1997. How doctors and patients discuss routine clinical decisions: Informed decision making in the outpatient setting. *Journal of General Internal Medicine* 12(6):339–345.

Braun, S. 2003. The history of breast cancer advocacy. *Breast Journal* 9:S101–S103.

Breslau, E. S., W. W. Davis, L. Doner, E. J. Eisner, N. R. Goodman, H. I. Meissner, B. K. Rimer, and J. E. Rossouw. 2003. The hormone therapy dilemma: Women respond. *Journal of the American Medical Women's Association* 58(1):33–43.

Burton, B., and A. Rowell. 2003. Unhealthy spin. *British Medical Journal* 326(7400):1205–1207.

Bush, T. M., A. E. Bonomi, L. Nekhlyudov, E. J. Ludman, S. D. Reed, M. T. Connelly, L. C. Grothaus, A. Z. LaCroix, and K. M. Newton. 2007. How the Women's Health Initiative (WHI) influenced physicians' practice and attitudes. *Journal of General Internal Medicine* 22(9):1311–1316.

California Health Interview Survey. 2010. *Ask CHIS: 2007 California health survey.* http://www.chis.ucla.edu/main/DQ3/output.asp?_rn=0.2069513 (accessed August 16, 2010).

Cancer Institute Proposes Limits on Breast X-Rays. 1976. *New York Times (1923–Current file)*, 12.

Charo, R. A. 2007. Politics, parents, and prophylaxis—mandating HPV vaccination in the United States. *New England Journal of Medicine* 356(19):1905–1908.

Chauhan, M. S., K. K. Ho, D. S. Baim, R. E. Kuntz, and D. E. Cutlip. 2005. Effect of gender on in-hospital and one-year outcomes after contemporary coronary artery stenting. *American Journal of Cardiology* 95(1):101–104.

Chlebowski, R. T., S. L. Hendrix, R. D. Langer, M. L. Stefanick, M. Gass, D. Lane, R. J. Rodabough, M. A. Gilligan, M. G. Cyr, C. A. Thomson, J. Khandekar, H. Petrovitch, and A. McTiernan. 2003. Influence of estrogen plus progestin on breast cancer and mammography in healthy post-menopausal women: The Women's Health Initiative randomized trial. *Journal of the American Medical Association* 289(24):3243–3253.

Chlebowski, R. T., L. H. Kuller, R. L. Prentice, M. L. Stefanick, J. E. Manson, M. Gass, A. K. Aragaki, J. K. Ockene, D. S. Lane, G. E. Sarto, A. Rajkovic, R. Schenken, S. L. Hendrix, P. M. Ravdin, T. E. Rohan, S. Yasmeen, G. Anderson, and the WHI Investigators. 2009. Breast cancer after use of estrogen plus progestin in postmenopausal women. *New England Journal of Medicine* 360(6):573–587.

Christian, A. H., W. Rosamond, A. R. White, and L. Mosca. 2007. Nine-year trends and racial and ethnic disparities in women's awareness of heart disease and stroke: An American Heart Association national study. *Journal of Women's Health (2002)* 16(1):68–81.

Corbett, J. B., and M. Mori. 1999. Medicine, media, and celebrities: News coverage of breast cancer, 1960–1995. *Journalism and Mass Communication Quarterly* 76(2):229–249.

Cunningham, M. P. 1997. The breast cancer detection demonstration project 25 years later. *CA: A Cancer Journal for Clinicians* 47(3):131–133.

Cuzick, J., T. Powles, U. Veronesi, J. Forbes, R. Edwards, S. Ashley, and P. Boyle. 2003. Overview of the main outcomes in breast-cancer prevention trials. *Lancet* 361(9354):296–300.

Destouet, J. M., L. W. Bassett, M. J. Yaffe, P. F. Butler, and P. A. Wilcox. 2005. The ACR's mammography accreditation program: Ten years of experience since MQSA. *Journal of the American College of Radiology* 2(7):585–594.

Donohue, G. A., P. J. Tichenor, and C. N. Olien. 1975. Mass media and the knowledge gap: A hypothesis reconsidered. *Communication Research* 2(1):3–23.

Dunwoody, S. 1999. Scientists, journalists, and the meaning of uncertainty. In *Communicating Uncertainty: Media Coverage of New and Controversial Science*, edited by S. M. Friedman, S. Dunwoody and C. L. Rogers. Mahwah, NJ: L. Erlbaum Associates. Pp. 59–79.

Estabrook, L. S., E. G. Witt, and H. Rainie. 2007. *Information Searches That Solve Problems: How People Use the Internet, Libraries, and Government Agencies When They Need Help.* Washington, DC: Pew Internet and American Life Project.

Fallows, D. 2005. *How Women and Men Use the Internet: Women Are Catching Up to Men in Most Measures of Online Life; Men Like the Internet for the Experiences It Offers, While Women Like It for the Human Connections It Promotes.* http://www.pewinternet.org/~/media//Files/Reports/2005/PIP_Women_and_Men_online.pdf.pdf (accessed December 8, 2009).

Farquhar, C., R. Basser, S. Hetrick, A. Lethaby, and J. Marjoribanks. 2003. High dose chemotherapy and autologous bone marrow or stem cell transplantation versus conventional chemotherapy for women with metastatic breast cancer. *Cochrane Database of Systematic Reviews* 1:CD003142.

FDA (US Food and Drug Administration). 1998. The oncologist news bulletin. *Oncologist* 3(6):452–454.

Finkel, M. L. 2005. *Understanding the Mammography Controversy: Science, Politics, and Breast Cancer Screening.* Westport, CT: Praeger.

Fisher, B., J. P. Costantino, D. L. Wickerham, C. K. Redmond, M. Kavanah, W. M. Cronin, V. Vogel, A. Robidoux, N. Dimitrov, J. Atkins, M. Daly, S. Wieand, E. Tan-Chiu, L. Ford, and N. Wolmark. 1998. Tamoxifen for prevention of breast cancer: Report of the National Surgical Adjuvant Breast and Bowel Project P-1 Study. *Journal of the National Cancer Institute* 90(18):1371–1388.

Fogel, J., S. M. Albert, F. Schnabel, B. A. Ditkoff, and A. I. Neugut. 2002. Use of the internet by women with breast cancer. *Journal of Medical Internet Research* 4(2):E9.

Foster, R. S. J., and M. C. Costanza. 1984. Breast self-examination practices and breast cancer survival. *Obstetrical & Gynecological Survey* 39(6):404.

Fox, S. 2006. *Online Health Search 2006.* Washington, DC: Pew Internet and American Life Project.

Franklin, L., J. Belkora, S. O'Donnell, D. Elsbree, J. Hardin, B. Ingle, and N. Johnson. 2009. Consultation support for rural women with breast cancer: Results of a community-based participatory research study. *Patient Education and Counseling* 80(1):80–87.

French, L. M., M. A. Smith, J. S. Holtrop, and M. Holmes-Rovner. 2006. Hormone therapy after the Women's Health Initiative: A qualitative study. *BMC Family Practice* 7:61.

Galkin, B. M., S. A. Feig, and H. D. Muir. 1988. The technical quality of mammography in centers participating in a regional breast cancer awareness program. *Radiographics* 8(1):133–145.

Gandy, O. H. 1982. *Beyond Agenda Setting: Information Subsidies and Public Policy, Communication and Information Science; Variation: Communication and Information Science.* Norwood, NJ: Ablex.

Garbe, E., and S. Suissa. 2004. Issues to debate on the Women's Health Initiative (WHI) Study: Hormone replacement therapy and acute coronary outcomes: Methodological issues between randomized and observational studies. *Human Reproduction* 19(1):8–13.

Gold, R. H. 1992. The evolution of mammography. *Radiologic Clinics of North America* 30(1): 1–19.

Goodman, R. M., M. R. Seaver, S. Yoo, S. Dibble, R. Shada, B. Sherman, F. Urmston, N. Milliken, and K. M. Freund. 2002. A qualitative evaluation of the national centers of excellence in women's health program. *Womens Health Issues* 12(6):291–308.

Gorringe, R., M. M. Lee, and A. Voda. 1978. The mammography controversy: A case for breast self-examination. *Journal of Obstetric, Gynecologic & Neonatal Nursing* 7(4):7–12.

Grady, D., L. Chaput, and M. Kristof. 2003. Results of systematic review of research on diagnosis and treatment of coronary heart disease in women. In *Evidence Report/Technology Assessment*. No. 80. (Prepared by the University of California, San Francisco—Stanford Evidence-based Practice Center under Contract No 290-97-0013.) AHRQ Publication No. 03-0035. Rockville, MD: Agency for Healthcare Research and Quality.

Green, B. B., and S. H. Taplin. 2003. Breast cancer screening controversies. *Journal of the American Board of Family Practice* 16(3):233–241.

Haas, J., B. Geller, D. L. Miglioretti, D. S. Buist, D. E. Nelson, K. Kerlikowske, P. A. Carney, E. S. Breslau, S. Dash, M. K. Canales, and R. Ballard-Barbash. 2006. Changes in newspaper coverage about hormone therapy with the release of new medical evidence. *Journal of General Internal Medicine* 21(4):304–309.

Haas, J., D. Miglioretti, B. Geller, D. Buist, D. Nelson, K. Kerlikowske, P. Carney, S. Dash, E. Breslau, and R. Ballard-Barbash. 2007. Average household exposure to newspaper coverage about the harmful effects of hormone therapy and population-based declines in hormone therapy use. *Journal of General Internal Medicine* 22:68–73.

Harman, S. M., F. Naftolin, E. A. Brinton, and D. R. Judelson. 2005. Is the estrogen controversy over? Deconstructing the Women's Health Initiative Study: A critical evaluation of the evidence. *Annals of the New York Academy of Sciences* 1052:43–56.

Harris Interactive. 2008a. *Four Out of Five Adults Now Use the Internet.* http://www.harrisinteractive.com/harris_poll/index.asp?PID973 (accessed April 15, 2009).

———. 2008b. *Number of "Cyberchondriacs"—Adults Going Online for Health Information—Has Plateaued or Declined.* http://www.harrisinteractive.com/harris_poll/index.asp?PID937 (accessed April 25, 2009).

Hausauer, A., T. Keegan, E. Chang, S. Glaser, H. Howe, and C. Clarke. 2009. Recent trends in breast cancer incidence in US white women by county-level urban/rural and poverty status. *BMC Medicine* 7(1):31.

Heiss, G., R. Wallace, G. Anderson, A. Aragaki, S. Beresford, R. Brzyski, R. Chlebowski, M. Gass, A. LaCroix, J. Manson, R. Prentice, J. Rossouw, and M. L. Stefanick. 2008. Health risks and benefits 3 years after stopping randomized treatment with estrogen and progestin. *Journal of the American Medical Association* 299(9):1036–1045.

Henson, R. M., S. W. Wyatt, and N. C. Lee. 1996. The National Breast and Cervical Cancer Early Detection Program: A comprehensive public health response to two major health issues for women. *Journal of Public Health Management and Practice* 2(2):36–47.

Herbst, A. L., and D. Anderson. 1990. Clear cell adenocarcinoma of the vagina and cervix secondary to intrauterine exposure to diethylstilbestrol. *Seminars in Surgical Oncology* 6(6):343–346.

Herxheimer, A. 2003. Relationships between the pharmaceutical industry and patients' organisations. *British Medical Journal* 326(7400):1208–1210.

HHS (US Department of Health and Human Services). 2002a. *NHLBI Stops Trial of Estrogen Plus Progestin Due to Increased Breast Cancer Risk, Lack of Overall Benefit.* Washington, DC.

———. 2002b. *News Release: NCI Statement on Mammography Screening, Edited by National Cancer Institute.* Washington, DC: Department of Health and Human Services.

———. 2004. *NHLBI Advisory for Physicians on the WHI Trial of Conjugated Equine Estrogens Versus Placebo.* http://www.nhlbi.nih.gov/whi/e-a_advisory.htm (accessed April 12, 2010).

————. 2010. *About the Heart Truth Campaign.* http://www.nhlbi.nih.gov/educational/hearttruth/ about/index.htm (accessed March 17, 2010).

Hilgartner, S., and C. L. Bosk. 1988. The rise and fall of social problems: A public arenas model. *American Journal of Sociology* 94(1):53–78.

Hoffmann, M., M. Hammar, K. I. Kjellgren, L. Lindh-Astrand, and J. Brynhildsen. 2005. Changes in women's attitudes towards and use of hormone therapy after HERS and WHI. *Maturitas* 52(1):11–17.

Hsia, J., R. J. Rodabough, J. E. Manson, S. M. Liu, M. S. Freiberg, W. Graettinger, M. C. Rosal, B. Cochrane, D. Lloyd-Jones, J. G. Robinson, B. V. Howard, and Women's Health Initiative Research Group. 2010. Evaluation of the American Heart Association cardiovascular disease prevention guideline for women. *Circulation-Cardiovascular Quality and Outcomes* 3(2):128–134.

IOM (Institute of Medicine). 1993. *An Assessment of the NIH Women's Health Initiative.* Washington, DC. National Academy Press.

————. 2000. *To Err Is Human: Building a Safer Health System.* Edited by L. T. Kohn, J. Corrigan and M. S. Donaldson. Washington, DC: National Academy Press.

————. 2001a. *Crossing the Quality Chasm: A New Health System for the 21st Century.* Washington, DC: National Academy Press.

————. 2001b. *Science and Risk Communication: A Mini-Symposium Sponsored by the Roundtable on Environmental Health Sciences, Research, and Medicine.* Edited by C. M. Coussens and B. Fischhoff. Washington, DC: National Academy Press.

————. 2002a. *The Future of the Public's Health in the 21st Century.* Washington, DC: The National Academies Press.

————. 2002b. *Speaking of Health: Assessing Health Communication Strategies for Diverse Populations.* Edited by Committee on Communication for Behavior Change in the 21st Century: Improving the Health of Diverse Populations. Washington, DC: The National Academies Press.

————. 2005. *Improving Breast Imaging Quality Standards.* Washington, DC: The National Academies Press.

————. 2006a. *Examining the Health Disparities Research Plan of the National Institutes of Health: Unfinished Business.* Edited by G. E. Thomson, F. Mitchell and M. Williams. Washington, DC: The National Academies Press.

————. 2006b. *Improving the Quality of Health Care for Mental and Substance-Use Conditions: Quality Chasm Series.* Edited by Committee on Crossing the Quality Chasm: Adaptation to Mental Health and Addictive Disorders. Washington, DC: The National Academies Press.

————. 2008. *Cancer Care for the Whole Patient: Meeting Psychosocial Health Needs.* Edited by N. E. Adler and A. Page. Washington, DC: The National Academies Press.

————. 2009. *America's Uninsured Crisis: Consequences for Health and Health Care.* Washington, DC: The National Academies Press.

Jagsi, R., N. Sheets, A. Jankovic, A. R. Motomura, S. Amarnath, and P. A. Ubel. 2009. Frequency, nature, effects, and correlates of conflicts of interest in published clinical cancer research. *Cancer* 115(12):2783–2791.

Jemal, A., E. Ward, and M. J. Thun. 2007. Recent trends in breast cancer incidence rates by age and tumor characteristics among US women. *Breast Cancer Research* 9(3):R28.

Justin, R. G. 1977. Annual physical examination and detection of breast cancer. *Journal of the American Medical Association* 238(5):397–398.

Keefe, R. H., S. D. Lane, and H. J. Swarts. 2006. From the bottom up: Tracing the impact of four health-based social movements on health and social policies. *Journal of Health and Social Policy* 21(3):55–69.

Kerlikowske, K., D. L. Miglioretti, D. S. M. Buist, R. Walker, and P. A. Carney. 2007. Declines in invasive breast cancer and use of postmenopausal hormone therapy in a screening mammography population. *Journal of the National Cancer Institute* 99(17):1335–1339.

Kitzinger, J., and J. Reilly. 1997. The rise and fall of risk reporting: Media coverage of human genetics research, "false memory syndrome" and "mad cow disease." *European Journal of Communication* 12(3):319–350.

Klemm, P., K. Reppert, and L. Visich. 1998. A nontraditional cancer support group. The internet. *Computers in Nursing* 16(1):31–36.

Koch, D. D. 2003. Industry support for physician education. *Journal of Cataract and Refractive Surgery* 29(3):419.

Kolker, E. S. 2004. Framing as a cultural resource in health social movements: Funding activism and the breast cancer movement in the US 1990–1993. *Sociology of Health and Illness* 26(6):820–844.

Kreuter, M. W., and R. J. Wray. 2003. Tailored and targeted health communication: Strategies for enhancing information relevance. *American Journal Health Behavior* 27 (Suppl. 3):S227–S232.

Krieger, N., J. T. Chen, and P. D. Waterman. 2010. Decline in US breast cancer rates after the Women's Health Initiative: Socioeconomic and racial/ethnic differentials. *American Journal of Public Health* 100(S1):S132–S139.

Lansky, A. J., J. S. Hochman, P. A. Ward, G. S. Mintz, R. Fabunmi, P. B. Berger, G. New, C. L. Grines, C. G. Pietras, M. J. Kern, M. Ferrell, M. B. Leon, R. Mehran, C. White, J. H. Mieres, J. W. Moses, G. W. Stone, and A. K. Jacobs. 2005. Percutaneous coronary intervention and adjunctive pharmacotherapy in women: A statement for healthcare professionals from the American Heart Association. *Circulation* 111(7):940–953.

Lerner, B. H. 2002. Breast cancer activism: Past lessons, future directions. *Nature Reviews Cancer* 2(3):225–230.

Lewis, J. P. 2007. An interpretation of the EBCTCG data. *Oncologist* 12(5):505–509.

Lexchin, J., and D. W. Light. 2006. Commercial influence and the content of medical journals. *British Medical Journal* 332(7555):1444–1447.

Lobo, R. A., S. Belisle, W. T. Creasman, N. R. Frankel, N. E. Goodman, J. E. Hall, S. L. Ivey, S. Kingsberg, R. Langer, R. Lehman, D. B. McArthur, V. Montgomery-Rice, M. Notelovitz, G. S. Packin, R. W. Rebar, M. Rousseau, R. S. Schenken, D. L. Schneider, K. Sherif, and S. Wysocki. 2006. Should symptomatic menopausal women be offered hormone therapy? *Medscape General Medicine* 8(3):40.

Long, T., A. M. Taubenheim, J. Wayman, S. Temple, and B. A. Ruoff. 2008. The heart truth: Using the power of branding and social marketing to increase awareness of heart disease in women. *Social Marketing Quarterly* 14(3):3–29.

MacLennan, A.H., A.W. Taylor, and D.H. Wilson. 2004. Hormone therapy use after the Women's Health Initiative. *Climacteric* 7(2):138–142.

Mamounas, E. P., J. Bryant, B. Lembersky, L. Fehrenbacher, S. M. Sedlacek, B. Fisher, D. L. Wickerham, G. Yothers, A. Soran, and N. Wolmark. 2005. Paclitaxel after doxorubicin plus cyclophosphamide as adjuvant chemotherapy for node-positive breast cancer: Results from NSABP B-28. *Journal Clinical Oncology* 23(16):3686–3696.

Mandelblatt, J. S., K. A. Cronin, S. Bailey, D. A. Berry, H. J. de Koning, G. Draisma, H. Huang, S. J. Lee, M. Munsell, S. K. Plevritis, P. Ravdin, C. B. Schechter, B. Sigal, M. A. Stoto, N. K. Stout, N. T. van Ravesteyn, J. Venier, M. Zelen, and E. J. Feuer. 2009. Effects of mammography screening under different screening schedules: Model estimates of potential benefits and harms. *Annals of Internal Medicine* 151(10):738–747.

Marcus, S. M., E. A. Young, K. B. Kerber, S. Kornstein, A. H. Farabaugh, J. Mitchell, S. R. Wisniewski, G. K. Balasubramani, M. H. Trivedi, and A. J. Rush. 2005. Gender differences in depression: Findings from the STAR*D study. *Journal of Affective Disorders* 87(2-3):141–150.

McCombs, M. E., and D. L. Shaw. 1977. *The Emergence of American Political Issues: The Agenda Setting Function of the Press (The West Series in Journalism).* St. Paul, MN: West Publishing.

———. 1993. The evolution of agenda-setting research: Twenty-five years in the marketplace of ideas. *Journal of Communication* 43(2):58–67.

McGlynn, E. A., E. A. Kerr, and S. M. Asch. 1999. New approach to assessing clinical quality of care for women: The QA Tool system. *Women's Health Issues* 9(4):184–192.

McIntosh, J., and S. J. Blalock. 2005. Effects of media coverage of women's health initiative study on attitudes and behavior of women receiving hormone replacement therapy. *American Journal of Health-System Pharmacy* 62(1):69–74.

McKinley, E. D., J. W. Thompson, J. Briefer-French, L. S. Wilcox, C. S. Weisman, and W. C. Andrews. 2002. Performance indicators in women's health: Incorporating women's health in the Health Plan Employer Data and Information Set (HEDIS). *Women's Health Issues* 12(1):46–58.

McLelland, R., R. Hendrick, M. Zinninger, and P. Wilcox. 1991. The American College of Radiology Mammography Accreditation Program. *American Journal of Roentgeneology* 157(3):473–479.

Mieres, J. H., L. J. Shaw, A. Arai, M. J. Budoff, S. D. Flamm, W. G. Hundley, T. H. Marwick, L. Mosca, A. R. Patel, M. A. Quinones, R. F. Redberg, K. A. Taubert, A. J. Taylor, G. S. Thomas, and N. K. Wenger. 2005. Role of noninvasive testing in the clinical evaluation of women with suspected coronary artery disease: Consensus statement from the Cardiac Imaging Committee, Council on Clinical Cardiology, and the Cardiovascular Imaging and Intervention Committee, Council on Cardiovascular Radiology and Intervention, and American Heart Association. *Circulation* 111(5):682–696.

Mosca, L., J. E. Manson, S. E. Sutherland, R. D. Langer, T. Manolio, and E. Barrett-Connor. 1997. Cardiovascular disease in women: A statement for healthcare professionals from the American Heart Association. Writing group. *Circulation* 96(7):2468–2482.

Mosca, L., S. M. Grundy, D. Judelson, K. King, M. Limacher, S. Oparil, R. Pasternak, T. A. Pearson, R. F. Redberg, S. C. Smith, Jr., M. Winston, and S. Zinberg. 1999. Guide to preventive cardiology for women. *Circulation* 99(18):2480–2484.

Mosca, L., L. J. Appel, E. J. Benjamin, K. Berra, N. Chandra-Strobos, R. P. Fabunmi, D. Grady, C. K. Haan, S. N. Hayes, D. R. Judelson, N. L. Keenan, P. McBride, S. Oparil, P. Ouyang, M. C. Oz, M. E. Mendelsohn, R. C. Pasternak, V. W. Pinn, R. M. Robertson, K. Schenck-Gustafsson, C. A. Sila, S. C. Smith, Jr., G. Sopko, A. L. Taylor, B. W. Walsh, N. K. Wenger, and C. L. Williams. 2004a. Evidence-based guidelines for cardiovascular disease prevention in women. *Circulation* 109(5):672–693.

Mosca, L., A. Ferris, R. Fabunmi, and R. M. Robertson. 2004b. Tracking women's awareness of heart disease: An American Heart Association national study. *Circulation* 109(5):573–579.

Mosca, L., A. H. Linfante, E. J. Benjamin, K. Berra, S. N. Hayes, B. W. Walsh, R. P. Fabunmi, J. Kwan, T. Mills, and S. L. Simpson. 2005. National study of physician awareness and adherence to cardiovascular disease prevention guidelines. *Circulation* 111(4):499–510.

Mosca, L., H. Mochari, A. Christian, K. Berra, K. Taubert, T. Mills, K. A. Burdick, and S. L. Simpson. 2006. National study of women's awareness, preventive action, and barriers to cardiovascular health. *Circulation* 113(4):525–534.

Mosca, L., C. L. Banka, E. J. Benjamin, K. Berra, C. Bushnell, R. J. Dolor, T. G. Ganiats, A. S. Gomes, H. L. Gornik, C. Gracia, M. Gulati, C. K. Haan, D. R. Judelson, N. Keenan, E. Kelepouris, E. D. Michos, L. K. Newby, S. Oparil, P. Ouyang, M. C. Oz, D. Petitti, V. W. Pinn, R. F. Redberg, R. Scott, K. Sherif, S. C. Smith, Jr., G. Sopko, R. H. Steinhorn, N. J. Stone, K. A. Taubert, B. A. Todd, E. Urbina, N. K. Wenger; Expert Panel/Writing Group; American Heart Association; American Academy of Family Physicians; American College of Obstetricians and Gynecologists; American College of Cardiology Foundation; Society of Thoracic Surgeons; American Medical Women's Association; Centers for Disease Control and Prevention; Office of Research on Women's Health; Association of Black Cardiologists; American College of Physicians; World Heart Federation; National Heart, Lung, and Blood Institute; and American College of Nurse Practitioners. 2007. Evidence-based guidelines for cardiovascular disease prevention in women: 2007 update. *Circulation* 115(11):1481–1501. [erratum appears in circulation. 2007 Apr 17;115(15):E407].

Mosca, L., H. Mochari-Greenberger, R. J. Dolor, L. K. Newby, and K. J. Robb. 2010. Twelve-year follow-up of American women's awareness of cardiovascular disease risk and barriers to heart health. *Circulation: Cardiovascular Quality and Outcomes* 3(2):120–127.

Moynihan, R. 2003. Who pays for the pizza? Redefining the relationships between doctors and drug companies. 2: Disentanglement. *British Medical Journal* 326(7400):1193–1196.

National Task Force on Breast Cancer Control. 1982. Mammography 1982: A statement of the American Cancer Society. *CA: A Cancer Journal for Clinicians* 32:226–230.

NCQA (National Committee for Quality Assurance). 2010. *HEDIS 2010 Measures.* http://www.ncqa. org/tabid/59/Default.aspx (accessed March 23, 2010).

Nelkin, D. 1995. *Selling Science: How the Press Covers Science and Technology.* Rev. ed. New York: W.H. Freeman.

Nelson, H. D., K. Tyne, A. Naik, C. Bougatsos, B. K. Chan, and L. Humphrey. 2009. Screening for breast cancer: An update for the US Preventive Services Task Force. *Annals of Internal Medicine* 151(10):727–737.

NIH (National Institutes of Health). 2010. *Clinical and Translational Science Awards.* http://www. ncrr.nih.gov/clinical_research_resources/clinical_and_translational_science_awards/ (accessed March 24, 2010).

O'Connor, A. M., A. Rostom, V. Fiset, J. Tetroe, V. Entwistle, H. Llewellyn-Thomas, M. Holmes-Rovner, M. Barry, and J. Jones. 1999. Decision aids for patients facing health treatment or screening decisions: Systematic review. *British Medical Journal* 319(7212):731–734.

O'Connor, A. M., C. Bennett, D. Stacey, M. J. Barry, N. F. Col, K. B. Eden, V. Entwistle, V. Fiset, M. Holmes-Rovner, S. Khangura, H. Llewellyn-Thomas, and D. R. Rovner. 2007. Do patient decision aids meet effectiveness criteria of the international patient decision aid standards collaboration? A systematic review and meta-analysis. *Medical Decision Making* 27(5):554–574.

Olsen, O., and P. C. Gotzsche. 2001. Cochrane review on screening for breast cancer with mammography. *Lancet* 358(9290):1340–1342.

Paine, B. J., N. P. Stocks, E. N. Ramsay, P. Ryan, and A. H. MacLennan. 2004. Use and perception of hormone therapy following media reports of the Women's Health Initiative: A survey of Australian WISDOM participants. *Climacteric* 7(2):143–152.

Pepine, C. J., R. S. Balaban, R. O. Bonow, G. A. Diamond, B. D. Johnson, P. A. Johnson, L. Mosca, S. E. Nissen, G. M. Pohost, and Endorsed by the American College of Cardiology Foundation. 2004. Women's ischemic syndrome evaluation: Current status and future research directions: Report of the National Heart, Lung And Blood Institute Workshop: October 2–4, 2002: Section 1: Diagnosis of Stable Ischemia and Ischemic Heart Disease. *Circulation* 109(6):e44–e46.

Picard, J. D. 1998. [History of mammography]. *Bulletin de l'Académie Nationale de Médicine* 182(8):1613–1620.

Power, M. L., J. Baron, and J. Schulkin. 2008. Factors associated with obstetrician-gynecologists' response to the Women's Health Initiative Trial of combined hormone therapy. *Medical Decision Making* 28(3):411–418.

Powles, T., R. Eeles, S. Ashley, D. Easton, J. Chang, M. Dowsett, A. Tidy, J. Viggers, and J. Davey. 1998. Interim analysis of the incidence of breast cancer in the Royal Marsden Hospital Tamoxifen Randomised Chemoprevention Trial. *Lancet* 352(9122):98–101.

Prentice, R. L., and G. L. Anderson. 2008. The Women's Health Initiative: Lessons learned. *Annual Review of Public Health* 29:131–150.

Rettig, R. A., P. D. Jacobson, C. Farquhar, and W. M. Aubry. 2007. *False Hope: Bone Marrow Trasnplantation for Breast Cancer.* New York, New York Oxford Univestiy Press.

Rich-Edwards, J. W., J. E. Manson, C. H. Hennekens, and J. E. Buring. 1995. The primary prevention of coronary heart disease in women. *New England Journal of Medicine* 332(26):1758–1766.

Rogers, E. M. 1995. Lessons for guidelines from the diffusion of innovations. *Joint Commission Journal on Quality Improvement* 21(7):324–328.

Rogers, N. 2003. Into our own hands: The women's health movement in the United States, 1969–1990. *Journal of the History of Medicine and Allied Sciences* 58(2):244–246.

Rymer, J., R. Wilson, and K. Ballard. 2003. Making decisions about hormone replacement therapy. *British Medical Journal* 326(7384):322–326.

Scheufele, D. A., and D. Tewksbury. 2007. Framing, agenda setting, and priming: The evolution of three media effects models. *Journal of Communication* 57(1):9–20, http://dx.doi.org/10.1111/j.0021-9916.2007.00326.x (accessed December 10, 2009).

Schonberg, M. A., R. B. Davis, and C. C. Wee. 2005. After the Women's Health Initiative: Decision making and trust of women taking hormone therapy. *Women's Health Issues* 15(4):187–195.

Schwartz, B., A. Ward, J. Monterosso, S. Lyubomirsky, K. White, and D. R. Lehman. 2002. Maximizing versus satisficing: Happiness is a matter of choice. *Journal of Personality and Social Psychology* 83(5):1178–1197.

Sepucha, K. R., J. K. Belkora, S. Mutchnick, and L. J. Esserman. 2002. Consultation planning to help breast cancer patients prepare for medical consultations: Effect on communication and satisfaction for patients and physicians. *Journal of Clinical Oncology* 20(11):2695–2700.

Sharf, B. F. 1997. Communicating breast cancer on-line: Support and empowerment on the internet. *Women and Health* 26(1):65–84.

Singer, N. 2009. Medical papers by ghostwriters pushed therapy. *New York Times*, August 4. P. A1.

Slade, B. A., L. Leidel, C. Vellozzi, E. J. Woo, W. Hua, A. Sutherland, H. S. Izurieta, R. Ball, N. Miller, M. M. Braun, L. E. Markowitz, and J. Iskander. 2009. Postlicensure safety surveillance for quadrivalent human papillomavirus recombinant vaccine. *Journal of the American Medical Association* 302(7):750–757.

Smith, R. A., S. W. Duffy, R. Gabe, L. Tabar, A. M. Yen, and T. H. Chen. 2004. The randomized trials of breast cancer screening: What have we learned? *Radiologic Clinics of North America* 42(5):v, 793–806.

Steele, W. R., F. Mebane, K. Viswanath, and J. Solomon. 2005. News media coverage of a women's health controversy: How newspapers and tv outlets covered a recent debate over screening mammography. *Women and Health* 41(3):83–97.

Subak-Sharpe, G. 1976. Is mammography safe? Yes, no and maybe. *New York Times Magazine*, October 24. Pp. 42–44.

Suleiman, O. H., D. C. Spelic, J. L. McCrohan, G. R. Symonds, and F. Houn. 1999. Mammography in the 1990s: The United States and Canada. *Radiology* 210(2):345–351.

Sundar, S. S., R. J. Gornall, and S. T. Kehoe. 2005. Advances in the management of cervical cancer. *Menopause International* 11(3):91–95.

Theroux, R. 2005. Evaluating its impact. The Women's Health Initiative. *Association of Women's Health, Obstetric and Neonatal Nurses* 9(2):140–145.

———. 2008. Postmenopausal hormone use: What does the latest evidence show? *Nursing for Women's Health* 12(1):56–61.

Trivedi, A., W. Rakowski, and J. Ayanian. 2008. Effect of cost sharing on screening mammography in Medicare health plans. *New England Journal of Medicine* 358(4):375.

Tu, H. T., and G. R. Cohen. 2008. *Tracking Report: Results from the Community Tracking Study*. Washington, DC: Center for Studying Health System Change.

US Preventive Services Task Force. 2009. Screening for breast cancer: US Preventive Services Task Force recommendation statement. *Annals of Internal Medicine* 151(10):716–726.

Veronesi, U., P. Maisonneuve, A. Costa, V. Sacchini, C. Maltoni, C. Robertson, N. Rotmensz, and P. Boyle. 1998. Prevention of breast cancer with tamoxifen: Preliminary findings from the Italian randomised trial among hysterectomised women. *Lancet* 352(9122):93–97.

Veronesi, U., P. Maisonneuve, N. Rotmensz, B. Bonanni, P. Boyle, G. Viale, A. Costa, V. Sacchini, R. Travaglini, G. D'Aiuto, P. Oliviero, F. Lovison, G. Gucciardo, M. R. del Turco, M. G. Muraca, M. A. Pizzichetta, S. Conforti, and A. Decensi. 2007. Tamoxifen for the prevention of breast cancer: Late results of the Italian randomized tamoxifen prevention trial among women with hysterectomy. *Journal of the National Cancer Institute* 99(9):727–737.

Viswanath, K., and J. Finnegan. 1996. The knowledge gap hypothesis: Twenty five years later. In *Communication Yearbook. Volume 19*, edited by B. R. Burleson and A. W. Kunkel. Thousand Oaks, CA: Sage Publications. Pp. 187–227.

———. 2002. Community health campaigns and secular trends: insights from the Minnesota Heart Health Program and community trials in heart disease prevention. In *Public Health Communication: Evidence for Behavior Change*, edited by R. C. Hornik. Mahwah, NJ: L. Erlbaum Associates. Pp. 289–312.

Watkins, C., L. Moore, I. Harvey, P. Carthy, E. Robinson, and R. Brawn. 2003. Characteristics of general practitioners who frequently see drug industry representatives: National Cross Sectional Study. *British Medical Journal* 326(7400):1178–1179.

Wegienka, G., S. Havstad, and J. L. Kelsey. 2006. Menopausal hormone therapy in a health maintenance organization before and after Women's Health Initiative hormone trials termination. *Journal of Women's Health* 15(4):369–378.

Weisman, C. S. 2000. Advocating for gender-specific health care: A historical perspective. *Journal of Gender-Specific Medicine* 3(3):22–24.

Williams, R. S., D. Christie, and C. Sistrom. 2005. Assessment of the understanding of the risks and benefits of hormone replacement therapy (HRT) in primary care physicians. *American Journal of Obstetrics and Gynecology* 193(2):551–556; discussion 556–558.

Woolf, S. H. 2010. The 2009 breast cancer screening recommendations of the US Preventive Services Task Force. *Journal of the American Medical Association* 303(2):162–163.

Writing Group for the Women's Health Initiative Investigators. 2002. Risks and benefits of estrogen plus progestin in healthy postmenopausal women: Principal results from the Women's Health Initiative randomized controlled trial. *Journal of the American Medical Association* 288(3):321–333.

6

Synthesis, Findings, and Recommendations

As discussed in Chapter 1, the committee developed a series of questions to focus its deliberations and to ensure that it responded to its charge (see Box 1-4). In this chapter, the committee synthesizes the previous chapters of the report in response to those questions and presents its key findings and recommendations.

The committee approached women's health as a concept that has expanded beyond a narrow focus on the female reproductive system to encompass other conditions that create a significant burden in women's lives. The committee focused on health conditions that are specific to women, are more common or more serious in women, have distinct causes or manifestations in women, or have different outcomes or treatments in women. Numerous conditions could be included in such a list. The committee could not review all such conditions and, therefore, highlights a number of such conditions as examples that are specific to women because of differences in prevalence, severity, preferred treatment, or understanding or because the condition is prominent in women or there is a research need regarding women, whether or not there are sex differences.

IS WOMEN'S HEALTH RESEARCH STUDYING THE MOST APPROPRIATE AND RELEVANT DETERMINANTS OF HEALTH?

The committee noted the growing understanding of the full spectrum of determinants of health and illness that has resulted from research over the last 20 years. Determinants can be related to a woman's biologic makeup, behaviors, and the social, cultural, and environmental contexts in which genetic vulnerabilities and individual traits and behaviors are developed and expressed. As discussed in Chapter 2, the committee concluded that more attention should be given to the

273

social and behavioral determinants of health than has been given in the past to achieve greater gains in women's health.

The committee initially planned to discuss health determinants in relation to each separate condition under consideration. However, the pervasive impact of social and behavioral determinants became apparent in that the same risk factors (such as smoking, eating habits, lack of physical activity, sexual risk behavior, and alcohol use) played a role in most of the conditions under consideration; therefore, the committee reviewed them in a separate chapter and provided evidence of their associations with a variety of conditions. For example, there is substantial evidence of links between smoking, alone and in conjunction with oral contraceptive use, and breast cancer, lung cancer, and cardiovascular disease (Burkman et al., 2004). There is growing evidence, from large cohort studies of women, on the role of eating habits and physical activity in the health of women.

As highlighted in the ecologic model presented in Chapter 2, smoking, eating habits, physical activity, and other behaviors are shaped by cultural and social contexts, including factors associated with social disadvantage. The marked differences in condition prevalence and mortality in women who experience social disadvantage are associated with race and ethnicity, lack of education, low income, and other factors such as differential exposure to stressors and violence, which are more common in more disadvantaged communities. Such exposures are related to outcomes as varied as injury and trauma, depression, arthritis, asthma, heart disease, human immunodeficiency virus (HIV) infection, and other sexually transmitted infections (Campbell et al., 2002; Coker et al., 2000; Ozer and Weinstein, 2004; Tjaden and Thoennes, 1998). Although the impact of social and community factors has been documented, little research on how to modify these factors to improve women's health has been conducted. Even less research has been conducted on the effects of those social and community factors in specific groups of women.

Greater support for research on social and behavioral determinants is needed, particularly research on how to modify them to improve health. Social and behavioral factors are important determinants of health for men as well as women, but the underlying factors probably differ by sex, and interventions tailored to women may be more effective than general treatments. For example, some studies show that women have a more difficult time with smoking cessation than men (Gritz et al., 1996) and face unique barriers to cessation (Schnoll et al., 2007). Smoking-cessation treatments designed to address barriers specific to women may be more effective, but they require empirical validation. Many intervention programs show promise, but most have not been well tested, and the health effects of smoking, such as cardiovascular disease and lung cancer, are still the leading killers of women. Similarly, interventions to improve eating habits, increase physical activity, decrease sexual risk behavior, and decrease substance abuse have not been as successful as they need to be to improve women's health.

IS WOMEN'S HEALTH RESEARCH FOCUSED ON THE MOST APPROPRIATE AND RELEVANT DISEASES, DISORDERS, CONDITIONS, OUTCOMES, AND END POINTS?

Several issues surfaced with the assessment of the question of whether women's health research has focused on the most appropriate and relevant health conditions. One was whether to look at progress in relation to women's overall health and well-being rather than listing progress by condition. Although the committee preferred the former, much of the knowledge regarding women's health has been conceptualized and conducted in relation to specific conditions. That approach reflects the organization of the National Institutes of Health (NIH), health-professions schools, specialties, and professional organizations. As a result, the committee examined progress in individual conditions in Chapter 3.

A second issue was the selection of conditions to discuss. Which conditions fall under the heading of women's health, and which conditions should the committee discuss? A narrow view would include only conditions that are unique to women. Although those are important, such a narrow view defines women primarily by their reproductive function. The committee chose a broader perspective: to consider all conditions that affect women disproportionately, that have different risk factors or that present differently in women, or that are treated differently in women and men. Applying the broader definition includes almost all conditions. The committee could not review all such conditions and, therefore, highlights a number of such conditions as examples that are specific to women because of differences in prevalence, severity, preferred treatment, or understanding or because the condition is prominent in women or there is a research need regarding women, whether or not there are sex differences.

Chapter 3 reviews and categorizes the progress in some of the most prevalent and problematic of the conditions for women, and they are presented in Table 6-1. A large amount of research on those conditions has been conducted, and progress has been made, especially with respect to some of the leading killers of women. That progress, however, has not been seen for all conditions, in particular for nonfatal conditions that affect women's quality of life. Women's health research has been focused on some appropriate and relevant health conditions, but more conditions need to be studied. Some of the research findings and the progress that has been made against a number of conditions are summarized briefly below.

Conditions on Which Research Has Contributed to Major Progress

Through its review of the literature, the committee identified three conditions in which scientific research led to major progress with respect to improvements in prevention, diagnosis, or treatment that resulted in substantial reductions in incidence or mortality: breast cancer, cardiovascular disease, and cervical cancer.

Research advances in breast cancer resulted in a decrease in mortality over

TABLE 6-1 Conditions Discussed by Committee, Categorized by Extent of
Progress

Conditions on Which Research Has Contributed to Major Progress
Breast Cancer
Cardiovascular Disease
Cervical Cancer

Conditions on Which Research Has Contributed to Some Progress
Depression
HIV/AIDS
Osteoporosis

Conditions on Which There Has Been Little Progress
Unintended Pregnancy
Maternal Morbidity and Mortality
Autoimmune Diseases
Alcohol and Drug Addiction
Lung Cancer
Gynecological Cancers Other than Cervical Cancer
Non-Malignant Gynecological Disorders
Alzheimer's Disease

the last 20 years. Consumer demand and involvement and increased funding
activity spurred research that elucidated key elements of the underlying pathophysiology of breast cancer, that developed more sensitive detection methods,
that increased identified biomarkers used in diagnosis and selection of targeted
treatments, that characterized risk factors, and that improved treatment options.
A substantial drop in breast-cancer incidence occurred following the reporting of
the findings from the Women's Health Initiative (WHI) and the later reduction in
the use of menopausal hormone therapy, which had both harmful and beneficial
effects. The WHI demonstrated that a given drug or treatment—in this case, conjugated equine estrogen with or without progestin—could have adverse effects on
some conditions (for example, breast cancer, stroke, embolism, and gall bladder
disease) while having beneficial effects on others (for example, reducing the risk
of bone fracture) and that women needed to balance risks and benefits, taking
into account a variety of outcomes.

Mammography provides another example of the need to balance risks and
benefits. Recent mammography guidelines try to balance the benefit of early detection in reducing mortality with the risks of overtreatment and anxiety caused
by false positives. The risk–benefit information is potentially useful to women in
making decisions about the use of mammography, but problems in communicating the findings have decreased its impact.

Research on breast cancer at the molecular, cellular, and animal levels in conjunction with clinical trials and observational studies in women have combined to improve outcomes, including quality of life after treatment. Disparities remain, however, in that black women have a higher mortality from breast cancer than white women despite a lower incidence; this highlights the need for research on groups of women that have the highest risks.

Although cardiovascular disease remains the leading cause of death of women and of men, women's age-adjusted mortality from coronary heart disease declined from 263.3 to 134.4 deaths per 100,000 from 1980 to 2000 (Ford et al., 2007). The first major breakthrough was the recognition that women are susceptible to cardiovascular disease just as men are. Sex differences in the underlying physiology and manifestation of cardiovascular disease have been documented. Data from women-only studies have contributed to the knowledge base of cardiovascular disease in women. The decline in mortality from cardiovascular disease occurred first in men and later in women. About half the decline in women is attributable to behavior change, including a drop in smoking, and the other half is attributable to new clinical treatments that emerged from research, such as secondary preventive therapy and initial treatment for acute myocardial infarction or revascularization (Ford et al., 2007). Major progress has been made in increasing awareness of cardiovascular disease in women through increasing physician's awareness of cardiovascular disease in women and through public-health campaigns. However, the long period during which cardiovascular disease was studied only in men has delayed greater progress. The lack of effective interventions for changing risk factors in women has limited decreases in the incidence of and mortality from cardiovascular disease in women.

Reductions in the incidence of and mortality from cervical cancer began in the 1960s and has continued as diagnosis and screening have improved further. In addition, a major transformation in research on cervical cancer and in the approach to cancer in general occurred with the development of a vaccine that prevents infection by several strains of human papilloma virus (HPV) that cause most cervical cancers. The vaccine was developed by using the findings of research on the basic biology of the virus and its relationship to cervical cancer in human cells and animals, and of studies of cervical cancer's etiology. Success with that multipronged approach highlights how information from different types of research builds and combines to yield progress against a condition. Although overall gains have been seen in mortality from cervical cancer, rates remain higher in black and Hispanic women than in white and Asian women. The differences highlight the need to focus translation and communication activities to the populations at greatest risk for the condition.

Conditions on Which Research Has Contributed to Some Progress

The committee identified depression, HIV/acquired immunodeficiency syndrome (AIDS), and osteoporosis as conditions on which some progress has been made through women's health research.

The incidence of depression is about twice as high in women as in men, and the consequences of depression, such as reduced educational attainment, are greater in women (Berndt et al., 2000). Some aspects of depression, such as postpartum depression, are more common to women. Advances have been made in the treatment of depression in the last 20 years (such as the development of combination norepinephrine-uptake inhibitors and serotonin-receptor antagonists with nonpharmaceutical interpersonal psychotherapy and cognitive–behavioral therapy) although their impact has not been maximized because of inadequate translation, particularly in relation to primary providers and the fragmentation of mental health services from other health-care delivery.

There have been advances in the treatment of HIV/AIDS in the last 20 years, including a decline in maternal–fetal transfer of HIV/AIDS because of treatment of pregnant women with antiretroviral agents. Much of the treatment research has been in men. The rapid development of treatments has benefited women despite the focus of the research on men, but the predominance of male-focused studies has limited some of the benefits for women. For example, issues related to the toxicity of treatments in women are only now being identified through women-based research. HIV/AIDS is becoming much more a women's issue, especially in black women, who make up 64% of the women living with HIV/AIDS.

Over the last 20 years there have been advances in the knowledge of the basic science underlying osteoporosis and in the diagnosis and treatment of osteoporosis. That includes the identification of genes whose expression affects the risk of osteoporosis (Huang and Kung, 2006). Recent trends show a decrease in the incidence of hip factures in the United States and Canada (Brauer et al., 2009; Leslie et al., 2009). Osteoporosis remains, however, a condition that greatly impacts the quality-of-life of a large number of women, particularly as they age.

Conditions on Which Little Progress Has Been Made

The committee identified a number of conditions on which little progress has been made in reducing incidence, morbidity, or mortality. Unintended pregnancy and autoimmune disease are highlighted below as examples of conditions on which there has been little progress.

Effective contraceptives are available to prevent pregnancy, and research has identified several risk factors for unintended pregnancy, but rates of unintended pregnancy have remained steady for decades. That unintended pregnancy continues to occur at a high rate points to the need for research on how to improve knowledge of and compliance with contraceptive regimens, the need to develop contraceptives that are more acceptable to cultures in which unintended pregnancy occurs with greater frequency, and the need for social and community-level interventions to decrease unintended pregnancy.

Another common condition in women that has seen little progress is autoimmune disease, which constitutes about 50 diseases. Most of the diseases are more common in women than in men, and as a group they are the leading cause of morbidity in women, greatly affecting quality of life. Despite their prevalence and morbidity and the availability of drugs to treat some of the symptoms, little progress has been made in understanding the conditions better, in identifying the risk factors, or in developing diagnostic tools, better treatments, or cures.

Looking at the set of conditions on which little progress has been made—including unintended pregnancy; autoimmune diseases; alcohol- and drug-addiction disorders; lung, ovarian, endometrial, and colorectal cancer; nonmalignant gynecologic disorders; and Alzheimer's disease—the committee tried to identify characteristics or explanations for the lack of progress. Several of the conditions have not had much attention and research, but other conditions have had considerable research. For example, there has been little progress in lung cancer despite a large amount of research, including some research on sex differences. The committee identified a number of potential reasons for the lack of progress, including degree of attention from government agencies, consumer advocate groups, and Congress and resulting research funding; availability of interested researchers trained in a given field; adequacy of understanding of the underlying pathophysiology and natural history of a condition; adequacy of understanding of behavioral factors associated with decreased risk; availability of sensitive and specific diagnostic tests and screening programs to identify individuals who are at risk for or have a condition; and nonmedical barriers associated with political or social concerns. Many of those reasons played a role in connection with specific conditions, but none emerged as a potent force that affected all the conditions. The committee did note, however, that many of the conditions that showed less progress were associated with morbidity and not mortality.

IS WOMEN'S HEALTH RESEARCH STUDYING THE MOST RELEVANT GROUPS OF WOMEN?

Women are not a homogeneous group, and differences—such as in age, race, ethnicity, social class, education, and area of residence—could lead to different health profiles and needs. Even when there has been progress in women's health, groups of women often have not improved or have shown more modest gains. More often, even when women are analyzed separately, there is no analysis of differences among groups of women, and groups of women at higher risk of having or dying from a condition (for example, those of lower socioeconomic status and members of racial and ethnic minorities) are the least represented in the studies. In the present report, when data were available, the committee pointed out disparities in knowledge regarding women of diverse backgrounds in determinants of health (Chapter 2), in progress in relation to specific conditions (Chapter 3), and in communication approaches (Chapter 5). The problems of adequate representation of women in research, discussed in Chapter 4, are compounded by challenges in having sufficient power to analyze groups of women separately. Not every study can have adequate numbers to allow such analysis, but the portfolio of studies funded by an agency should contain sufficient data to inform the understanding of vulnerable populations.

ARE THE MOST APPROPRIATE RESEARCH METHODS BEING USED TO STUDY WOMEN'S HEALTH?

In addition to reviewing the determinants and conditions that have been researched and have led to advances in women's health, the committee looked more broadly at the characteristics of research to evaluate whether particular methods or approaches yielded information that resulted in more progress and whether any particular components have contributed more to improving women's health.

Research can broadly be categorized as basic research, which involves the study of cellular and molecular components in animal and in vitro systems; population-based or observational studies; clinical research, which is conducted in human subjects; and health-services and health-policy research. Studies vary in size and complexity. Methods can be observational or experimental (such as randomized clinical trials), and the focus of research can range from cells to populations to cultural and societal factors. Chapters 2 and 3 demonstrate the diversity of women's health research and how the diverse research portfolio has contributed to progress in improving women's health, as in the cases of breast and cervical cancer.

The committee found that observational studies of women's health have provided information for identifying associations and are especially useful for generating hypotheses for further testing. Observational studies—such as the dietary component of the WHI, the Nurses' Health Study, and the Study of Women's Health Across the Nation (SWAN)—are sometimes coordinated in multiple research centers to accrue large and diverse samples. The postmenopausal hormone therapy and the calcium and vitamin D components of the WHI were randomized clinical trials that were based on the findings from such observational research. In addition, the observational studies led to animal and in vitro studies aimed at elucidating the pathophysiology of conditions and identifying potential treatments.

Different study types have different strengths and limitations, and results from diverse study designs can combine to provide extremely useful information that is directly relevant to the health of women and that has led to clear improvements in women's health. The committee recognizes that there are drawbacks to different study types. For example, observational and clinical studies can be expensive, can have subject attrition, can be of long duration, and, in the case of observational epidemiologic studies, can have difficulty in finding appropriate comparison populations and in controlling for potential confounders. Large human studies, such as the WHI, are further hindered by complex study designs and associated pitfalls. Despite those drawbacks, the committee concluded that information from large, complex observational and clinical studies could not be obtained with other study designs and are integral to progress in women's health. New study designs that yield similar levels of certainty would be valuable. Smaller studies, in contrast, provide different information, can often be better controlled, and are potentially faster (depending on the end points studied) and less expensive. Internal validity (for example, the ability to establish causal relationships) is generally stronger in such studies, but this may be at the cost of external validity (that is, generalizability). Smaller studies are important to provide information on which to base large studies and to test specific hypotheses.

Although women are now routinely included in clinical research, persistent problems limit the usefulness of the data and their applicability to women's health. Too often, the initial design is not optimal for obtaining data on women, because of problems in the inclusion criteria and end points assessed that may be less relevant to women's health given what is known about sex differences in the etiology and symptoms of disease. Sample size and the ability to recruit women in studies in numbers that are adequate for appropriate analyses can be a challenge. Notably, there is a continuing lack of analysis and reporting of data by sex to determine whether there are sex differences.

Methods and techniques that could facilitate sex-specific or group analysis should be explored. New analytic techniques, such as Bayesian analysis, appear promising and should be investigated and refined and expanded as appropriate. As outlined in NIH guidelines, clinical research should take advantage of previous epidemiologic studies, smaller human studies, and available incidence, prevalence, and mortality data to identify where sex, racial, and ethnic differences have been documented (NIH, 2001). Research should focus on groups at the highest risk for morbidity and mortality from a condition.

To improve women's health, sex- and gender-specific analyses must be published and used in drug development and clinical guidelines. Even when sex-specific analyses are conducted by researchers, the results of the analyses are often not included in publications, because of page limitations and journal restrictions. Such practices are a barrier to progress in women's health.

Women tend to report worse overall health than do men and tend to rank quality of life as very important when considering their health (Rieker and Bird, 2005). Nevertheless, the end points assessed in studies are often incidence and 5-year survival rates; a smaller number of studies look either at morbidity or quality-of-life end points after treatment and survival or at diseases, such as autoimmune disease and benign gynecologic disorders, that result in morbidity and affect quality of life rather than resulting in death. Health-related quality of life

(HRQoL) encompasses morbidity and functioning and is affected by a variety of factors, including limitations attributable to specific symptoms, the constellation of symptoms associated with a specific condition, and the combined effects on overall well-being. Although the effect of treatments on women's HRQoL is increasingly recognized as an important outcome, the ability to infer that effect is limited by the ability to compare measures among trials, treatments, and conditions, especially in a sex-specific manner. Often, health and treatment decisions are driven by HRQoL considerations, so having unifying metrics for the assessment of quality of life that can be used to compare clinical interventions across the spectrum of conditions and patients is important. Including a common metric for women's health HRQoL in studies would be an important first step in comparing treatments and interventions and would assist women in making health-related decisions.

ARE THE RESEARCH FINDINGS BEING TRANSLATED IN A WAY THAT AFFECTS PRACTICE?

Although it is not unique to women's health, there is clearly a major problem in the translation of research findings into practice; many findings take 1 of 2 decades to be incorporated into practice (Bansal and Barnes, 2008; Sussman et al., 2006). There are some instances of success in women's health. Notably, a decrease in the incidence of breast cancer has been attributed to the decrease in prescriptions for hormone-replacement therapy after the WHI trial (Jemal et al., 2007). It is partly attributable to effective processes for translating findings to practice, but the decrease in use also resulted from effective communication of the findings directly to women, who then questioned their doctors about the risks posed by using the medication (Bluming and Tavris, 2009).

Such success is the exception rather than the rule. More commonly, research findings are not translated into practice quickly or effectively. The problem of inadequate translation reflects the whole set of obstacles to optimal health care that occur in the current system. The committee identified a number of barriers to the translation of research on women's health, of which some are more of a problem for women and others are problems in all health research. The nature of scientific research is itself a barrier to translation. The advancement of scientific knowledge is an iterative process in which one research result builds on previous work and inconsistent or contradictory results are often published before a clear picture emerges from a multitude of different types of studies. Inconsistent results can lead to uncertainty in best practices, including contradictory guidelines and suspicion of new practices, and can delay adoption of scientific findings.

Social and cultural factors can be barriers to the translation of scientific findings regardless of scientific consensus, especially in connection with sexual mores, as occurred with a vaccine against HPV that has the potential to prevent most cases of cervical cancer. Socioeconomic status, immigration status, and language barriers can delay the adoption of research findings in some populations of women.

Health-care providers themselves and quality of care can be barriers to the translation of new findings. A particular concern for women with respect to health-care providers is the fragmentation of care that results when women see multiple providers for different health concerns; primarily care is often provided by an obstetrician or gynecologist during their reproductive years. The health-care systems in place in the United States can also present barriers to the translation of results of women's health research. Performance measures (such as the Healthcare Effectiveness Data and Information Set) used to evaluate the quality of care do not include many conditions that are more common to women, and sex-based differences in care are rarely analyzed (Bird et al., 2007; McKinley et al., 2002; Weisman, 2000), so incentives to include the latest research findings on women might not be present. In addition, in the case of both men and women, if new treatments or practices are not reimbursed by government and private insurers, they are less likely to be adopted into widespread practice. Patients themselves can be barriers to adoption of research findings. Faced with a multitude of research findings and complex decisions related to their own health, patients can have a difficult time in weighing new options.

ARE THE RESEARCH FINDINGS BEING COMMUNICATED EFFECTIVELY TO WOMEN?

As is the case with translation, the problems of communication are not limited to women's health issues. Communication of research findings in women's health, however, is facilitated by women's tendency to seek health-related information, including engagement in more health-related online activities than men (Fallows, 2005). The complexity of results and the sometimes inconsistent or contradictory results present challenges to the communication of findings and highlight the importance of having a clear, concise message. The emergence of the Internet and the World Wide Web has increased the amount of and access to health-related information for the general public but has also added to the confusion about findings and to concerns about the validity of the available information (Arora et al., 2008). Communication is further complicated by competing forces, especially when some health messages are competing with the marketing forces of industries.

Lessons learned from the WHI, mammography, and cardiovascular disease highlight both the challenges to and the successes in the translation and communication of research findings. The results of the WHI were disseminated to women, both study participants and the general public, through the mass media and health-care providers. The findings quickly translated into changes in prescribing practices, but that occurred amid much confusion (French et al., 2006). Cardiovascular disease was long thought to be a male disease despite being the leading cause of death of women. Increased research into cardiovascular disease has provided information specific to the prevention and treatment of heart disease in women. Concerted efforts by government agencies and nonprofit organizations to disseminate information, including research findings, on cardiovascular disease in women have improved awareness of cardiovascular disease in women and helped in the translation of the research findings into practice, including the development of women-specific guidelines. The combination of all those efforts has contributed to decreased mortality from cardiovascular disease in women. The broad availability of affordable screening, the effectiveness of mammography screening in reducing breast-cancer mortality, and more recently the most effective age and frequency for that screening have been controversial issues. Advocacy groups have played a large role in successfully pushing Congress and government agencies to fund screening programs and to increase the awareness of breast cancer in the general public. And the implementation of mandated national standards for mammography improved the quality of mammography and patient care.

GAPS IN WOMEN'S HEALTH RESEARCH

In addition to the many successes in women's health research, the committee identified gaps, including inadequate study of some conditions and at-risk populations, insufficient focus on determinants of specific health outcomes or conditions and of general health, inadequate attention to function and quality of life, and gaps in the translation of research findings into practice and in communication of the findings to the public. With respect to specific conditions, there are few data on ovarian and endometrial cancer, for which effective screening methods are lacking, and little is known about the causes and prevention of preeclampsia during pregnancy, which is a major cause of maternal morbidity and mortality. Conditions that affect elderly women, including frailty, have received relatively little attention. Research on prevention of and treatment for Alzheimer's disease, obesity, and diabetes has rarely examined sex differences. There is little information on autoimmune diseases that affect women disproportionately, such as rheumatoid arthritis, lupus, and other potentially related immune system disorders. And conditions that affect women's quality of life—such as endometriosis, chronic pain, chronic fatigue syndrome, and fibroids—are under studied.

Even in the case of health outcomes in which research has enabled advances, such as cardiovascular disease and breast and cervical cancer, challenges remain. New guidelines for the care of women have been developed, but there are still questions. Health-services research can address questions of implementation, such as whether the specialty of a clinician (for example, cardiologist vs internist) or the type of care facility (for example, women's health center vs general clinic) affects the likelihood or quality of implementation. Among the unresolved issues in breast cancer are explanations of differential risk of onset, treatment success, and survival among different groups of women.

Some of the identified gaps apply to many or most of the conditions that affect women. There has been relatively little attention to the causes and treatment of comorbidities. The issue of co-occurring conditions and the need to evaluate risk and benefit tradeoffs among multiple outcomes and end points cut across both mental and physical conditions. Large-scale studies—such as the WHI, which included both observational and experimental arms and considered multiple end points—provided some of the needed data from that perspective. Its overall history demonstrates the limitations of using only observational studies even if they are based on a good understanding of the molecular and cellular basis of sex differences, and also shows their synergistic value in developing targeted prevention and treatment strategies

Genetic and pathophysiologic studies are increasingly providing information on risk factors for conditions and potential treatment options on an individual level. Clinicians now need better tools to make personalized decisions about prevention, screening, and treatment. Those issues are not peculiar to women's health but are relevant to conditions that affect women especially.

Although genetic information is useful, it will not map perfectly onto health without accounting for environmental exposures that can affect gene expression in addition to affecting health directly. More information on factors in the physical and social environment is needed, including an understanding of how they may result in health disparities for disadvantaged groups. Research has provided more information on sex differences in the pathophysiology of conditions than on gender or sex differences in social determinants of health and illness. Both types of knowledge are necessary to prevent conditions in women and treat them. Social factors also play a role in the translation of knowledge into practice by health professionals and by women themselves. In some cases, particularly reproductive health, strong data supporting the safety and efficacy of treatments may be insufficient to fuel their use if there is social or political opposition on nonmedical grounds. Advances in women's health may require attention to such obstacles in addition to those inherent in the research.

Having evaluated progress in women's health research and considering whether the research has looked at the right determinants, has studied the right outcomes with the right methods, and has translated the resulting knowledge into practice and communicated it to women, the committee agreed on a set of primary findings and recommendations.

COMMITTEE'S KEY FINDINGS AND RECOMMENDATIONS

Substantial progress has been made since the expansion of investment in women's health research. Research findings have changed the practice of medicine and public-health recommendations in several prominent contexts, including changes in standards of care for women. There have also been decreases in mortality in women from breast cancer, heart disease, and cervical cancer. In other contexts, however, there has been less progress, including research on other conditions that affect women and identification of ways to reduce disparities among subpopulations of women.

Several barriers to further progress in improving the health status of women were identified. For example, there has been inadequate attention to the social and environmental factors that, along with biologic risk factors, influence health. There also has been inadequate enforcement of requirements that representative numbers of women be included in clinical trials and that women's results be reported. A lack of taking account of sex and gender differences in the design and analysis of studies, and a lack of reporting on sex and gender differences has hindered identification of potentially important sex differences and slowed progress in women's health research and its translation to clinical practice. The committee recommends that all published scientific reports that receive federal funding and all medical product evaluations by the Food and Drug Administration present efficacy and safety data separately for men and women.

Poor communication of the results of women's health research has in many cases led to substantial confusion and may affect the care of women adversely. Research findings will have a greater impact if they are coupled with a well thought-out plan for communication and dissemination. Development of a plan for communication and dissemination should be a standard component of federally sponsored women's health research and the clinical recommendations that are made on the basis of that research.

The committee's specific findings and recommendations follow.

Finding 1

Investment in women's health research has afforded substantial progress and led to improvements in women's health with respect to such important conditions as some cancers and heart disease. Greater progress in women's health has occurred in conditions characterized by multipronged research involving molecular, animal, and cellular data; in observational studies to identify effects in the overall population; and in clinical trials or intervention studies from which evidence-based conclusions on treatment effectiveness can be drawn.

Recommendation 1

US government agencies and other relevant organizations should sustain and strengthen their focus on women's health, including the spectrum of research that includes genetic, behavioral, and social determinants of health and how they change during one's life. In addition to conducting women-only research as appropriate, a goal should be to integrate women's health research into all health research—that is, to mainstream women's health research—in such a way that differences between men and women and differences between subgroups of men and women are routinely assessed in all health research. Relevant US government agencies include the Department of Health and Human Services and its institutes and agencies—especially the National Institutes of Health, the Centers for Disease Control and Prevention, the Food and Drug Administration, the Agency for Healthcare Research and Quality, and the Substance Abuse and Mental Health Services Administration—and such others as the Department of Veterans Affairs, the Department of Defense, and the Environmental Protection Agency.

Finding 2

Women who experience social disadvantage as a result of race or ethnicity, low income, or low educational level suffer disproportionate disease burdens, adverse health outcomes, and barriers to care but have not been well represented in studies of behavior and health.

Recommendation 2

The National Institutes of Health, the Agency for Healthcare Research and Quality, and the Centers for Disease Control and Prevention should develop targeted initiatives to increase research on the populations of women that have the highest risks and burdens of disease.

Finding 3

The incidence, prevalence, morbidity, or mortality associated with a number of conditions—for example, unintended pregnancy, maternal mortality and morbidity, nonmalignant gynecologic disorders, alcohol- and drug-addiction disorders, autoimmune diseases, and lung, ovarian, and endometrial cancer—have not improved. Most of those conditions substantially affect the quality of life of those who experience them. The major focus of health research has been on reducing mortality; a singular focus on mortality, however, can divert attention from other health outcomes despite the high value that women place on quality of life.

Recommendation 3

Research should include the promotion of wellness and quality of life in women. Research on conditions that have high morbidity and affect quality of life should be increased. Research should include the development of better measures or metrics to compare effects of health conditions, interventions, and treatments on quality of life. The end points examined in studies should include quality-of-life outcomes (for example, functional status or functionality, mobility, and pain) in addition to mortality.

Finding 4

Social factors and health-related behaviors and their interactions with genetic and cellular factors contribute to the onset and progression of multiple diseases; they act as pathways that are common to multiple outcomes. Considerable progress has been made in understanding the behavioral determinants of women's health, but less is known about how to change them and about the broader determinants of women's health that involve social, community, and societal factors.

Recommendation 4
Cross-institute initiatives in the National Institutes of Health—such as those in the Division of Program Coordination, Planning, and Strategic Initiatives—should support research on common determinants and risk factors that underlie multiple diseases and on interventions on those determinants that will decrease the occurrence or progression of diseases in women. The National Institutes of Health's Office of Research on Women's Health should increase collaborations with the Office of Behavioral and Social Sciences Research to design and oversee such research initiatives.

Finding 5

Limitations in the design, analysis, and scientific reporting of health research have slowed progress in women's health. Inadequate enforcement of recruitment of women and of reporting data by sex has fostered suboptimal analysis and reporting of data on women from clinical trials and other research. That failure has limited possibilities for identifying potentially important sex or gender differences. New methods and approaches are needed to maximize advances in promoting women's health.

Recommendation 5
- Government and other funding agencies should ensure adequate participation of women, analysis of data by sex, and reporting of sex-stratified analyses in health research. One possible mechanism would be expansion of the role of data safety monitoring boards to monitor participation, efficacy, and adverse outcomes by sex.
- Given the practical limitations in the size of research studies, research designs and statistical techniques should be explored that facilitate analysis of data on sociodemographic subgroups without substantially increasing the overall size of a study population. Conferences or meetings with a specific goal of developing consensus guidelines or recommendations for such study methods (for example, the use of Bayesian statistics and the pooling of data across study groups) should be convened by the National

Institutes of Health, other federal agencies, and relevant professional organizations.

- To gain knowledge from existing studies that individually do not have sufficient numbers of female subjects for separate analysis, the director of the Office of the National Coordinator for Health Information Technology in the Department of Health and Human Services should support the development and application of mechanisms for the pooling of patient and subject data to answer research questions that are not definitively answered by single studies.
- For medical products (drugs, devices, and biologics) that are coming to market, the Food and Drug Administration should enforce compliance with the requirement for sex-stratified analyses of efficacy and safety and should take those analyses into account in regulatory decisions.
- The International Committee of Medical Journal Editors and other editors of relevant journals should adopt a guideline that all papers reporting the outcomes of clinical trials report on men and women separately unless a trial is of a sex-specific condition (such as endometrial or prostatic cancer). The National Institutes of Health should sponsor a meeting to facilitate establishment of the guidelines.

Finding 6

The translation of research findings into practice can be delayed or precluded by various barriers—the complexity of science and research and challenges in communicating understandable and actionable messages, social or political opposition to advances for nonmedical reasons, fragmentation of health-care delivery, health-care policies and reimbursement, consumer confusion and apprehension, and so on. Many of those barriers are seen in connection with translation of research in general, but some have aspects that are peculiar to women, and few studies have been conducted to examine how to increase the speed or extent of the translation of findings related specifically to women's health into clinical practice. Methods of translation that have been used and that warrant evaluation for translating research findings in women include clinical-practice guidelines, mandatory standards, reimbursement practices, laws (including public-health laws), health-professions school curricula, and continuing education.

Recommendation 6
Research should be conducted on how to translate research findings on women's health into clinical practice and public-health policies rapidly. Research findings should be incorporated at the practitioner level and at the overall public-health systems level through, for example, the use of education programs targeted to practitioners and the development of guidelines.

As programs and guidelines are developed and implemented, they should be evaluated to ensure effectiveness.

Finding 7

The public is confused by conflicting findings and opposing recommendations that emerge from health research, including women's health research. Conflicting results and work to resolve disagreements are part of the scientific process, but that iterative aspect of scientific discovery is not clearly conveyed to, or understood by, the public. The resulting uncertainty and distrust of research may affect women's care adversely. Relevant knowledge from studies of communication often is not used by researchers, funders, providers, and public-health professionals to target health messages and information to women.

Recommendation 7

The Department of Health and Human Services should appoint a task force to develop evidence-based strategies to communicate and market health messages that are based on research results to women. In addition to content experts in relevant departments and agencies, the task force should include mass-media and targeted-messaging and marketing experts. The strategies should be designed to communicate to the diverse audience of women; to increase awareness of women's health issues and treatments, including preventive and intervention strategies; and to decrease confusion regarding complex and sometimes conflicting findings. The goals of the task force should be to facilitate and improve the communication of research findings by researchers to women. Strategies for the task force to consider or explore might include

- requiring a plan for the communication and dissemination of findings in federally funded studies to the public, providers, and policy makers; and
- establishing a national media advisory panel of experts in women's health that would be readily available to provide context to reporters, scientists, clinicians, and policy makers at the time of release of new research reports.

REFERENCES

Arora, N. K., B. W. Hesse, B. K. Rimer, K. Viswanath, M. L. Clayman, and R. T. Croyle. 2008. Frustrated and confused: The American public rates its cancer-related information-seeking experiences. *Journal of General Internal Medicine* 23(3):223–228.

Bansal, A. T., and M. R. Barnes. 2008. Genomics in drug discovery: The best things come to those who wait. *Current Opinion in Drug Discovery and Development* 11(3):303–310.

Berndt, E. R., L. M. Koran, S. N. Finkelstein, A. J. Gelenberg, S. G. Kornstein, I. M. Miller, M. E. Thase, G. A. Trapp, and M. B. Keller. 2000. Lost human capital from early-onset chronic depression. *American Journal of Psychiatry* 157(6):940–947.

Bird, C. E., A. M. Fremont, A. S. Bierman, S. Wickstrom, M. Shah, T. Rector, T. Horstman, and J. J. Escarce. 2007. Does quality of care for cardiovascular disease and diabetes differ by gender for enrollees in managed care plans? *Women's Health Issues* 17(3):131–138.

Bluming, A. Z., and C. Tavris. 2009. Hormone replacement therapy: Real concerns and false alarms. *Cancer Journal* 15(2):93–104.

Brauer, C. A., M. Coca-Perraillon, D. M. Cutler, and A. B. Rosen. 2009. Incidence and mortality of hip fractures in the United States. *Journal of the American Medical Association* 302(14):1573–1579.

Burkman, R., J. J. Schlesselman, and M. Zieman. 2004. Safety concerns and health benefits associated with oral contraception. *American Journal of Obstetrics and Gynecology* 190(4 Suppl.): S5–S22.

Campbell, J., A. S. Jones, J. Dienemann, J. Kub, J. Schollenberger, P. O'Campo, A. C. Gielen, and C. Wynne. 2002. Intimate partner violence and physical health consequences. *Archives of Internal Medicine* 162(10):1157–1163.

Coker, A. L., P. H. Smith, L. Bethea, M. R. King, and R. E. McKeown. 2000. Physical health consequences of physical and psychological intimate partner violence. *Archives of Family Medicine* 9(5):451–457.

Fallows, D. 2005. *How Women and Men Use the Internet: Women Are Catching Up to Men in Most Measures of Online Life; Men Like the Internet for the Experiences It Offers, While Women Like It for the Human Connections It Promotes.* http://www.pewinternet.org/~/media//Files/Reports/2005/PIP_Women_and_Men_online.pdf.pdf (accessed August 15, 2009).

Ford, E. S., U. A. Ajani, J. B. Croft, J. A. Critchley, D. R. Labarthe, T. E. Kottke, W. H. Giles, and S. Capewell. 2007. Explaining the decrease in US deaths from coronary disease, 1980–2000. *New England Journal of Medicine* 356(23):2388–2398.

French, L. M., M. A. Smith, J. S. Holtrop, and M. Holmes-Rovner. 2006. Hormone therapy after the Women's Health Initiative: A qualitative study. *BMC Family Practice* 7:61.

Gritz, E. R., I. R. Nielsen, and L. A. Brooks. 1996. Smoking cessation and gender: The influence of physiological, psychological, and behavioral factors. *Journal of the American Medical Women's Association* 51(1-2):35–42.

Huang, Q. Y., and A. W. C. Kung. 2006. Genetics of osteoporosis. *Molecular Genetics and Metabolism* 88:295–306.

Jemal, A., E. Ward, and M. J. Thun. 2007. Recent trends in breast cancer incidence rates by age and tumor characteristics among US women. *Breast Cancer Research* 9(3):R28.

Leslie, W. D., S. O'Donnell, S. Jean, C. Lagace, P. Walsh, C. Bancej, S. Morin, D. A. Hanley, and A. Papaioannou. 2009. Trends in hip fracture rates in Canada. *Journal of the American Medical Association* 302(8):883–889.

McKinley, E. D., J. W. Thompson, J. Briefer-French, L. S. Wilcox, C. S. Weisman, and W. C. Andrews. 2002. Performance indicators in women's health: Incorporating women's health in the Health Plan Employer Data and Information Set (HEDIS). *Women's Health Issues* 12(1):46–58.

NIH (National Institutes of Health). 2001. *NIH Policy and Guidelines on the Inclusion of Women and Minorities as Subjects in Clinical Research—Amended, October, 2001.* http://grants.nih.gov/grants/funding/women_min/guidelines_amended_10_2001.htm (accessed August 15, 2009).

Ozer, E. J., and R. S. Weinstein. 2004. Urban adolescents' exposure to community violence: The role of support, school safety, and social constraints in a school-based sample of boys and girls. *Journal of Clinical Child and Adolescent Psychology* 33(3):463–476.

Rieker, P. P., and C. E. Bird. 2005. Rethinking gender differences in health: Why we need to integrate social and biological perspectives. *Journals of Gerontology Series B Journal of Gerontology: Psychological Sciences and the Journal of Gerontology: Social Sciences* 60(Special Issue 2): S40–S47.

Schnoll, R. A., F. Patterson, and C. Lerman. 2007. Treating tobacco dependence in women. *Journal of Women's Health (2002)* 16(8):1211–1218.

Sussman, S., T. W. Valente, L. A. Rohrbach, S. Skara, and M. A. Pentz. 2006. Translation in the health professions: Converting science into action. *Evaluation and the Health Profession* 29(1):7–32.

Tjaden, P. G., and N. Thoennes. 1998. *Prevalence, Incidence, and Consequences of Violence Against Women: Findings from the National Violence Against Women Survey, Research in Brief.* Washington, DC: US Department of Justice, Office of Justice Programs, National Institute of Justice.

Weisman, C. S. 2000. Advocating for gender-specific health care: A historical perspective. *Journal of Gender-Specific Medicine* 3(3):22–24.

Agendas for Public Meetings

AGENDA

Tuesday, February 24, 2009
National Academy of Sciences Building,
2100 C Street, N.W., Washington, DC

1:00-1:10 PM   **Introductory Remarks and Introduction of Committee
Members**
Nancy E. Adler, Ph.D., Chair, Committee on Women's
Health Research

1:10-1:40 PM   **Presentation of Study Charge**
Wanda Jones, Dr.P.H., Deputy Assistant Secretary for
Health (Women's Health), Office on Women's Health,
US Department of Health and Human Services

1:40-2:40 PM   **Perspectives from Department of Health and Human
Services Offices and Programs on Women's Health**

        1:40-2:00   *Vivian Pinn*, M.D., Associate Director
for Research on Women's Health, National
Institutes of Health

        2:00-2:20   *Kathleen Uhl*, M.D., Director, Office of
Women's Health, Assistant Commissioner for
Women's Health, Food and Drug Administration

2:20-2:40   *Shakeh Kaftarian*, Ph.D., Senior Advisor,
             Women's Health and Gender Research, Agency
             for Healthcare Research and Quality

2:40-2:55 PM   **Break**

2:55-3:55 PM   **Perspectives from Women's Health Organizations**

2:55-3:15   *Phyllis Greenberger*, M.S.W., President and
             Chief Executive Officer, Society for Women's
             Health Research

3:15-3:35   *Diana Zuckerman*, Ph.D., President, National
             Research Center for Women and Families

3:35-3:55   *Cindy Pearson*, National Women's Health
             Network

3:55-4:10 PM   **Open Microphone for Statements from the Floor**

4:10-4:30 PM   **Comments on Study Charge**
             Mona Shah, J.D., M.P.H., Professional Staff Member,
             Office of Senator Barbara Mikulski (MD), United States
             Senate Committee on Health, Education, Labor, and Pensions

4:30-5:00 PM   **Open Microphone for Statements from the Floor**

5:00 PM   **Adjourn Open Session**

AGENDA

Thursday, May 7, 2009
The National Academies Keck Center, Washington, DC

1:00-1:10 PM   **Introductory Remarks and Introduction of Committee
             Members**
             Nancy E. Adler, Ph.D., Chair, Committee on Women's Health
             Research

1:10-1:30 PM   **Priorities for Women's Health Research**
             Kerri D. Schuiling, Ph.D., CNM, WHNP-BC, FACNM,
             Senior Staff Researcher, American College of
             Nurse-Midwives

1:30-1:50 PM   **Research on Women Veterans**
             Linda Lipson, M.A., Scientific Program Manager, Women's
             Health, Equity and Rural Health, Health Services Research
             and Development Service, Department of Veterans Affairs

Elizabeth Yano, Ph.D., M.S.P.H., Deputy Director, Department of Veterans Affairs Greater Los Angeles Health Services Research and Design, Center of Excellence for the Study of Healthcare Provider Behavior

1:50-2:20 PM **Physical and Mental Health Effects of Intimate Partner Violence and Areas of Needed Research**
Jacquelyn C. Campbell, Ph.D., R.N., FAAN, Anna D. Wolf Chair, The Johns Hopkins University School of Nursing

2:20-2:50 PM **Research on Obesity and Eating Disorders**
Madelyn Fernstrom, Ph.D., CNS, Professor of Psychiatry, Epidemiology, and Surgery; Director, Weight Management Center, University of Pittsburgh Medical Center

2:50-3:05 PM **Break**

3:05-3:35 PM **The Problem with Individualized Prevention**
Beverly Rockhill Levine, Ph.D., M.A., Department of Public Health Education, University of North Carolina, Greensboro

3:35-4:05 PM **Measures of Health-Related Quality of Life**
Dennis G. Fryback, Ph.D., Professor of Population Health Sciences and Industrial Engineering, Department of Population Health Sciences, University of Wisconsin, Madison

APPENDIX

B

Mortality Statistics

OVERALL CAUSES OF DEATH

Overall causes of death in men and women in 2006, not adjusted for age, are presented in Table B-1. The committee used the information from these tables to identify those diseases that cause the greatest mortality in women and those that affect more women than men. Heart disease and cancer each accounted for close to one-fourth of deaths in women in the United States in 2006. They were the leading causes of death in US women residents and in US residents overall in 2006, the year on which most recent data are available. Heart disease led to more deaths in women in 2006 than did cancer, and slightly more women than men died of heart disease in that year. Men were somewhat more likely than women to die of cancer. Men and women differed substantially with respect to deaths due to stroke and unintentional injuries: stroke was the third-leading cause of death in women in 2006 (and accounted for almost 30,000 more deaths in women than in men), and unintentional injuries (for example, those due to motor-vehicle crashes and firearms) were the third-leading cause of death in men. Suicide was the seventh-leading cause of death in men but was not among the 10 leading causes of death in women. More than 4% of deaths in women and 1.7% of deaths in men were due to Alzheimer's disease; the difference may be attributable in part to women's longer life expectancy.

With respect to causes of death in younger women, unintentional injury was the leading cause of death in young women 15–34 years old in 2006, and homicide and suicide were the second- and third-leading causes of death in young women 15–24 years old. Cancer and heart disease were other major causes of death in young women in 2006. Human immunodeficiency virus (HIV) was

TABLE B-1 Leading Causes of Female and Male Deaths in the United States in 2006 (estimated number of deaths, estimated percentage of deaths)[a]

Rank	Females	Males
1	Heart disease (315,930, 25.8%)	Heart disease (315,706, 26.3%)
2	Malignant neoplasm (cancer) (269,819, 22%)	Malignant neoplasm (cancer) (290,069, 24.1%)
3	Cerebrovascular disease (stroke) (82,595, 6.7%)	Unintentional injury (78,941, 6.6%)
4	Chronic lower respiratory disease (65,323, 5.3%)	Chronic lower respiratory disease (59,260, 4.9%)
5	Alzheimer's disease (51,281, 4.2%)	Cerebrovascular disease (stroke) (54,524, 4.5%)
6	Unintentional injury (42,658, 3.5%)	Diabetes mellitus (36,006, 3%)
7	Diabetes mellitus (36,443, 3%)	Suicide (26,308, 2.2%)
8	Influenza and pneumonia (30,676, 2.5%)	Influenza and pneumonia (25,650, 2.1%)
9	Nephritis (kidney inflammation) (23,250, 1.9%)	Nephritis (kidney inflammation) (22,094, 1.8%)
10	Septicemia (blood poisoning) (18,712, 1.5%)	Alzheimer disease (21,151, 1.8%)
Total deaths (all causes)	1,224,322	1,201,942

[a]Data are not age-adjusted.
DATA SOURCE: CDC (2009a).

among the 10 leading causes of death in women 15–54 years old in 2006. Women 35–44 years old, in whom HIV ranked as the fifth-leading cause of death, had the highest proportion of deaths from HIV in that year.

Table B-2 summarizes the leading causes of death from cancer in women by race and ethnicity. Lung cancer and colorectal cancer were estimated to be the leading and third-leading causes of cancer deaths in both women and men in 2008 on the basis of projections from trends in cancer deaths in previous years (ACS, 2008).[1] The second-leading cause of cancer deaths in women and men was

---

[1]Each year, the American Cancer Society estimates the number of new cancer cases and deaths expected in the United States in the current year on the basis of the most recent data on cancer incidence, mortality, and survival from the National Cancer Institute, the Centers for Disease Control and Prevention, and the North American Association of Central Cancer Registries and mortality data from the National Center for Health Statistics.

TABLE B-2 Leading Causes of Cancer Death in Women in the United States by Race or Ethnicity, 2006[a]

	Estimated Number (Percentage) Cancer Deaths				
	All Women	Non-Hispanic White	Non-Hispanic Black	Asian and Pacific Islander	American Indian and Alaska Native	Hispanic
All cancers	269,819	219,585	30,222	5,810	1,230	12,777
Trachea, bronchus, and lung	69,385 (25.7)	59,723 (27.2)	6,622 (21.9)	1,081 (18.6)	296 (24.1)	1,609 (12.6)
Breast	40,821 (15.1)	32,114 (14.6)	5,631 (18.6)	830 (14.3)	160 (13)	2,054 (16.1)
Colon and rectum	26,628 (9.9)	21,183 (9.6)	3,419 (11.3)	595 (10.2)	106 (8.6)	1,312 (10.3)

[a]Data are not age-adjusted.
SOURCE: CDC (2009b).

expected to be breast cancer and prostatic cancer, respectively. Lung, breast, and colorectal cancer combined were expected to account for over half the cancer deaths in women in 2008: lung cancer, 26.2%, breast cancer, 14.9%, and colorectal cancer, 9.5%. Pancreatic cancer and ovarian cancer were also estimated to be major causes of cancer deaths in women in 2008.

Trends

Heart disease, cancer, and stroke were the leading causes of deaths in women each year from 1989 to 2006 (CDC, 2001, 2009a) (Table B-3). Two notable changes over that period were the gradual decline in the proportion of deaths in women from heart disease and the increase in the proportion of deaths in women from Alzheimer's disease. Deaths from unintentional injuries have also increased somewhat. The proportion of deaths from stroke appears to have declined from 1999 to 2006, but this change may be related partially to a disease-coding rule change that resulted in assignment to vascular dementia (*International Classification of Diseases 10th Revision [ICD-10]* code F01) and to unspecified dementia (*ICD-10* code F03) of some deaths that previously would have been assigned to stroke (CDC, 2009b). Proportions of deaths in women from cancer of any type were very consistent, accounting for 21.6–23.3% of deaths in women each year from 1989 to 2006, whereas deaths from respiratory disease gradually increased during this period. The proportion of deaths in women from diabetes mellitus remained generally stable but its standing in the 10 leading causes of death relative to Alzheimer's disease and unintentional injuries changed. In recent years,

TABLE B-3 Trends in Causes of Death in Women: Leading Causes of Deaths in Women, 1989–2006

	Percentage of Deaths in Women from Given Health Outcome (Rank Among Causes of Death in Women)																	
	1989	1990	1991	1992	1993	1994	1995	1996	1997	1998	1999	2000	2001	2002	2003	2004	2005	2006
Heart disease	35.3 (1)	34.7 (1)	34.5 (1)	34.2 (1)	34 (1)	33.2 (1)	33 (1)	32.4 (1)	32 (1)	31.4 (1)	30.7 (1)	29.9 (1)	29.3 (1)	28.6 (1)	28 (1)	27.2 (1)	26.5 (1)	25.8 (1)
Malignant neoplasm (cancer)	22.5 (2)	22.9 (2)	23.1 (2)	23.3 (2)	22.6 (2)	22.7 (2)	22.5 (2)	22.4 (2)	22.3 (2)	22 (2)	21.7 (2)	21.8 (2)	21.6 (2)	21.6 (2)	21.6 (2)	22 (2)	21.7 (2)	22 (2)
Cerebrovascular disease (stroke)	8.5 (3)	8.4 (3)	8.9 (3)	8.3 (3)	8.2 (3)	8.3 (3)	8.5 (3)	8.5 (3)	8.4 (3)	8.2 (3)	8.5 (3)	8.4 (3)	8.1 (3)	8 (3)	7.7 (3)	7.5 (3)	7 (3)	6.7 (3)
Chronic lower respiratory disease[a]	3.5 (5)	3.6 (5)	3.8 (4)	3.9 (4)	4.2 (4)	4.3 (4)	4.3 (4)	4.5 (4)	4.6 (4)	4.7 (4)	5.1 (4)	5.1 (4)	5.1 (4)	5.2 (4)	5.3 (4)	5.2 (4)	5.5 (4)	5.3 (4)
Diabetes mellitus	2.6 (7)	2.6 (7)	2.7 (7)	2.7 (7)	2.8 (6)	2.9 (6)	2.9 (6)	3 (6)	3 (6)	3 (6)	3.1 (5)	3.1 (5)	3.1 (5)	3.1 (6)	3.1 (6)	3.1 (7)	3.1 (7)	3 (7)
Influenza and pneumonia	3.9 (4)	4.1 (4)	4 (5)	3.8 (5)	4.1 (5)	4 (5)	4 (5)	4 (5)	4.1 (5)	4.3 (5)	3 (6)	3 (6)	2.8 (8)	3 (8)	2.9 (8)	2.7 (8)	2.8 (8)	2.5 (8)
Alzheimer's disease	N/A	N/A	N/A	N/A	N/A	1.1 (8)	1.2 (8)	1.3 (8)	1.3 (8)	1.3 (8)	2.6 (8)	2.9 (7)	3.1 (6)	3.4 (5)	3.6 (5)	3.9 (5)	4.1 (5)	4.2 (5)
Unintentional injury	3 (6)	2.9 (6)	2.8 (6)	2.7 (6)	2.7 (7)	2.8 (7)	2.8 (7)	2.9 (7)	2.9 (7)	2.9 (7)	2.8 (7)	2.8 (8)	2.9 (7)	3 (7)	3.1 (7)	3.3 (6)	3.3 (6)	3.5 (6)
Nephritis (kidney inflammation)	1 (10)	1 (9)	1 (9)	1.1 (8)	1.1 (8)	1.1 (9)	1.1 (9)	1.1 (9)	1.1 (9)	1.2 (9)	1.5 (9)	1.6 (9)	1.7 (9)	1.7 (9)	1.8 (9)	1.8 (9)	1.8 (9)	1.9 (9)
Septicemia (blood poisoning)	1 (9)	1 (10)	1.1 (8)	1.1 (9)	1.1 (9)	1 (10)	1.1 (10)	1.1 (10)	1.1 (10)	1.1 (10)	1.4 (10)	1.4 (10)	1.5 (10)	1.5 (10)	1.5 (10)	1.5 (10)	1.5 (10)	1.5 (10)
All other causes	14	14.2	17.7	17.9	18.3	18.6	19	19	19.3	19.7	19.7	20.2	20.8	20.9	21.4	21.8	22.5	23.5

NOTE: The ranking of the given health outcome for cause of death in women is presented in parenthesis.
N/A (not applicable) indicates that health outcome was not in top 10 leading causes of death.
[a] Chronic obstructive pulmonary diseases and allied conditions, 1989–1998.
SOURCES: CDC (2001, 2009a).

a smaller proportion of deaths in women were due to influenza and pneumonia than during the 1990s (CDC, 2001, 2009a).

Racial and Ethnic Disparities

The leading causes of deaths in women differ in important ways by race and ethnicity. For instance, diabetes mellitus was the fourth-leading cause of death in non-Hispanic black, Hispanic, and American Indian and Alaska Native women and the seventh-leading cause in non-Hispanic white women in 2006 (Table B-4). Markedly higher proportions of Asian and Pacific Islander women than women in other racial and ethnic groups died from cancer (27.2% vs 22% overall) and stroke (9.5% vs 6.7% overall). American Indian and Alaska Native women experienced the highest proportion of deaths due to unintentional injury (8% vs 3.5% overall). Nephritis was the cause of more than 3% of non-Hispanic black women deaths compared with 1.9% overall.

There are also a number of racial and ethnic disparities in causes of cancer deaths in women. Lung, breast, and colorectal cancer were the three leading

TABLE B-4 10 Leading Causes of Female Death by Race or Ethnicity, 2006

Cause of Death	Estimated Percentage (Rank)					
	All Women	Non-Hispanic White	Non-Hispanic Black	Hispanic[a]	Asian and Pacific Islander	American Indian and Alaska Native[b]
Heart disease	25.8 (1)	26 (1)	25.5 (1)	22.8 (1)	22.7 (2)	18.8 (2)
Malignant neoplasm (cancer)	22 (2)	22 (2)	21.6 (2)	21.7 (2)	27.2 (1)	19.2 (1)
Cerebrovascular disease (stroke)	6.7 (3)	6.7 (3)	6.8 (3)	6.4 (3)	9.3 (3)	4.9 (5)
Chronic lower respiratory disease	5.3 (4)	5.8 (4)	2.5 (7)	2.7 (6)	2.4 (7)	4.3 (6)
Alzheimer's disease	4.2 (5)	4.5 (5)	2.3 (9)	2.7 (7)	2.2 (8)	1.7 (10)
Unintentional injury	3.5 (6)	3.5 (6)	3.1 (6)	5 (5)	3.8 (4)	8.1 (3)
Diabetes mellitus	3 (7)	2.7 (7)	5 (4)	5.4 (4)	3.8 (5)	7 (4)
Influenza and pneumonia	2.5 (8)	2.6 (8)	2 (10)	2.6 (8)	3 (6)	2 (9)
Nephritis (kidney inflammation)	1.9 (9)	1.7 (9)	3.2 (5)	2.2 (10)	2 (9)	2.4 (8)
Septicemia (blood poisoning)	1.5 (10)	1.4 (10)	2.4 (8)	N/A	N/A	N/A

NOTE: N/A (not applicable) indicates that given health outcome is not in top 10 leading causes of death in the racial or ethnic group noted.

[a]The ninth-leading cause of death in Hispanic females was perinatal conditions.

[b]The seventh-leading cause of death in American Indian and Alaska Native females was chronic liver disease and cirrhosis (4.2% of deaths in 2006).

SOURCE: CDC (2009a).

causes of cancer death in women of all racial and ethnic groups in 2006 (CDC, 2009a). However, although breast cancer was the leading cause of cancer deaths in Hispanic women in 2006, it was the second-leading cause of cancer deaths in each of the other groups (Table B-2). Asian American and Pacific Islander women had a notably lower proportion of deaths from lung cancer, perhaps because of this population's lower prevalence of smoking.[2] Lymphoma, ovarian cancer, and pancreatic cancer were also leading causes of cancer death in women in each racial and ethnic category in 2006 (CDC, 2009a).

Besides breast cancer, there are notable racial and ethnic disparities in other female-specific cancers. For example, about 1.2% of cancer deaths in non-Hispanic white women in 2006 were due to cervical cancer compared with 2.1% in American Indian and Alaska Native, 2.5% in non-Hispanic black, 2.6% in Asian and Pacific Islander, and 3.6% in Hispanic women. The highest proportion of uterine-cancer deaths was in non-Hispanic black women (4% of cancer deaths vs 2.7% overall) (CDC, 2009b).

A few things should be noted about changes and differences in leading causes of death in women in specific racial and ethnic populations in 1999–2006.[3] Deaths from heart disease and stroke declined in women of all racial and ethnic categories, although Asian and Pacific Islander women had the highest proportion of deaths from stroke in that period. Proportions of deaths from cancer and diabetes did not decline much in any group, but diabetes consistently led to more deaths among in American Indian and Alaska Native, non-Hispanic black, and Hispanic women than in other groups. In 1999–2002, a higher proportion of deaths in non-Hispanic black women were from HIV (the 10th-leading cause of death in non-Hispanic black women during that period) than from Alzheimer's disease or influenza and pneumonia (which by 2006 were the 9th-leading and 10th-leading causes of death in black women). Deaths from Alzheimer's disease have increased in each group. Deaths from unintentional injury have also gone up in general except in American Indian and Alaska Native women, in whom the proportion of deaths from unintentional injury remained relatively stable (an average of 8.4% of deaths each year in 1999–2006).

REFERENCES

ACS (American Cancer Society). 2008. *Cancer Facts and Figures. 2008.* http://www.cancer.org/acs/groups/content/@nho/documents/document/2008cafffinalsecuredpdf.pdf (accessed August 3, 2010).

ALA (American Lung Association). 2008. *Smoking and Asian Americans/Pacific Islanders Fact Sheet.* http://www.lungusa.org/site/pp.asp?c=dvLUK9OOE&b=36001 (accessed April 27, 2009).

---

[2]In 2006, 10.3% of Asian Americans, 32.2% of American Indians and Alaskan Natives, 22.6% of non-Hispanic blacks, 21.8% of non-Hispanic whites, and 15.1% of Hispanics smoked (ALA, 2008).

[3]Racial and ethnic group-specific data for the period 1989–1999 are not available.

CDC (Centers for Disease Control and Prevention). 2001. *Leading Causes of Death, 1900–1998.* http://www.cdc.gov/nchs/data/dvs/lead1900_98.pdf (accessed August 3, 2010)
———. 2009a. *WISQARS Leading Causes of Death Reports, 1999–2006.* http://webappa.cdc.gov/ sasweb/ncipc/leadcaus10.html (accessed April 27, 2009).
———. 2009b. *Deaths: Final Data for 2006. National Vital Statistics Reports.* Volume 57, Number 14.

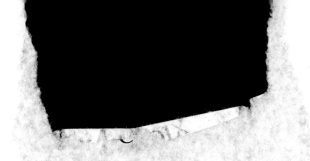

Selected Studies of Women's Health

The contents of Appendix C are provided on the CD in the back of the book and are available online at http://www.nap.edu/catalog.php?record_id=12908.